Current Progress in Dermatology

Current Progress in Dermatology

Edited by **Deb Willis**

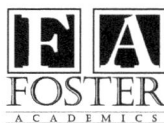

FOSTER ACADEMICS

New Jersey

Published by Foster Academics,
61 Van Reypen Street,
Jersey City, NJ 07306, USA
www.fosteracademics.com

Current Progress in Dermatology
Edited by Deb Willis

International Standard Book Number: 978-1-63242-458-7 (Hardback)

Printed in the United States of America.

Contents

Preface

Over the recent decade, advancements and applications have progressed exponentially. This has led to the increased interest in this field and projects are being conducted to enhance knowledge. The main objective of this book is to present some of the critical challenges and provide insights into possible solutions. This book will answer the varied questions that arise in the field and also provide an increased scope for furthering studies.

Dermatology is a field of medical study which deals with diagnosing and treating disorders related to skin, nails, hair and also treats cosmetic problems related to the same. It has many branches like cosmetic dermatology, dermatopathology, immunodermatology, pediatric dermatology, teledermatology, dermatoepidemiology, etc. Dermatologists use many therapies to cure diseases such as laser therapy, photodynamic therapy, tumescent liposuction, cryosurgery, radiation therapy, etc. This book talks in detail about the progress made in therapies and applications related to this field. It will provide case studies from around the world to give a better understanding to the readers. For someone with an interest and eye for detail, this book will provide the most significant topics about new researches and discoveries in dermatology. It will serve as a beneficial guide for researchers and students alike.

I hope that this book, with its visionary approach, will be a valuable addition and will promote interest among readers. Each of the authors has provided their extraordinary competence in their specific fields by providing different perspectives as they come from diverse nations and regions. I thank them for their contributions.

Editor

Hypertrichotic Giant Nevus Spilus Tardivus and Neurofibroma of the Tongue in Sporadic von Recklinghausen's Disease

Prabhath Ramakrishnan,[1] Vijay Sylvester,[1] Prathima Sreenivasan,[1] Janisha Vengalath,[1] and Smruthi Valambath[2]

[1] *Department of Oral Medicine and Radiology, Kannur Dental College, Anjarakandy, Kannur, Kerala 670612, India*
[2] *Department of Physiology, SDM College of Medical Sciences, Dharwad, Karnataka 580009, India*

Correspondence should be addressed to Prabhath Ramakrishnan; prabathrk@gmail.com

Academic Editor: Akimichi Morita

Solitary neurofibromas are rare, benign tumours of nonodontogenic origin. The presentation of a solitary neurofibroma on the tongue is an uncommon occurrence and we present such a case here which was discovered in concomitance with multiple neurofibromatosis type 1 (von Recklinghausen's disease). Such a rare presentation seen in this case is a diagnostic challenge and often clinched only with the aid of histopathological and immunohistochemical examination. This work also discusses the various differential diagnoses that can be considered in similar cases. The presence of a hypertrichotic "giant" nevus spilus tardivus (Becker's nevus) is also a rare finding in this particular case. We present such a case which will be of interest to the budding dental practitioner. The lesion was excised and the patient followed up without any evidence of malignant transformation.

1. Introduction

Neurofibromas are benign nerve sheath tumors originating from the peripheral nerves and are the hallmark presentation in von Recklinghausen's disease or neurofibromatosis type 1 [1].

Neurofibromatosis is a rare disease that includes two variants that is divided into neurofibromatosis type 1 (NF1) and type 2 (NF2). NF1 is the most common of these two types with a frequency of 90%, compared with 10% for NF2. Among these the NF1 is also called the peripheral neurofibromatosis, popularly called von Recklinghausen's disease with a reported prevalence of 1:5000 in the population and a birth incidence of 1 in 2500–3300 [2]. There are clinical criteria suggested by the National Institute of Health (NIH) Consensus Development Conference to classify a patient as having NF1. The patient has to have 6 or more café au lait spots equal to or larger than 0.5 cm in prepubertal individuals and equal to or larger than 1.5 cm in postpubertal individuals; 2 or more neurofibromas of any type or 1 or more plexiform neurofibroma; inguinal or axillary freckling (Crowe's sign); an optical nerve glioma; 2 or more benign iris hamartomas

(or Lisch nodules); a distinctive osseous lesion: dysplasia of the sphenoid bone, dysplasia or thinning of long bone cortex with or without pseudarthrosis, and a first degree relative with NF1 [3–5].

Neurofibromatosis is an autosomal dominant disorder and sporadic incidences are not very uncommon (30–50%). The genetic mutation is located on the NF1 gene and can be traced to chromosome 17q11.2. Gene mutations usually cause a deficiency of a tumour suppressor protein product called neurofibromin. So, there is uncontrolled cell proliferation that results in the growth of a tumour. The penetrance of NF1 gene is 100% in adults, but, there is a high variance in expression [5]. The neurofibromas in the oral cavity most commonly involve the tongue, followed by lips, palate, buccal mucosa, gingiva, floor of the mouth, or the pharynx [6].

Although there are numerous reports of the incidence of plexiform neurofibromas involving the oral cavity and head and neck regions, solitary plexiform neurofibromas of the tongue are rare lesions and one does not usually come across them in day to day practice; however, in most cases their coexistence with von Recklinghausen's disease has been quite well established as seen from reports around the world. A

TABLE 1: Isolated plexiform neurofibromas of the tongue case reports over the past 15 years [7–13].

Location	Age/sex	Year	Authors
Tongue	39/M	2014	Present case
Tongue	11/F	2013	Sharma et al. [7]
Tongue	34/F	2012	Iyer et al. [8]
Tongue	5/F	2010	Sirinoglu et al. [9]
Tongue	3/F	2006	Guneri et al. [10]
Tongue	24/F	2006	Marocchio et al. [11]
Tongue	35/F	2006	Bongiorno et al. [12]
Tongue	5/F	2006	Guclu et al. [13]

search of the reported cases in the past 15 years was conducted and to the best of our knowledge this is the very first case of a plexiform neurofibroma of the tongue reported in a male patient in literature (Table 1) [7–13].

The differentiation between neurofibroma and the plexiform variety is usually clinched with histopathological and immunohistochemical diagnosis. This case report presents with a solitary plexiform neurofibroma involving the tongue which is not a very common presentation with sporadic neurofibromatosis type 1. It is also interesting because the case presents with a hypertrichotic giant nevus spilus tardivus in von Recklinghausen's disease involving the right arm which has very rarely been reported in literature.

2. Case Presentation

A 39-year-old Asian male presented to our department with a chief complaint of a painless swelling involving the left lateral border of the tongue. History revealed that the growth began as a pea-sized nodule and gradually increased in size to its present state over a period of 4 months.

The past medical history did not reveal any cardiovascular, respiratory, genitourinary, gastrointestinal, endocrine, haematological, neurological, or any other medical history of relevance. The past dental or familial history was not of any consequence to our particular case. A complete blood count was performed and no abnormality was detected. No history of trauma, bleeding, pain, or paresthesia was present. There were no signs of any cervical lymphadenopathy noted. Orthopantomographic examination did not reveal any bony abnormalities. Extraoral examination revealed multiple soft cutaneous nodules involving either side of the face, back, trunk, and the lower and upper extremities. They were round to oval in shape and were of various sizes ranging from a few millimetres to centimetres across. On palpation they were found to be sessile and some pedunculated also, soft to firm in consistency, nontender, and noncompressible and showed no signs of fixity. Around 15 café au lait (coffee in milk) macules were present over 15 mm in diameter throughout the body with increased prevalence in the back and trunk. The largest one among these was located over the right arm measuring a whopping 22 × 13 cm across with smooth borders. It was roughly ovoid in shape and there was a brownish macule with long thick dark hair involving the surface of the lesion and it extended from the acromioclavicular joint all the way down

to the upper arm (Figure 1). The distribution of the lesion did not follow the lines of Blaschko. Rubbing the affected area exhibited a pseudo-Darier sign which consisted of a transient piloerection. Neither axillary freckling (Crowe's sign) nor Lisch nodules were noted in our case.

Intraoral examination revealed a sessile lesion with a lobulated appearance and measured 2 × 1.5 cm in greatest dimensions. It was roughly ovoid in shape with irregular borders and exhibited a smooth surface. The periphery was non-erythematous in appearance. On palpation it was found to be nontender, firm in consistency, and fixed to the underlying tissue. It was noncompressible, nonreducible, and nonpulsatile in nature (Figure 2). The slow-growing, asymptomatic nature of the lesion with the presence of well circumscribed margins led us to give a provisional diagnosis of a benign lesion. Based on the positive clinical features in our extra- and intraoral assessment of the patient, a provisional diagnosis of a neurofibroma was considered, taking into consideration the fact that the patient revealed pathognomonic signs of neurofibromatosis type 1 extraorally.

Considering the clinical presentation and localization of the lesion, we included a neurofibroma, schwannoma, neurilemmoma, granular cell tumour, reactive lesions like a giant cell fibroma or focal fibrous hyperplasia, leiomyoma, rhabdomyoma, hemangioma, lymphangioma, lipoma, and benign salivary gland tumours among differential diagnosis taking into account the peripheral exophytic nature of the lesion.

Routine haematological examination revealed a normal blood profile and no other imaging findings for soft tissue analysis like ultrasonography or MRI were performed considering the miniscule proportions of the lesion and its benign presentation. Patient was also referred to the adjacent medical college to rule out the possibility of any internal lesions. Excisional biopsy of the tumour mass on the tongue was performed in toto and primary closure achieved with a single interrupted Vicryl suture. The patient was prescribed an NSAID medication and asked to use povidone-iodine mouth rinse.

Histopathological examination which is the investigation of choice in peripheral exophytic lesions involving the tongue revealed a section with densely collagenous stroma with proliferation of spindle cells as fascicles with thin wavy nuclei in irregular pattern. Numerous plump fibroblasts were present and there were many vascular channels. Connective tissue is lined by stratified squamous epithelium (Figure 3). The specimen further underwent immunohistochemical analysis, which can be considered a gold standard, and was found to be immunoreactive for S-100 stain which was positive for the spindle cells, thereby, signifying its origin from neural crest tissue and confirming our diagnosis of a neurofibroma (Figure 4). The lesion on the shoulder underwent an incisional biopsy and on histopathological examination revealed numerous elongated rete ridges with melanin pigmentation of the basal layer with no increase in the number of melanocytes. The specimen tested negative for S-100 protein (Figure 5).

The postoperative healing was uneventful and patient was followed up after two weeks and subsequently after 6 months.

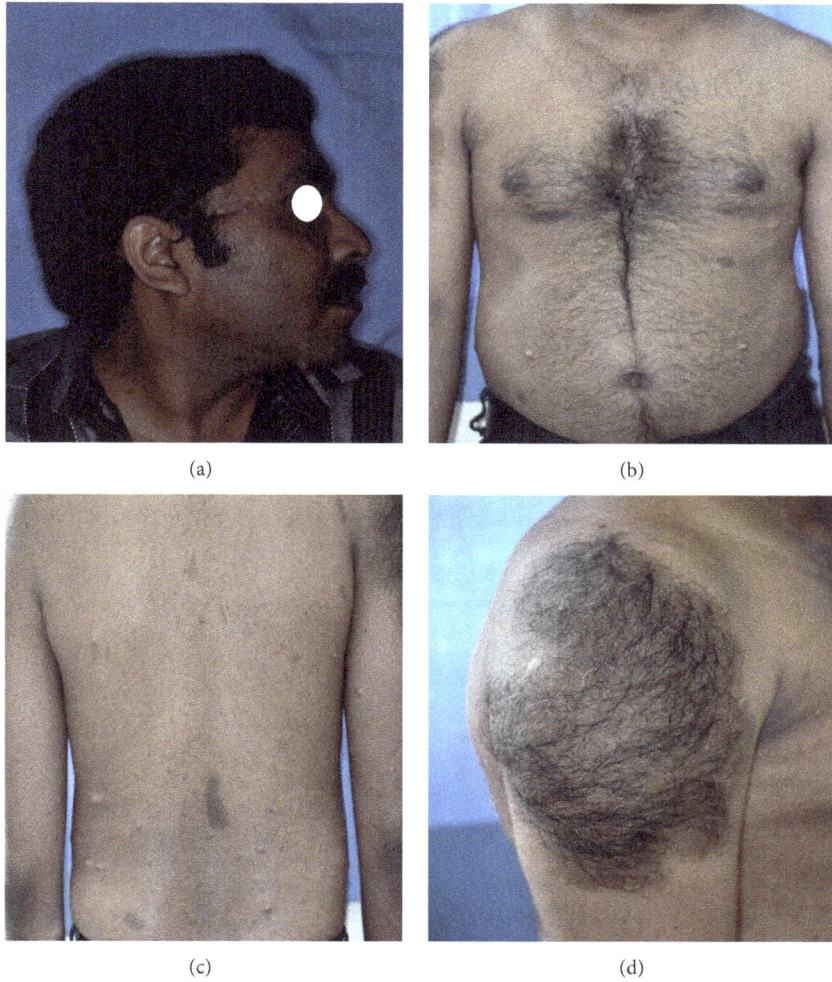

FIGURE 1: (a) Right profile view revealing multiple cutaneous nodules. (b) Multiple cutaneous nodules and café au lait macules on the trunk. (c) Multiple cutaneous nodules and café au lait macules on the back. (d) Hypertrichotic giant café au lait macule on the right arm.

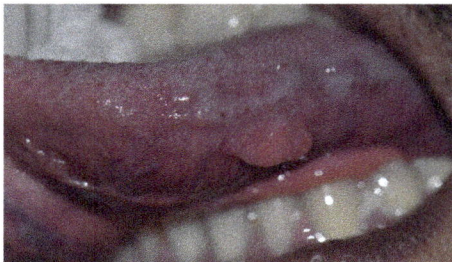

FIGURE 2: Nodular growth on the left lateral border of tongue.

The patient was also advised to report for periodic follow-up visits due to the potential for neurofibromas to undergo malignant transformation.

3. Discussion

A neurofibroma is a benign tumour arising from the cells of neural sheath origin. Although an uncommon benign tumour, we found it prudent to place the diagnosis of a neurofibroma with a higher ranking in our list of differential

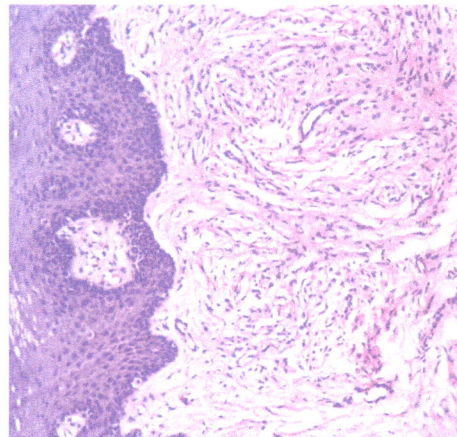

FIGURE 3: Photomicrograph revealing spindle cells as fascicles with thin wavy nuclei.

diagnoses considering the fact that our patient exhibited other extraoral features of neurofibromatosis type 1. It usually

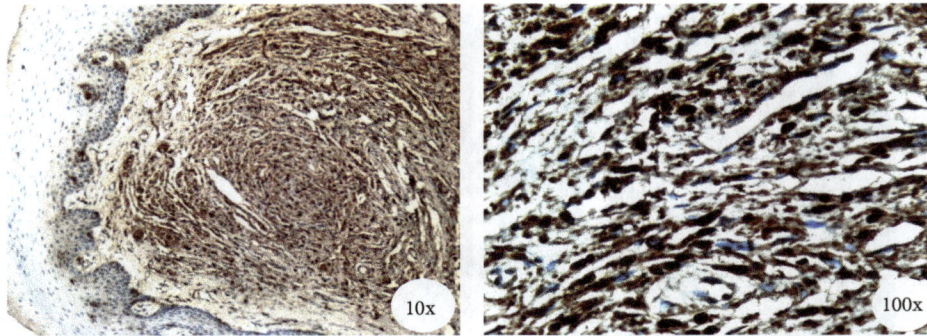

FIGURE 4: Photomicrograph exhibiting immunoreactivity for S-100 protein in spindle cells. (10x) and most of the tumour cells are positive for S-100 protein (100x).

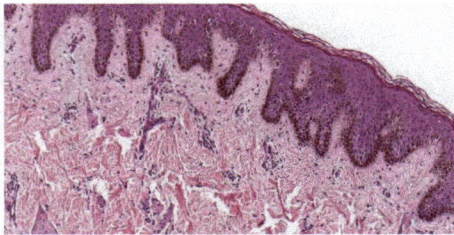

FIGURE 5: Photomicrograph reveals elongated rete ridges and pigmentation of the basal layer with no increase in the number of melanocytes.

presents on the tongue and also occasionally on the buccal mucosa, gingiva and involves the lips very rarely [1–3]. The expression of the condition shows a wide variation. Some individuals may have thousands of neurofibromas on the body whereas some may have few like our patient. The neurofibromas involving the tongue are almost always nodular in nature as was present in our case. The patient presented to us with a complaint of a slow growing mass involving the left lateral border of the tongue. The patient was educated and aware about the condition developing on his tongue and wanted expert consultation. It is important that the general public is made aware regarding the importance of having such lumps and swellings examined by a clinician and the possibility of malignancy ruled out. The differential diagnosis of enlarging tongue masses includes schwannoma, granular cell tumour, reactive lesions like a giant cell fibroma or focal fibrous hyperplasia, leiomyoma, rhabdomyoma, hemangioma, lymphangioma, lipoma, and benign salivary gland tumours among differential diagnosis taking into account the peripheral exophytic nature of the lesion.

A neurilemmoma or a schwannoma is an encapsulated tumour mass that is present submucosally. They are not very common in the oral cavity, but if present, the tongue is the most common location for the lesion. They appear nodular and sometimes may grow to fantastic sizes. Confirmatory diagnosis is by conducting a biopsy [14].

Granular cell tumour, also called the Abrikossoff's, may occur anywhere in the body but has a marked predilection for the tongue when it occurs in the oral cavity. Usually it presents

in the fourth to sixth decades of life. In over 50% of the cases tongue shows pseudoepitheliomatous hyperplasia, but, IHC can help in diagnosis with the aid of S-100 immunoreactivity in the mesenchymal tissues [15].

Another reactive lesion, namely, the focal fibrous hyperplasia (irritation fibroma), typically presents as a smooth nodule. It is usually 1.5 cm or smaller in diameter. Prevalence is greater in individuals above 40 yrs of age [16].

Oral leiomyomas are benign smooth muscle tumours that are rarely noticed in the oral cavity and most of them, if present, arise from the smooth muscles of the underlying vasculature. They generally present as tiny, slow growing, solitary nodular masses located principally on the tongue, lips, palate, and buccal mucosa. Although asymptomatic, they may present with symptoms such as pain, tooth mobility, or difficulty in chewing [17, 18].

Rhabdomyomas are striated muscle tumours which may occur on the mucosal surfaces as well. They are usually very rare and diagnosis can be confirmed by normal H&E staining. However, they have to be biopsied to evaluate the presence of its extremely malignant counterpart, the rhabdomyosarcoma [19].

Hemangioma of the tongue is highly unusual occurrences and is more common in the 1st decade of life. Intramuscular tumours are nonmetastasizing benign congenital tumours. Most of them also increase in size in 2nd-3rd decades of life. They are usually not life threatening entities [20].

Lymphangioma is a benign proliferation of lymphatic vessels and is often hamartomatous transformations of malformed lymphatics. They may present as localised growths and their limited extension facilitates easy surgical removal. They are difficult to diagnose based on the clinical appearance alone and are mainly caused because of the difficulty in drainage of the lymph which causes a localised collection in the area [21].

Lipoma is a painless benign mesenchymal tumor that is well circumscribed. It may be present in any site but is rare in the oral cavity. Possible causes include infection, chronic irritation, hormonal imbalance, and trauma. Histopathological analysis is the gold standard for diagnosis and they are composed of mature far cells with fibrous connective tissue which is often hyalinised with or without the capsule and/or fibrous septa [22].

The majority of salivary gland tumours are benign in nature, with pleomorphic adenoma accounting for 60% of them. The involvement of the tongue is very rare for a pleomorphic adenoma and is hence ranked the last [23, 24].

There is still some controversy regarding the presence of Lisch nodules associated with neurofibromatosis type 1, which was not present in our case, which certain authors think are asymptomatic and not correlated with visual impairment or severe optic nerve involvement [25]. Our case also revealed a giant nevus spilus tardivus macule. They histologically reveal increased melanin deposition by the underlying basal keratinocytes and the melanocytes [26]. The lesion on his tongue was excised under local anaesthesia. An incisional biopsy of the lesion on his shoulder was performed and subjected to histopathological examination which revealed several elongated rete ridges with pigmentation of the basal layer. To the best of our knowledge hypertrichosis involving a giant café au lait macule has never before been reported in literature and is a novel finding in our case. The café au lait spots produced in neurofibromatosis type 1 are individually indistinguishable from nevus spilus or in this case with the overlying hypertrichosis. In fact when multiple nevus spilus is seen, there is a possibility of café au lait spots of neurofibromatosis type 1. They can be ideally differentiated only by performing immunohistochemical analysis for S-100 protein [27]. In our case, the sample from the shoulder tested negative for the S-100 protein. Although it has been proven that café au lait spots are associated with von Recklinghausen's disease, we require more case reports with immunohistochemical analysis to associate these kinds of hypertrichotic giant nevus spilus with NF1. In this case, the patient revealed that he remembers the nevus was not congenital, appearing at the age of 12, and gradually grew in size and became hypertrichotic over a period of 5 years.

As was in our case, most of the time, neurofibromas are usually not with significant clinical consequences; a feared complication of neurofibromas is the probability for malignant transformation which is the reason why it is most prudent to perform biopsies of the tumour masses, as we have done. The incidence of sarcomatous transformation has been placed at 15% of all cases by Preston and coworkers. Fibrosarcoma, spindle cell sarcoma, and neurogenic sarcoma are some of these. In addition, Preston and coworkers have also mentioned other pathological lesions, mental disorders, osseous defects, and congenital defects which were not seen in our case [28]. In the specimen we excised, we obtained immunohistochemical analysis for S-100 protein, which was adequate for the diagnosis of neurofibromas. However, if they do not show positive immunoreactivity or if there is difficulty in differentiation between different neural tumours we can apply other staining tests like epithelial membrane antigen (EMA), factor XIIIa, CD34 or CD68, or type IV collagen [29]. Since our patient is showing other signs of multiple neurofibromatosis regular follow-up visits are required to detect any features of malignant transformation. Rarely, cases like this present us with a unique opportunity to diagnose neurofibromatosis. Although the oral manifestations of von Recklinghausen's disease are well documented, it may not be at the forefront of the inexperienced clinician's mind while diagnosing nodules of the tongue. Extraoral examination of all the patients who visit the dental operatory is of paramount importance as this case suggests, for one may miss the "bigger" picture if we as dental practitioners concentrated only on the oral findings of a particular condition. It is also important considering the fact that neurofibromas have a rare malignant transformation potential.

Conflict of Interests

The authors declare that there is no conflict of interests regarding the publication of this paper.

References

[1] E. M. Jouhilahti, V. Visnapuu, T. Soukka et al., "Oral soft tissue alterations in patients with neurofibromatosis," *Clinical Oral Investigations*, vol. 16, no. 2, pp. 551–558, 2012.

[2] S. W. Weiss and J. R. Goldblum, "Benign tumors of peripheral nerves," in *Enzinger and Weiss's Soft Tissue Tumors*, S. W. Weiss and J. R. Goldblum, Eds., pp. 1111–1207, Mosby, St. Louis, Mo, USA, 2001.

[3] T. M. Lynch and D. H. Gutmann, "Neurofibromatosis 1," *Neurologic Clinics*, vol. 20, no. 3, pp. 841–865, 2002.

[4] National Institutes of Health Consensus Development Conference, "Neurofibromatosis," *Archives of Neurology*, vol. 45, pp. 575–578, 1988.

[5] Y. Inoue, Y. Nemoto, T. Tashiro, K. Nakayama, T. Nakayama, and H. Daikokuya, "Neurofibromatosis Type 1 and Type 2: review of the central nervous system and related structures," *Brain and Development*, vol. 19, no. 1, pp. 1–12, 1997.

[6] P. Vabres, F. Otsuka, and T. Kawashima, "Absence of Lisch nodules in sporadic neurofibromatosis type 1 may reflect somatic mosaicism," *Archives of Dermatology*, vol. 138, no. 6, pp. 839–840, 2002.

[7] A. Sharma, P. Sengupta, and K. R. A. Das, "Isolated plexiform neurofibroma of the tongue," *Journal of Laboratory Physicians*, vol. 5, no. 2, pp. 127–129, 2013.

[8] V. H. Iyer, P. Ramalingam, and E. Nagadevan, "Neurofibroma of tongue: solitary lesion," *International Journal of Laser Dentistry*, vol. 2, no. 2, pp. 56–58, 2012.

[9] H. Sirinoglu and M. Bayramicli, "Isolated plexiform neurofibroma of the tongue," *Journal of Craniofacial Surgery*, vol. 21, no. 3, pp. 926–927, 2010.

[10] E. A. Güneri, E. Akoğlu, S. Sütay, K. Ceryan, Ö. Sağol, and U. Pabuçcuoğlu, "Plexiform neurofibroma of the tongue: a case report of a child," *Turkish Journal of Pediatrics*, vol. 48, no. 2, pp. 155–158, 2006.

[11] L. S. Marocchio, M. C. Pereira, C. T. Soares, and D. T. Oliveira, "Oral plexiform neurofibroma not associated with neurofibromatosis type I: case report," *Journal of Oral Science*, vol. 48, no. 3, pp. 157–160, 2006.

[12] M. R. Bongiorno, G. Pistone, and M. Aricò, "Manifestations of the tongue in Neurofibromatosis type 1," *Oral Diseases*, vol. 12, no. 2, pp. 125–129, 2006.

[13] E. Guclu, A. Tokmak, F. Oghan, O. Ozturk, and E. Egeli, "Hemimacroglossia caused by isolated plexiform neurofibroma: a case report," *Laryngoscope*, vol. 116, no. 1, pp. 151–153, 2006.

[14] C. Moreno-García, M. A. Pons-García, R. González-Garcí, and F. Monje-Gil, "Schwannoma of tongue," *Journal of Oral and Maxillofacial Surgery*, vol. 13, no. 2, pp. 217–221, 2014.

[15] G. Suchitra, K. N. Tambekar, and K. P. Gopal, "Abrikossoff's tumor of tongue: report of an uncommon lesion," *Journal of Oral and Maxillofacial Pathology*, vol. 18, no. 1, pp. 134–136, 2014.

[16] M. Toida, T. Murakami, K. Kato et al., "Irritation fibroma of the oral mucosa: a clinicopathological study of 129 lesions in 124 cases," *Oral Medicine & Pathology*, vol. 6, pp. 91–94, 2001.

[17] E. Baden, J. L. Doyle, and D. A. Lederman, "Leiomyoma of the oral cavity: a light microscopic and immunohistochemical study with review of the literature from 1884 to 1992," *European Journal of Cancer Part B: Oral Oncology*, vol. 30, no. 1, pp. 1–7, 1994.

[18] W. Burford, L. Ackerman, and H. Robinson, "Leiomyoma of the tongue," *The American Journal of Orthodontics and Oral Surgery*, vol. 30, p. 395, 1944.

[19] O. Sangueza, P. Sangueza, J. Jordan, and C. R. White Jr., "Rhabdomyoma of the tongue," *The American Journal of Dermatopathology*, vol. 12, no. 5, pp. 492–495, 1990.

[20] S. K. Nayak and P. Nayak, "Intramuscular hemangioma of the oral cavity—a case report," *Journal of Clinical and Diagnostic Research*, vol. 8, no. 8, pp. ZD41-ZD42, 2014.

[21] M. Goswami, S. Singh, S. Gokkulakrishnan, and A. Singh, "Lymphangioma of tongue," *National Journal of Maxillofacial Surgery*, vol. 2, no. 1, pp. 86–88, 2011.

[22] R. Kaur, S. Kler, and A. Bhullar, "Intra oral lipoma: report of 3 cases," *Dental Research Journal*, vol. 8, no. 1, pp. 48–51, 2011.

[23] K. Subhashraj, "Salivary gland tumors: a single institution experience in India," *British Journal of Oral and Maxillofacial Surgery*, vol. 46, no. 8, pp. 635–638, 2008.

[24] A. Buchner, P. W. Merrell, and W. M. Carpenter, "Relative frequency of intra-oral minor salivary gland tumors: a study of 380 cases from northern California and comparison to reports from other parts of the world," *Journal of Oral Pathology and Medicine*, vol. 36, no. 4, pp. 207–214, 2007.

[25] G. Zuccoli, F. Ferrozzi, G. Tognini, and A. Troiso, "Enlarging tongue masses in neurofibromatosis type 1MR findings of two cases," *Clinical Imaging*, vol. 25, no. 4, pp. 268–271, 2001.

[26] K. N. Shah, "The diagnostic and clinical significance of cafe au lait macules," *Pediatric Clinics of North America*, vol. 57, no. 5, pp. 1131–1153, 2010.

[27] H. Shimizu, *Shimizu's Textbook of Dermatology*, chapter 20, Hokkaidu University Press, Hokkaidu, Japan, 1st edition, 2007.

[28] F. W. Preston, W. S. Walsh, and T. H. Clarke, "Cutaneous neurofibromatosis (Von Recklinghausen's disease); clinical manifestation and incidence of sarcoma in sixty-one male patients," *A.M.A. Archives of Surgery*, vol. 64, no. 6, pp. 813–827, 1952.

[29] E. Chrysomali, S. I. Papanicolaou, N. P. Dekker, and J. A. Regezi, "Benign neural tumors of the oral cavity: a comparative immunohistochemical study," *Oral Surgery, Oral Medicine, Oral Pathology, Oral Radiology, and Endodontics*, vol. 84, no. 4, pp. 381–390, 1997.

Bilateral Paget's Disease of the Breast—Case Report of Long-Time Misdiagnosed Tumors with Underlying Ductal Carcinomas and Review of the Literature

Dietrich Barth

Hautarztpraxis Leipzig/Borna, Rudolf Virchow Straße, Borna, 04552 Leipzig, Germany

Correspondence should be addressed to Dietrich Barth; barthri@hotmail.com

Academic Editors: M. Jinnin and J.-H. Lee

Paget's disease of the breast is often misdiagnosed. We report on a 72-year old patient with a history of 2.5 years without any malignant findings, followed by the identification of a bilateral Paget's disease with bilateral breast cancers. This case underlines how important histological examinations even in unusual clinical pictures are.

1. Introduction

Paget's disease (PD) of the breast can be a diagnostic challenge. It might take years until the diagnosis. If the skin changes are intended to be benign but do not respond to topical therapy, a biopsy has to be performed to exclude malignancies. Almost all cases are single sided. We observed one of the rare cases of bilateral PD.

2. A Case Report

A 72-year-old woman (para 1) was seen with erythematous and eczematous patches that developed simultaneously on both nipples and had been present for 2.5 years (Figures 1(a) and 1(d)). No individual or familiar risk factors were known. She was extensively evaluated by gynecology and several investigations were performed (mammography, vacuum-punch biopsies, and cytological examination of breast fluid), but only minor dysplastic changes were detected in the breast fluid cytology. The patient was then treated with topical antimycotics, antibiotics, and corticosteroids.

After 2.5 years she was referred to dermatology, where we biopsied both nipples. The histopathology showed epidermal cells with hyperchromatic and polymorphic nuclei, intraepithelial gland cells (Figure 1(b)), and a high expression of cytokeratin 7 (Figure 1(c)), so-called Paget's cells. Cytokeratin 7 is a typical marker for glandular and transitional epithelia.

Because of an induration of the left mamma and the incidence of underlying carcinomas, the patient was evaluated again by gynecologists who decided to operate on both breasts. They identified a bifocal invasive ductal carcinoma and an intermediate grade ductal carcinoma in situ (DCIS) of the left breast and a low-grade DCIS of the right central breast. Sentinel lymph nodes were not involved. Following surgery, the patient received chemotherapy with 6 cycles FEC (5-fluorouracil, epirubicin, and cyclophosphamide), trastuzumab, because of positive Her-2 status, radiotherapy, and tamoxifen. At 1.5-year follow-up being maintained on tamoxifen, she showed no relapse.

3. Discussion

Between 1 and 4% of all breast cancers are Paget's diseases [1]. Bilateral synchronous tumors occur in about 1% of all breast cancers [2]. So far there are less than 10 reported women with synchronous bilateral PD. The age of these patients ranges from 45 to 74 years [3, 4]. This phenomenon has been described twice in men [5, 6].

The disease appears in three forms: (1) associated with an underlying ductal carcinoma in situ (DCIS), (2) associated

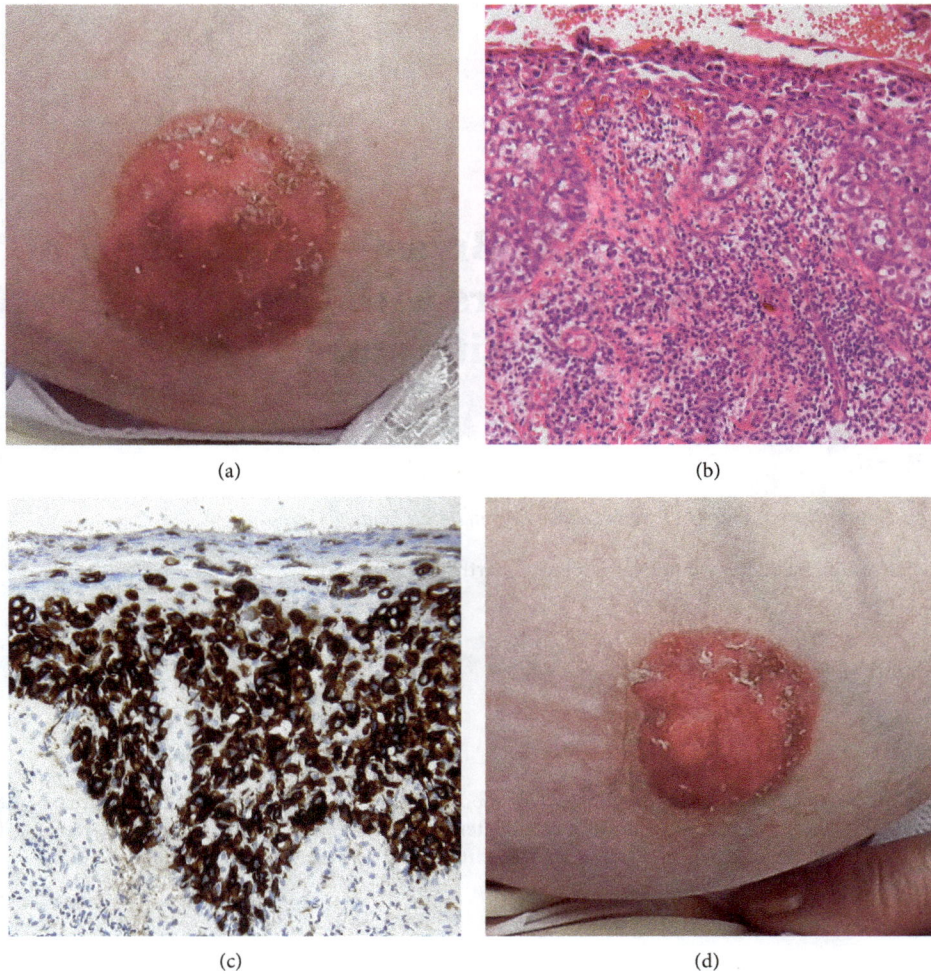

FIGURE 1: Clinical picture at time of first presentation and histological stains ((a) right breast, (b) cytokeratin 7 stain, (c) HE stain, and (d) left breast).

with an invasive carcinoma, or (3) without any underlying malignancy [7]. The majority of patients with PD have an underlying DCIS or even invasive carcinoma [8, 9].

For bilateral PD the limited data are controversial. Sahoo et al. [4] connected the PD of its patient to an underlying lobular CIS because of the immunohistochemical profile; Xie et al. [10] found no underlying tumor, whereas the patients of Anderson [11] and Franceschini et al. [12] as well as our patient had underlying ductal carcinomas.

It is still in discussion if the disease is the cause or consequence of an underlying malignancy. Most authors support the epidermotropism of malignant ductal gland cells into the epidermis. Some favor the migration of malignant keratinocytes from epidermis into deeper tissues, because in up to 50% of the cases no underlying tumors can be found [13].

Multiparous patients seem to have a reduced risk of ductal, lobular, tubular, and mucinous breast cancers. By contrast, the risk of medullary breast cancers increases with the number of pregnancies [14]. If similar findings for PD

are evident [15] should be subject for further investigations. One explanation could be the inflammatory processes and restructuring of the ductal network after lactation [16].

The cause for the bilateral form of PD remains uncertain as the number of patients is limited and the reported patients differ in age, gender, and ethnicity (see Table 1). Coincidences cannot be excluded.

The treatment options are mastectomy or breast-conserving strategies including nipple excision or central lumpectomy with a lymph node biopsy. There are reports of positive lymph nodes even without any underlying malignancies [8, 9]. If surgery is not possible, radiotherapy, laser therapy, photodynamic therapy, or chemotherapy, for example, with trastuzumab or imiquimod, can offer a therapeutic alternative.

Although radiological diagnostic tools have improved over the years, each suspicious skin lesion of the breast must be biopsied in order to avoid the progression of a malignancy. Our patient's history of 2.5 years without any findings underlines the importance of early histological examinations.

TABLE 1: Summary of all available cases of bilateral Paget's disease.

Age/gender	Associated cancer	Country	Author/reference
53/female	L: intraductal carcinoma	USA	Anderson 1979/[11]
Female	?	Netherlands	Knol and Voorhuis 1981/[17]
Female	?	India	Sinha and Prasad 1983/[18]
Male	?	India	Nagar 1983/[5]
74/female	?	Portugal	Fernandes et al. 1990/[3]
Female	?	Greece	Markopoulos et al. 1997/[19]
53/female	R: LCIS of the nipple, DCIS + microinvasive ductal carcinoma L: LCIS of the nipple, DCIS	USA	Sahoo et al. 2002/[4]
73/female	R: high-grade intraductal carcinoma L: micropapillary invasive carcinoma	Italy	Franceschini et al. 2005/[12]
74/male	R: infiltrative ductal carcinoma	Turkey	Ucar et al. 2008/[6]
45/female	None	China	Xie et al. 2012/[10]
72/female	R: low-grade DCIS L—intermediate DCIS, invasive ductal carcinoma	Germany	Barth 2014

L: left breast; R: right breast; DCIS: ductal carcinoma in situ; LCIS: lobular carcinoma in situ.

Conflict of Interests

The author declares that there is no conflict of interests regarding the publication of this paper.

References

[1] J. K. Marshall, K. A. Griffith, B. G. Haffty et al., "Conservative management of Paget disease of the breast with radiotherapy: 10- and 15-year results," *Cancer*, vol. 97, no. 9, pp. 2142–2149, 2003.

[2] Y. X. Shi, Q. Xia, R. J. Peng et al., "Comparison of clinico-pathological characteristics and prognoses between bilateral and unilateral breast cancer," *Journal of Cancer Research and Clinical Oncology*, vol. 138, no. 4, pp. 705–714, 2012.

[3] F. J. Fernandes, M. M. Costa, and M. Bernardo, "Rarities in breast pathology. Bilateral Paget's disease of the breast—a case report," *European Journal of Surgical Oncology*, vol. 16, no. 2, pp. 172–174, 1990.

[4] S. Sahoo, I. Green, and P. P. Rosen, "Bilateral Paget disease of the nipple associated with lobular carcinoma in situ: application of immunohistochemistry to a rare finding," *Archives of Pathology & Laboratory Medicine*, vol. 126, no. 1, pp. 90–92, 2002.

[5] R. C. Nagar, "Bilateral Paget's disease of the nipple in a male," *Journal of the Indian Medical Association*, vol. 81, no. 3-4, pp. 55–56, 1983.

[6] A. E. Ucar, B. Korukluoglu, E. Ergul, R. Aydin, and A. Kusdemir, "Bilateral Paget disease of the male nipple: first report," *Breast*, vol. 17, no. 3, pp. 317–318, 2008.

[7] C.-Y. Chen, L.-M. Sun, and B. O. Anderson, "Paget disease of the breast: changing patterns of incidence, clinical presentation, and treatment in the U.S.," *Cancer*, vol. 107, no. 7, pp. 1448–1458, 2006.

[8] M. Caliskan, G. Gatti, I. Sosnovskikh et al., "Paget's disease of the breast: the experience of the European institute of oncology and review of the literature," *Breast Cancer Research and Treatment*, vol. 112, no. 3, pp. 513–521, 2008.

[9] E. Siponen, K. Hukkinen, P. Heikkil, H. Joensuu, and M. Leidenius, "Surgical treatment in Paget's disease of the breast,"

The American Journal of Surgery, vol. 200, no. 2, pp. 241–246, 2010.

[10] B. Xie, H. Zheng, H. Lan, B. Cui, K. Jin, and F. Cao, "Synchronous bilateral Paget's disease of the breast: a case report," *Oncology letters*, vol. 4, no. 1, pp. 83–85, 2012.

[11] W. R. Anderson, "Bilateral Paget's disease of the nipple: case report," *American Journal of Obstetrics & Gynecology*, vol. 134, no. 8, pp. 877–878, 1979.

[12] G. Franceschini, R. Masetti, D. D'Ugo et al., "Synchronous bilateral Paget's disease of the nipple associated with bilateral breast carcinoma," *The Breast Journal*, vol. 11, no. 5, pp. 355–356, 2005.

[13] G. H. Sakorafas, K. Blanchard, M. G. Sarr, and D. R. Farley, "Paget's disease of the breast," *Cancer Treatment Reviews*, vol. 27, no. 1, pp. 9–18, 2001.

[14] G. K. Reeves, K. Pirie, J. Green, D. Bull, and V. Beral, "Reproductive factors and specific histological types of breast cancer: prospective study and meta-analysis," *British Journal of Cancer*, vol. 100, no. 3, pp. 538–544, 2009.

[15] G. Albrektsen, I. Heuch, and S. Ø. Thoresen, "Histological type and grade of breast cancer tumors by parity, age at birth, and time since birth: a register-based study in Norway," *BMC Cancer*, vol. 10, article 226, 2010.

[16] P. Schedin, J. O'Brien, M. Rudolph, T. Stein, and V. Borges, "Microenvironment of the involuting mammary gland mediates mammary cancer progression," *Journal of Mammary Gland Biology and Neoplasia*, vol. 12, no. 1, pp. 71–82, 2007.

[17] W. L. R. Knol and F. J. Voorhuis, "Paget's disease of the breast: a case of bilateral occurrence," *Nederlands Tijdschrift voor Geneeskunde*, vol. 125, no. 11, pp. 416–418, 1981.

[18] M. R. Sinha and S. B. Prasad, "Bilateral Paget's disease of the nipple," *Journal of the Indian Medical Association*, vol. 80, no. 2, pp. 27–28, 1983.

[19] C. Markopoulos, H. Gogas, F. Sampalis, and B. Kyriakou, "Bilateral Paget's disease of the breast," *European Journal of Gynaecological Oncology*, vol. 18, no. 6, pp. 495–496, 1997.

Crusted Demodicosis in an Immunocompetent Pediatric Patient

Guillermo Antonio Guerrero-González, Maira Elizabeth Herz-Ruelas, Minerva Gómez-Flores, and Jorge Ocampo-Candiani

Dermatology Department, Hospital Universitario "Dr. José Eleuterio González," Universidad Autónoma de Nuevo León, Avenida Francisco I. Madero Poniente s/n y Avenida Gonzalitos, Colonia Mitras Centro, 64460 Monterrey, NL, Mexico

Correspondence should be addressed to Jorge Ocampo-Candiani; jocampo2000@yahoo.com.mx

Academic Editor: Alireza Firooz

Demodicosis refers to the infestation by *Demodex* spp., a saprophytic mite of the pilosebaceous unit. Demodex proliferation can result in a number of cutaneous disorders including pustular folliculitis, pityriasis folliculorum, papulopustular, and granulomatous rosacea, among others. We report the case of a 7-year-old female presenting with pruritic grayish crusted lesions over her nose and cheeks, along with facial erythema, papules, and pustules. The father referred chronic use of topical steroids. A potassium hydroxide mount of a pustule scraping revealed several *D. folliculorum* mites. Oral ivermectin (200 μg/kg, single dose) plus topical permethrin 5% lotion applied for 3 consecutive nights were administered. Oral ivermectin was repeated every week and oral erythromycin plus topical metronidazole cream was added. The facial lesions greatly improved within the following 3 months. While infestation of the pilosebaceous unit by *Demodex folliculorum* mites is common, only few individuals present symptoms. Demodicosis can present as pruritic papules, pustules, plaques, and granulomatous facial lesions. To our knowledge, this is the first reported case of facial crusted demodicosis in an immunocompetent child. The development of symptoms in this patient could be secondary to local immunosuppression caused by the chronic use of topical steroids.

1. Introduction

Demodicosis refers to the infestation by *Demodex* spp., a saprophytic mite of the pilosebaceous unit. Colonization usually occurs starting adolescence or afterwards, when sebaceous glands mature and multiply. A high prevalence of Demodex (80–100%) by the age of 50 years is proposed [1], although few individuals develop symptoms. Demodex proliferation can result in a number of cutaneous disorders including pustular folliculitis, pityriasis folliculorum, and papulopustular and granulomatous rosacea [2]. Several factors may be implicated in the development of pathogenic forms, including increased density of the mite, immune system disorders such as HIV infection, and the use of corticosteroids.

2. Case Presentation

We report the case of a 7-year-old female patient presenting with pruritic grayish and yellowish crusted, scaly plaques over her nose and cheeks, along with diffuse facial erythema, papules, and pustules (Figure 1(a)). The father referred chronic use of topical hydrocortisone and betamethasone for over 4 months to treat facial eczematous lesions. The patient was otherwise healthy. A potassium hydroxide (KOH) mount of a pustule scraping revealed several *Demodex folliculorum* mites (Figure 1(b)). Oral ivermectin (200 μg/kg, single dose) plus topical permethrin 5% lotion applied for 3 consecutive nights were administered; afterwards, oral erythromycin 30 mg/kg/day, divided in three doses, plus metronidazole cream was added. Oral ivermectin was repeated every week for a total of 10 doses. Although lesions improved greatly within the following 3 months (Figure 2), oral erythromycin was maintained for 2 months to avoid a recurrence.

3. Discussion

Two species of Demodex have been identified in humans: *D. folliculorum*, with a cigar-shaped body usually found within hair follicles, and *D. brevis*, which is smaller and favors

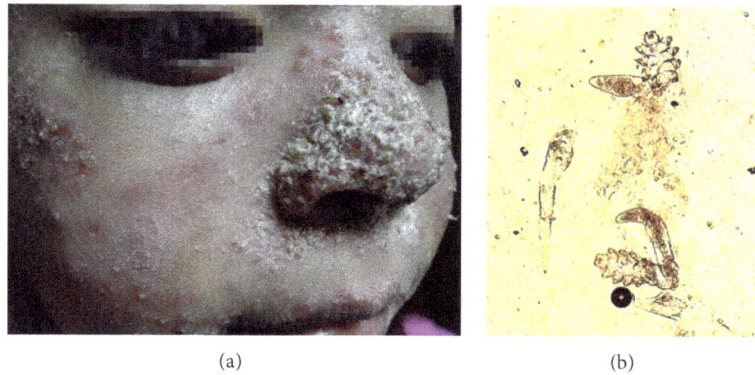

FIGURE 1: (a) Facial erythema, grayish crusted lesions, papules, and pustules. (b) Skin scraping revealing *D. folliculorum* mites.

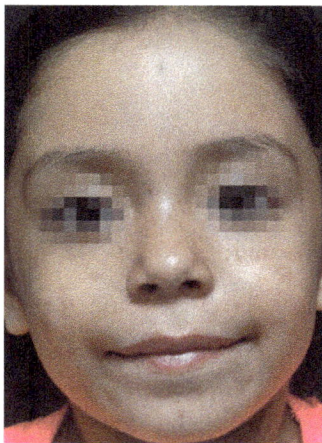

FIGURE 2: Clinical resolution after 3 months of treatment.

the sebaceous glands [3]. While inhabiting the pilosebaceous unit, they feed on sebum and bacteria. Infestation of the pilosebaceous unit by Demodex mites is common, mite density is low in healthy skin, and only few individuals present symptoms [4].

Demodicosis can be classified as primary, in the absence of other inflammatory dermatoses, having a sudden onset, or secondary when associated with other cutaneous or systemic diseases, developing gradually over existing dermatoses [5]. The latter is frequently found in severely immunosuppressed patients, including those using topical corticosteroids or calcineurin inhibitors [6]. Clinical presentation is heterogeneous and can include pruritic papules, vesicles, pustules, plaques, granulomatous, and even cystic facial lesions [5, 7]. Crusted exuberant lesions have already been reported in an adult with HIV infection and chronic use of steroids [8]. A case of demodicosis mimicking favus has been reported in an immunocompetent child [9].

Diagnosis can be made by standardized skin surface biopsy or skin scraping, usually considering abnormal anything more than 5 mites per cm^2 [6].

There are several treatment options with varied efficacy, although there is a strong lack of evidence-based literature.

Ivermectin (200 μg/kg single dose) is the current treatment of choice and can be combined with topical permethrin, benzyl benzoate, or metronidazole [6, 7]. The mechanism of action of antimicrobial agents remains to be fully elucidated, with reports of its efficacy being secondary to their anti-inflammatory effect or by reducing bacteria both living on the mite and that on which the mites feed on [2].

To our knowledge, this is the first reported case of facial crusted rosacea-like demodicosis in a pediatric patient. Usually, *Demodex* colonization is not significant in infants and children due to low sebum production [3].

The pathogenesis and immune response to mite invasion are not clearly understood; thus, the particularly severe clinical manifestations seen in this case could be attributed to local immunosuppression secondary to chronic use of topical steroids. Like the lesions observed in patients with Norwegian scabies, this particular clinical presentation of *D. folliculorum* infestation could be due to other unknown factors besides the local immunosuppression that led to a defective host-defense immune response resulting in a great increase in parasite population.

Conflict of Interests

The authors declare that there is no conflict of interests regarding the publication of this paper.

References

[1] R. Aylesworth and J. C. Vance, "Demodex folliculorum and Demodex brevis in cutaneous biopsies," *Journal of the American Academy of Dermatology*, vol. 7, no. 5, pp. 583–589, 1982.

[2] J. R. Vu and J. C. English, "Demodex folliculitis," *Journal of Pediatric and Adolescent Gynecology*, vol. 24, no. 5, pp. 320–321, 2011.

[3] P. A. Rather and I. Hassan, "Human demodex mite: the versatile mite of dermatological importance," *Indian Journal of Dermatology*, vol. 59, no. 1, pp. 60–66, 2014.

[4] B. Baima and M. Sticherling, "Demodicidosis revisited," *Acta Dermato-Venereologica*, vol. 82, no. 1, pp. 3–6, 2002.

[5] O. E. Akilov, Y. S. Butov, and K. Y. Mumcuoglu, "A clinico-pathological approach to the classification of human

demodicosis," *JDDG—Journal of the German Society of Dermatology*, vol. 3, no. 8, pp. 607–614, 2005.

[6] W. Chen and G. Plewig, "Human demodicosis: revisit and a proposed classification," *British Journal of Dermatology*, vol. 170, no. 6, pp. 1219–1225, 2014.

[7] J. C. Fichtel, A. K. Wiggins, and J. L. Lesher Jr., "Plaque-forming demodicidosis," *Journal of the American Academy of Dermatology*, vol. 52, no. 2, supplement 1, pp. S59–S61, 2005.

[8] C. S. Brutti, G. Artus, L. Luzzatto, R. R. Bonamigo, S. N. Balconi, and R. Vettorato, "Crusted rosacea-like demodicidosis in an HIV-positive female," *Journal of the American Academy of Dermatology*, vol. 65, no. 4, pp. e131–e132, 2011.

[9] A. García-Vargas, J. A. Mayorga-Rodríguez, and C. Sandoval-Tress, "Scalp demodicidosis mimicking favus in a 6-year-old boy," *Journal of the American Academy of Dermatology*, vol. 57, no. 2 supplement, pp. S19–S21, 2007.

Pemphigus Vulgaris Presented with Cheilitis

Zaheer Abbas,[1] Zahra Safaie Naraghi,[1] and Elham Behrangi[2]

[1] Department of Dermatology, Razi Hospital, Tehran University of Medical Sciences, Vahdate Eslami Square,
    Vahdate Eslami Avenue, Tehran 11996, Iran
[2] Department of Dermatology, Rasoul-e Akram Hospital, Iran University of Medical Sciences, Tehran, Iran

Correspondence should be addressed to Zaheer Abbas; drzaheerabbas@yahoo.com

Academic Editor: Bhushan Kumar

Background. Pemphigus vulgaris is an autoimmune blistering disease affecting the mucous membrane and skin. In 50 to 70% of cases, the initial manifestations of pemphigus vulgaris are oral lesions which may be followed by skin lesions. But it is unusual for the disease to present with initial and solitary persistent lower lip lesions without progression to any other location. *Main Observations*. We report a 41-year-old woman with dry crusted lesions only on the lower lip, clinically resembling actinic cheilitis and erosive lichen planus, but histopathological evaluation showed unexpected results of suprabasal acantholysis and cleft compatible with pemphigus vulgaris. We treated her with intralesional triamcinolone 10 mg/mL for 2 sessions and 2 g cellcept daily. Patient showed excellent response and lesions resolved completely within 2 months. In one-year follow-up, there was no evidence of relapse or any additional lesion on the other sites. *Conclusion*. Cheilitis may be the initial and sole manifestation of pemphigus vulgaris. Localized and solitary lesions of pemphigus vulgaris can be treated and controlled without systemic corticosteroids.

1. Introduction

Pemphigus vulgaris (PV) is an autoimmune intraepithelial blistering disease involving mucous membranes and the skin. The oral mucous membrane is frequently affected in PV patients; most of patients present with oral lesions as the first sign of PV [1, 2]. Lesions may occur anywhere on the oral mucosa, but the buccal mucosa is the most commonly affected site, followed by involvement of the palatal, lingual, labial mucosae, and the gingiva [3]. Here we present a case of PV manifested as persistent crusted lesions only on the lower lip.

2. Case Report

A 41-year-old woman was referred to the dermatology clinic of Razi Hospital, Tehran, Iran, with a 6-month history of erosions and crusts on lower lip accompanied by pain and burning sensation (Figure 1). Further physical examination did not reveal any lesion on the skin and mucosa. Multiple topical treatments had been used by the patient in this period but lesions did not improve.

Our initial differential diagnosis included actinic cheilitis and erosive lichen planus. Biopsy was performed to make definite diagnosis. Histopathological evaluation showed unexpected results of intraepithelial, suprabasal clefting along with keratinocyte acantholysis compatible with pemphigus vulgaris (Figures 2(a) and 2(b)). For the sake of confirmation, we performed rebiopsy and direct immunofluorescence (DIF) studies. DIF study revealed intercellular space deposits of IgG and C3 in the surface epithelium, proving the diagnosis of PV. Quantitative ELISA values of anti-Dsg 1 and anti-Dsg 3 (antidesmoglein 1 and 3) antibodies were 15 and 56 (positive > 20), respectively.

As the disease was mild and localized, we started cellcept 2 g daily along with 2 sessions of triamcinolone 10 mg/mL intralesional injections after performing initial necessary tests. Lesions were totally resolved within 2 months (Figure 3). After disease remission, treatment continued with cellcept 2 g daily for 1 year follow-up period. There was neither recurrence nor any new lesion elsewhere (Figure 4). Anti-Dsg 1 and anti-Dsg 3 values at the end of 6-month follow-up were 11 and 18.9 (positive >20), respectively.

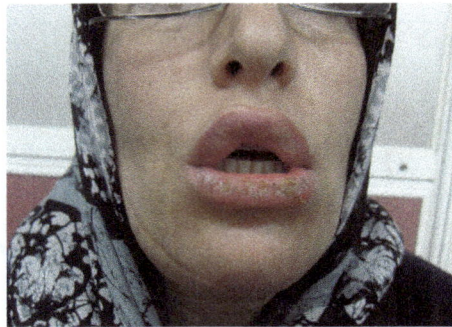

FIGURE 1: Scaly crusted lesions on lower lip (before biopsy).

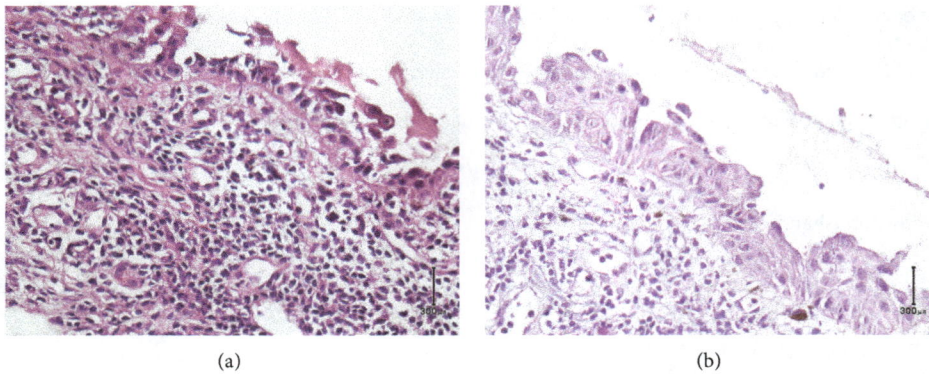

(a)   (b)

FIGURE 2: Lip mucosa showing suprabasal acantholysis, clefting, and retraction of tonofilaments.

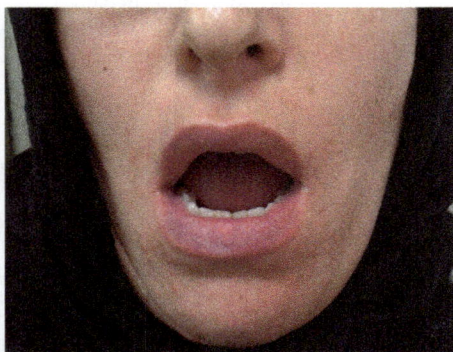

FIGURE 3: After 2-month follow-up (lesions resolved).

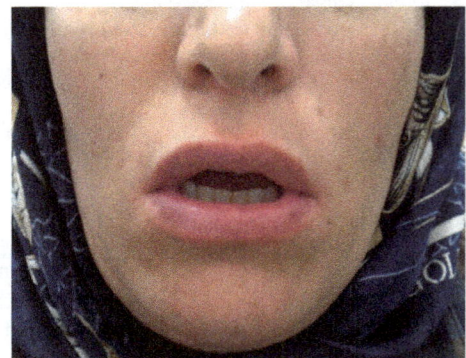

FIGURE 4: After one-year follow-up.

3. Discussion

PV is a chronic autoimmune blistering disease. PV almost always affects the mouth and it can be initial site of presentation in 50% of cases, before skin and other mucosal sites involvement [4]. Diagnosis is based on oral erosions, while confirmation is provided by histological findings, which show the intraepithelial acantholysis. DIF reveals IgG and C3 deposits in intercellular space [5].

In Iran, 62% of PV patients referred to skin clinics had oral lesions [6]. Intact bullae are rarely observed in the oral cavity; in fact, most patients present with irregular erosions with ill-defined borders that tend to heal very slowly and often extend [7]. These erosions are commonly detected in the buccal mucosa and the palate; some cases may progress to involve the pharynx and larynx, causing hoarseness and dysphagia. Other mucous membranes occasionally involved comprise the nasal mucosa, esophagus, conjunctiva, anus, penis, vagina, cervix, and labia [3, 7, 8].

In our patient, disease had some peculiar aspects: (1) the first and only site involved was the lower lip. (2) Disease was mild in such a way that PV was not suspected clinically. (3) Rapid response to intralesional steroid injections without oral steroids and cellcept was used alone in the maintenance phase.

There is only one such case report in the literature, presenting with sole persistent lesion on the lower lip [9] but lesions in our patient were very mild and without hemorrhagic erosions. Interestingly, our patient had positive disease activity shown by high circulating anti-Dsg 3 antibodies. The pathogenesis of pemphigus is thought to be related to the presence of autoantibodies against Dsgs [10–13]. Anti-Dsg antibodies cause disruption to intercellular adhesion in keratinocytes resulting in blister formation [14] but the exact mechanism of how the disease causes such localization in spite of high circulating anti-Dsg antibodies has yet to be determined.

Our patient showed rapid response to intralesional steroid injection and after remission cellcept 2 g daily continued for 1 year and circulating anti-Dsg 3 antibody was in normal range after a 6-month follow-up. Although PV is generally known as a lifetime fatal disease, exceptionally it can be mild and easily managed by steroid sparing agents along with intralesional steroid injection to avoid side effects of systemic corticosteroids.

4. Conclusions

This report describes the case of a patient presenting with a 6-month history of persistent crusted lesion on the lower lip, who was finally diagnosed as having PV. Although the main presentation of PV is oral lesions particularly on buccal, palate, and tongue that can extend to gingiva and lips, it is very rare for the disease to present only on the lower lip without involving any other site. We recommend that PV should be taken into account when persistent cheilitis was presented to make early diagnosis. Additionally, we may conclude that localized and solitary lesions of pemphigus vulgaris can be treated and controlled without systemic corticosteroids. Cellcept alone can be used safely and effectively as maintenance therapy in such cases.

Conflict of Interests

The authors declare that there is no conflict of interests regarding the publication of this paper.

References

[1] D. A. Sirois, M. Fatahzadeh, R. Roth, and D. Ettlin, "Diagnostic patterns and delays in pemphigus vulgaris: experience with 99 patients," *Archives of Dermatology*, vol. 136, no. 12, pp. 1569–1570, 2000.

[2] H. Endo, T. D. Rees, W. W. Hallmon et al., "Disease progression from mucosal to mucocutaneous involvement in a patient with desquamative gingivitis associated with pemphigus vulgaris," *Journal of Periodontology*, vol. 79, no. 2, pp. 369–375, 2008.

[3] C. Scully, O. Paes De Almeida, S. R. Porter, and J. J. H. Gilkes, "Pemphigus vulgaris: the manifestations and long-term management of 55 patients with oral lesions," *British Journal of Dermatology*, vol. 140, no. 1, pp. 84–89, 1999.

[4] C. Scully and S. J. Challacombe, "Pemphigus vulgaris: update on etiopathogenesis, oral manifestations, and management," *Critical Reviews in Oral Biology and Medicine*, vol. 13, no. 5, pp. 397–408, 2002.

[5] F. Femiano, F. Gombos, and C. Scully, "Pemphigus vulgaris with oral involvement: Evaluation of two different systemic corticosteroid therapeutic protocols," *Journal of the European Academy of Dermatology and Venereology*, vol. 16, no. 4, pp. 353–356, 2002.

[6] C. Chams-Davatchi, M. Valikhani, M. Daneshpazhooh et al., "Pemphigus: analysis of 1209 cases," *International Journal of Dermatology*, vol. 44, no. 6, pp. 470–476, 2005.

[7] F. Wojnarowska, V. A. Venning, and S. M. Burge, "Immunobullous diseases," in *Rook's Textbook of Dermatology*, T. Burns, S. Breathnach, N. Cox, and C. Griffiths, Eds., vol. 2, Blackwell, 7th edition, 2004.

[8] M. C. Udey and J. R. Stanley, "Pemphigus—diseases of antidesmosomal autoimmunity," *Journal of the American Medical Association*, vol. 282, no. 6, pp. 572–576, 1999.

[9] M. Shahidi Dadras, M. Qeisari, and S. Givrad, "Pemphigus vulgaris manifesting as a sole persistent lesion on the lower lip: a case report," *Dermatology Online Journal*, vol. 15, no. 6, article 7, 2009.

[10] M. Amagai, V. Klaus-Kovtun, and J. R. Stanley, "Autoantibodies against a novel epithelial cadherin in Pemphigus vulgaris, a disease of cell adhesion," *Cell*, vol. 67, no. 5, pp. 869–877, 1991.

[11] T. Hashimoto, M. M. Ogawa, A. Konohana, and T. Nishikawa, "Detection of pemphigus vulgaris and pemphigus foliaceus antigens by immunoblot analysis using different antigen sources," *Journal of Investigative Dermatology*, vol. 94, no. 3, pp. 327–331, 1990.

[12] T. Hashimoto, A. Konohana, and T. Nishikawa, "Immunoblot assay as an aid to the diagnoses of unclassified cases of pemphigus," *Archives of Dermatology*, vol. 127, no. 6, pp. 843–847, 1991.

[13] T. Hashimoto, M. Amagai, D. R. Garrod, and T. Nishikawa, "Immunofluorescence and immunoblot studies on the reactivity of pemphigus vulgaris and pemphigus foliaceus sera with desmoglein 3 and desmoglein 1," *Epithelial Cell Biology*, vol. 4, no. 2, pp. 63–69, 1995.

[14] K. Nishifuji, T. Olivry, K. Ishii, T. Iwasaki, and M. Amagai, "IgG autoantibodies directed against desmoglein 3 cause dissociation of keratinocytes in canine pemphigus vulgaris and paraneoplastic pemphigus," *Veterinary Immunology and Immunopathology*, vol. 117, no. 3-4, pp. 209–221, 2007.

Mixed Cutaneous Infection Caused by *Mycobacterium szulgai* and *Mycobacterium intermedium* in a Healthy Adult Female: A Rare Case Report

Amresh Kumar Singh,[1] **Rungmei S. K. Marak,**[2] **Anand Kumar Maurya,**[3] **Manaswini Das,**[2] **Vijaya Lakshmi Nag,**[3] **and Tapan N. Dhole**[2]

[1]*Department of Microbiology, BRD Medical College, Gorakhpur, Uttar Pradesh 273013, India*
[2]*Department of Microbiology, Sanjay Gandhi Post Graduate Institute of Medical Sciences, Lucknow 226014, India*
[3]*Department of Microbiology, All India Institute of Medical Sciences, Jodhpur 342005, India*

Correspondence should be addressed to Amresh Kumar Singh; amresh.sgpgi@gmail.com

Academic Editor: Kowichi Jimbow

Nontuberculous mycobacteria (NTMs) are ubiquitous and are being increasingly reported as human opportunistic infection. Cutaneous infection caused by mixed NTM is extremely rare. We encountered the case of a 46-year-old female, who presented with multiple discharging sinuses over the lower anterior abdominal wall (over a previous appendectomy scar) for the past 2 years. Microscopy and culture of the pus discharge were done to isolate and identify the etiological agent. Finally, GenoType Mycobacterium CM/AS assay proved it to be a mixed infection caused by *Mycobacterium szulgai* and *M. intermedium*. The patient was advised a combination of rifampicin 600 mg once daily, ethambutol 600 mg once daily, and clarithromycin 500 mg twice daily to be taken along with periodic follow-up based upon clinical response as well as microbiological response. We emphasize that infections by NTM must be considered in the etiology of nonhealing wounds or sinuses, especially at postsurgical sites.

1. Introduction

Nontuberculous mycobacteria (NTMs) also known as atypical mycobacteria or mycobacteria other than tuberculosis (MOTT) have been recognized since the late 19th century but being opportunists, these organisms did not gain much importance for a long time. However, presently the recovery of NTM from clinical specimens from sites where they have been proved to cause infections (called "other mycobacterioses") is of concern to microbiologists and physicians alike [1]. NTMs are ubiquitous organisms that are readily isolated from soil, water, domestic and wild animals, milk, and other items [2]. NTM on isolation was believed to represent environmental contamination or colonization for a long time; it was only during the late 1950s that NTMs were recognized as potential pathogens [3]. Nearly every pathogenic species of NTM may cause skin and soft tissue infections, but rapidly growing mycobacteria (*M. fortuitum, M. chelonae,*

and *M. abscessus*), *M. marinum* and *M. ulcerans*, are the ones most commonly involved. Many of these cutaneous mycobacteria, such as the rapidly growing mycobacteria, *M. marinum, M. avium* complex, *M. kansasii*, and *M. xenopi*, are distributed worldwide [4]. The incidence of NTM infection has increased manifold, so much so that these infections currently account for 10%–15% of all mycobacterial infections [5, 6]. While the *Mycobacterium avium* complex (MAC) and *M. kansasii* are responsible for more than 90% of cases of nontuberculous mycobacterial infection, number of clinically important *Mycobacterium* species have rapidly increased and now include species such as *M. szulgai* [7]. *M. szulgai* has been recovered from environmental sources, including a snail, aquarium water, swimming pool water, and tropical fish [8]. The environment is the suspected source of human NTM infection [9, 10]. *M. szulgai* is an uncommon mycobacterial pathogen of humans [11]. It causes pulmonary disease resembling the common type of *M. tuberculosis* infection, as well

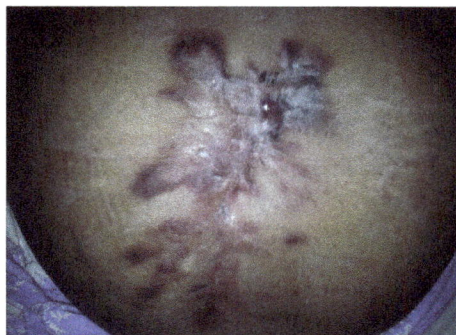

FIGURE 1: Clinical photograph showing discharging (serosanguinous as white arrow) sinuses present over previous-surgical scar with scarring and keloid formation on lower anterior abdominal wall.

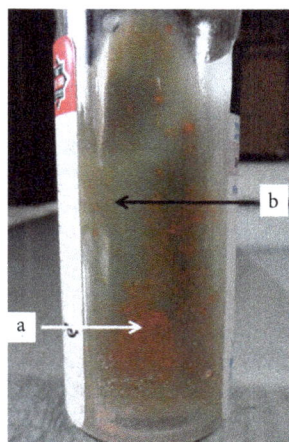

FIGURE 2: Showing numerous dry, rough, pigmented colonies of *M. szulgai* (a: bright orange as white arrow) and *M. intermedium* (b: pale/light yellow as black arrow) over Lowenstein-Jensen media slant.

as extrapulmonary infections. Cutaneous infection caused by *M. szulgai* was reported in one case which was seen after bone marrow transplantation [12], but mixed infection caused by two NTM species is extremely rare. *M. intermedium* is an intermediate to slow growing *Mycobacterium* that was first reported in 1993 [13]. We present here a case of an apparently immunocompetent patient with a history of previous surgery presenting with a mixed infection of the skin and soft tissue caused by *M. szulgai* and *M. intermedium*.

2. Case Report

A 46-year-old nondiabetic woman from a middle-class family, presented with discharging sinuses over the lower anterior abdominal wall for the past 2 years. There was no rise of temperature or weight loss. Her incision wound from laparoscopic appendectomy in 1998 did not heal properly and the surgical site was reopened after 1 month. There was no healing of the incision wound after reexcision. After that the whole area started to become erythematous and indurated and later on a keloid started developing over the scar. A large sinus developed over the operation scar and the other stitch sites also developed into sinuses discharging pus. However, there was no history of cough, haemoptysis, breathlessness, and anorexia. There was no history of intake of any immunosuppressive drugs/corticosteroids, any local trauma/injury, or tuberculosis. She had been treated off and on without having any definitive microbiological diagnosis with multiple injectable and oral antibiotics before consultation at this hospital. She did not have any contact with tuberculosis patients.

On examination, a previous-surgical scar was present over which a large keloid had formed, on the lower anterior abdominal wall in the midline (although a little more towards the right). There was no apparent mass over the abdomen, but 6 sinus openings were noted over the lower anterior abdominal wall (Figure 1). At the time of presentation a single sinus was discharging pus. On palpation, tenderness was noted over and around the sinuses. The sinus opening was bluish, wide, and undermined and it was discharging a serosanguinous exudate admixed with pus. Complete haemogram

and clinical chemistry were within normal limits including blood sugar. HIV ELISA negative by two kits, C-reactive protein normal and the ESR, was peaked at 22 mm. Pus from the discharging sinus was collected and processed using standard procedures. Gram stained smear showed plenty of pus cells with Gram variable bacilli (many of which were Gram positive) and on Ziehl–Neelsen staining numerous acid fast bacilli could be observed. The discharge was cultured on blood agar, MacConkey medium, and Lowenstein-Jensen medium and inoculated into a BacT/ALERT MP bottle, which was incubated in the BacT/ALERT 3D system (bioMerieux, USA). The blood agar and MacConkey medium were incubated under aerobic conditions at 37°C. The blood agar plate showed numerous dry, small nonhemolytic colonies after 72 hours but there was no growth on the MacConkey medium. The BacT/ALERT MP showed positive growth in 5 days for acid fast bacilli, which on further subculture onto L-J medium gave dry, rough, pigmented, and yellow to orange colonies after one-week period (Figure 2). They were found to be scotochromogenic at 37°C. Speciation for the isolate was confirmed by the GenoType Mycobacterium CM/AS assay based on Mycobacterium DNA strip technology (Hain Lifescience, Nehren, Germany), [14] following manufacturer's instructions. It showed a mixed infection caused by two NTM species, that is, *Mycobacterium szulgai* and *M. intermedium*. To confirm microbiological result, culture from repeat sample after one week showed the same dual infection caused by *Mycobacterium szulgai* and *M. intermedium* by the GenoType Mycobacterium CM/AS assay. Drug susceptibility testing (DST) was performed by standard disk diffusion method over Middlebrook 7H10 agar supplemented with OADC (oleic acid, dextrose, and citrate) and the following results were obtained: sensitive to linezolid, levofloxacin, clarithromycin, amikacin, and ciprofloxacin and found to be resistant to cotrimoxazole. DST for 1st and 2nd line antitubercular drugs were done by the GenoType MTBDR*plus* and MTBDR*sl* assay (Hain Lifescience, Nehren, Germany) which showed resistance to isoniazid and sensitive to rifampicin, fluoro-quinolones, aminoglycosides/cyclic peptides, and ethambutol.

The patient was advised a combination of rifampicin 600 mg once daily, ethambutol 600 mg once daily, and clarithromycin 500 mg twice daily to be taken along with periodic follow-up based upon clinical response as well as microbiological response.

She was advised to continue the therapy and when she presented to the hospital after one month, there was no pus discharge from the sinus. She was advised to continue the therapy and report to hospital after another month. Again after one month of therapy, there was no discharge present and the sinus was almost completely healed. Thereafter, she was advised to continue the same therapy for another two months. Thereafter, patient was completely all right with no such discharge after completion of two-month antibiotic therapy.

3. Discussion

Nontuberculous mycobacteria (NTMs) can be classified by their growth rate as slowly growing and rapidly growing species, by pigment production (pigmented and nonpigmented species) and optimal growth temperature requirement. *M. marinum*, *M. kansasii*, *M. avium-intracellulare*, *M intermedium*, and *M. szulgai* are examples of slow-growing mycobacteria. *M. fortuitum*, *M. chelonae*, and *M. abscessus* are examples of rapidly growing mycobacteria [4]. Diagnosis relies upon clinical presentations, microscopy, microbiological culture, and molecular detection of mycobacterial DNA to confirm species identification. NTMs have had a strong impact on human populations in both developing and industrialized countries [2]. Cutaneous infections caused by NTMs are still uncommon but their relative importance has changed during last decade and still further changes are expected. *M. szulgai* is a slow growing, scotochromogenic NTM, first identified in 1972 by a Polish microbiologist T Szulg. *M. intermedium* was first identified in 1993 and classified as a photochromogen, usually causing chronic bronchitis, dermatitis, and sometimes pulmonary infections. The name "intermedium" was used to denote its intermediate phylogenetic position between the slowly and rapidly growing mycobacteria [15]. The infection caused by *M. szulgai* is very rare and this bacterium accounts for 0.5% of all isolates obtained from human patients with NTM infection [16, 17]. *M. szulgai* when isolated is thought to be clinically significant unless proven otherwise and treatment should always be considered [18]. Only 27 cases of *M. szulgai* infection have been reported between 1989 and 2008 from Japan, most of which involved preexisting disease [19]. Cultures yielding *M. szulgai* usually have a pathologic significance, because this bacterium is rarely recovered from the environment [17, 18]. The acquisition of *M. szulgai* from the local environment especially water was already proven by different previous studies [9, 10, 20]. The sensitivity and specificity of the GenoType Mycobacterium CM strip have been shown to be 97.0–98.9% and 88.9–92.4% and of the AS strip 99.3–99.4 and 99.4–100%, respectively [21, 22]. Consequently, even one positive culture under appropriate clinical circumstances may suffice for diagnosing *M. szulgai* infection. In the present case, cultures of the sinus exudate from the anterior abdominal wall revealed mixed infection caused by *M. szulgai* and *M. intermedium*. The source of infection in the patient fits the pattern potentially resulting from introduction of mycobacteria during surgery, because it was present at the site of laparoscopic ports. However, the source of the infection could not be proved in this case because surgery was done in a private hospital setting and could not be accessed by the authors. *M. szulgai* can cause chronic nonhealing skin and soft tissue infection through iatrogenic spread. *M. intermedium* has been known to cause granulomatous dermatitis in a patient with hot tub exposure and appeared to be refractory to appropriate antimicrobial therapy because of repeated exposure to contaminated water [23]. *M. szulgai* infection causing nonhealing sinus is extremely rare but can be successfully treated with a combination of different antibiotics and antitubercular drugs.

Our case report highlights the paramount importance of eliciting adequate medical history in the diagnosis of NTM infection. The patient failed to respond to seemingly appropriate antibiotic therapy over a 2-year period due to the lack of definite microbiological diagnosis. In this case, the patient had undergone surgery for appendicitis and at that time she presented with nonhealing wound and was treated with off and on multiple antibiotics. The discharging sinuses developed later at the site of previous surgery and during that time no attempt was made for appropriate diagnosis. The reservoir for many mycobacterial species is generally municipal and hospital water supplies. These mycobacterial species are incredibly hardy and able to grow in tap water and distilled water, thrive at temperatures of 45°C or above (especially *M. xenopi* and *M. avium* complex), and resist the activity of organomercurials, chlorine, 2% concentrations of formaldehyde, and alkaline glutaraldehyde [24]. Perhaps in our patient, the nontuberculous mycobacteria were transmitted from a contaminated environmental source by the direct cutaneous route. Nevertheless, even in a healthy individual exposure to saprophytic mycobacteria may lead to infections, as described for *M. kansasii*. It is difficult to recognize and treat NTM infections, especially mixed infections caused by unusual pathogens like *M. szulgai* and *M. intermedium*. A high index of suspicion is warranted in these cases and prompt treatment should be initiated once adequate material for diagnosis has been secured.

We insist on strict adherence to standard sterilization procedures for surgical instruments, medical equipment, skin-marking solutions, water supplies, and proper preoperative skin cleansing, since all are important factors with a definite influence in the initiation of these infections. Finally, mycobacteria should be included in the differential diagnosis of nonhealing wound and soft tissue infections after surgical procedures.

Conflict of Interests

The authors declare that there is no conflict of interests regarding the publication of this paper.

References

[1] R. Narang, P. Narang, A. P. Jain et al., "*Mycobacterium avium* bacteremia and dual infection with mycobacterium avium and mycobacterium wolinskyi in the gut of an aids patient—first case report," *Indian Journal of Tuberculosis*, vol. 57, no. 3, pp. 148–151, 2010.

[2] J. O. Falkinham III, "Epidemiology of infection by nontuberculous mycobacteria," *Clinical Microbiology Reviews*, vol. 9, no. 2, pp. 177–215, 1996.

[3] A. Timpe and E. H. Runyon, "Classics in infectious diseases: the relationship of 'atypical' acid-fast bacteria to human disease: a preliminary report by Alice Timpe and Ernest H. Runyon," *Reviews of Infectious Diseases*, vol. 3, no. 5, pp. 1098–1103, 1981.

[4] S. Sungkanuparph, B. Sathapatayavongs, and R. Pracharktam, "Infections with rapidly growing mycobacteria: report of 20 cases," *International Journal of Infectious Diseases*, vol. 7, no. 3, pp. 198–205, 2003.

[5] J. A. McDonald, K. Suellentrop, L. J. Paulozzi, and B. Morrow, "Reproductive health of the rapidly growing Hispanic population: data from the pregnancy risk assessment monitoring system, 2002," *Maternal and Child Health Journal*, vol. 12, no. 3, pp. 342–356, 2008.

[6] J. Glassroth, "Pulmonary disease due to nontuberculous mycobacteria," *Chest*, vol. 133, no. 1, pp. 243–251, 2008.

[7] S. Kusunoki, T. Ezaki, M. Tamesada et al., "Application of colorimetric microdilution plate hybridization for rapid genetic identification of 22 Mycobacterium species," *Journal of Clinical Microbiology*, vol. 29, no. 8, pp. 1596–1603, 1991.

[8] J. van Ingen, M. J. Boeree, W. C. M. de Lange, P. E. W. de Haas, P. N. R. Dekhuijzen, and D. Van Soolingen, "Clinical relevance of *Mycobacterium szulgai* in The Netherlands," *Clinical Infectious Diseases*, vol. 46, no. 8, pp. 1200–1205, 2008.

[9] M. L. Abalain-Colloc, D. Guillerm, M. Saläun, S. Gouriou, V. Vincent, and B. Picard, "*Mycobacterium szulgai* isolated from a patient, a tropical fish and aquarium water," *European Journal of Clinical Microbiology and Infectious Diseases*, vol. 22, no. 12, pp. 768–769, 2003.

[10] F. Portaels, "Epidemiology of mycobacterial diseases," *Clinics in Dermatology*, vol. 13, no. 3, pp. 207–222, 1995.

[11] W. B. Schaefer, E. Wolinsky, P. A. Jenkins, and J. Marks, "Mycobacterium szulgai—a new pathogen. Serologic identification and report of five new cases," *The American Review of Respiratory Disease*, vol. 108, no. 6, pp. 1320–1326, 1973.

[12] P. Frisk, G. Boman, K. Pauksen, B. Petrini, and G. Lönnerholm, "Skin infection caused by *Mycobacterium szulgai* after allogeneic bone marrow transplantation," *Bone Marrow Transplantation*, vol. 31, no. 6, pp. 511–513, 2003.

[13] A. Meier, P. Kirschner, K. H. Schroder, J. Wolters, R. M. Kroppenstedt, and E. C. Bottger, "*Mycobacterium intermedium* sp. nov," *International Journal of Systematic Bacteriology*, vol. 43, no. 2, pp. 204–209, 1993.

[14] E. Richter, S. Rüsch-Gerdes, and D. Hillemann, "Evaluation of the genotype mycobacterium assay for identification of mycobacterial species from cultures," *Journal of Clinical Microbiology*, vol. 44, no. 5, pp. 1769–1775, 2006.

[15] E. Tortoli, "Mycobacterium kansasii, species or complex? Biomolecular and epidemiological insights," *Kekkaku*, vol. 78, no. 11, pp. 705–709, 2003.

[16] E. Tortoli, G. Besozzi, C. Lacchini, V. Penati, M. T. Simonetti, and S. Emler, "Pulmonary infection due to *Mycobacterium szulgai*, case report and review of the literature," *European Respiratory Journal*, vol. 11, no. 4, pp. 975–977, 1998.

[17] J. M. F. Sánchez-Alarcos, J. de Miguel-Díez, I. Bonilla, J. J. Sicilia, and J. L. Álvarez-Sala, "Pulmonary infection due to *Mycobacterium szulgai*," *Respiration*, vol. 70, no. 5, pp. 533–536, 2003.

[18] H. Ohta, E. Miyauchi, M. Ebina, and T. Nukiwa, "A case of cutaneous infection caused by *Mycobacterium szulgai* with progression to acute respiratory distress syndrome," *Clinical Medicine Insights: Case Reports*, vol. 4, pp. 29–33, 2011.

[19] A. Sekine, E. Hagiwara, T. Ogura et al., "Four cases of pulmonary infection due to *Mycobacterium szulgai* with a review of previous case reports in Japan," *Nihon Kokyuki Gakkai Zasshi*, vol. 46, no. 11, pp. 880–888, 2008.

[20] Q. Zhang, R. Kennon, M. A. Koza, K. Hulten, and J. E. Clarridge III, "Pseudoepidemic due to a unique strain of *Mycobacterium szulgai*: genotypic, phenotypic, and epidemiological analysis," *Journal of Clinical Microbiology*, vol. 40, no. 4, pp. 1134–1139, 2002.

[21] C. Russo, E. Tortoli, and D. Menichella, "Evaluation of the new GenoType Mycobacterium assay for identification of mycobacterial species," *Journal of Clinical Microbiology*, vol. 44, no. 2, pp. 334–339, 2006.

[22] A. S. Lee, P. Jelfs, V. Sintchenko, and G. L. Gilbert, "Identification of non-tuberculous mycobacteria: utility of the GenoType Mycobacterium CM/AS assay compared with HPLC and 16S rRNA gene sequencing," *Journal of Medical Microbiology*, vol. 58, no. 7, pp. 900–904, 2009.

[23] L. A. Carson, L. A. Bland, L. B. Cusick et al., "Prevalence of nontuberculous mycobacteria in water supplies of hemodialysis centers," *Applied and Environmental Microbiology*, vol. 54, no. 12, pp. 3122–3125, 1988.

[24] R. J. Wallace Jr., B. A. Brown, and D. E. Griffith, "Nosocomial outbreaks/pseudo-outbreaks caused by nontuberculous mycobacteria," *Annual Review of Microbiology*, vol. 52, pp. 453–490, 1998.

Omalizumab for Urticarial Vasculitis: Case Report and Review of the Literature

Misbah Nasheela Ghazanfar[1] and Simon Francis Thomsen[1,2]

[1]*Department of Dermatology, Bispebjerg Hospital, 2400 Copenhagen NV, Denmark*
[2]*Center for Medical Research Methodology, Department of Biomedical Sciences, University of Copenhagen, 2200 Copenhagen N, Denmark*

Correspondence should be addressed to Simon Francis Thomsen; simonfrancisthomsen@gmail.com

Academic Editor: Michihiro Hide

Urticarial vasculitis is characterised by inflamed itching or burning red patches or wheals that resemble urticaria but persist for greater than 24 hours. It is often idiopathic but is sometimes associated with collagen-vascular disease, particularly systemic lupus erythematosus. Treatment options include oral antihistamines, oral corticosteroids, dapsone, colchicine or hydroxychloroquine. We describe a male patient with urticarial vasculitis who was treated with omalizumab (anti-IgE) with convincing results and provide a review of previous reports of patients with urticarial vasculitis treated with omalizumab.

1. Introduction

Urticarial vasculitis is a variation of cutaneous vasculitis. Individual lesions appear as inflamed itching or burning red patches or wheals that resemble urticaria but persist for greater than 24 hours. Histopathologically, urticaritis presents as leukocytoclastic vasculitis with a perivascular mixed infiltrate of lymphocytes, neutrophils, and eosinophils, as well as fibrin deposits. Urticarial vasculitis is classified as normocomplementaemic or hypocomplementaemic based on the level of complement protein in blood. Although both subtypes are associated with typical symptoms such as angioedema, chest or abdominal pain, fever, and joint pain, the symptoms are more prominent in the hypocomplementaemic form, which is associated with systemic lupus erythematous. The majority of urticarial vasculitis cases are idiopathic [1, 2].

Recommended treatments for urticarial vasculitis are oral antihistamines and systemic immunosuppressant drugs such as oral corticosteroids, dapsone, colchicine, or hydroxychloroquine. While oral antihistamines might be useful for symptomatic relief of itch and for mild cutaneous disease without systemic involvement, most patients will need a course of oral corticosteroids to control exacerbation of cutaneous or systemic symptoms. Patients with hypocomplementaemic urticarial vasculitis with or without systemic lupus erythematous may have a more favourable response to dapsone, but the mechanism of action of dapsone is poorly understood and there are several adverse effects such as haemolysis, severe headache, and agranulocytosis. Monoclonal antibodies such as omalizumab (anti-IgE) have also been suggested for treatment of urticarial vasculitis [3]. An effective treatment for urticarial vasculitis is much needed as urticarial vasculitis impacts negatively the quality of life.

Omalizumab is a humanized anti-IgE monoclonal antibody that has recently been approved for treatment of chronic urticaria. Studies have shown that omalizumab significantly reduces the activity and symptoms of chronic urticaria. Also, omalizumab reduces the need for additional medication and improves quality of life. Clinical phases II and III studies have concluded that the ideal omalizumab dose for the treatment of chronic urticaria is 300 mg s.c. administered once every four weeks [4–6].

Herein, we describe a male patient with urticarial vasculitis who was treated with omalizumab with convincing results. Furthermore, we review previous reports of patients with urticarial vasculitis treated with omalizumab.

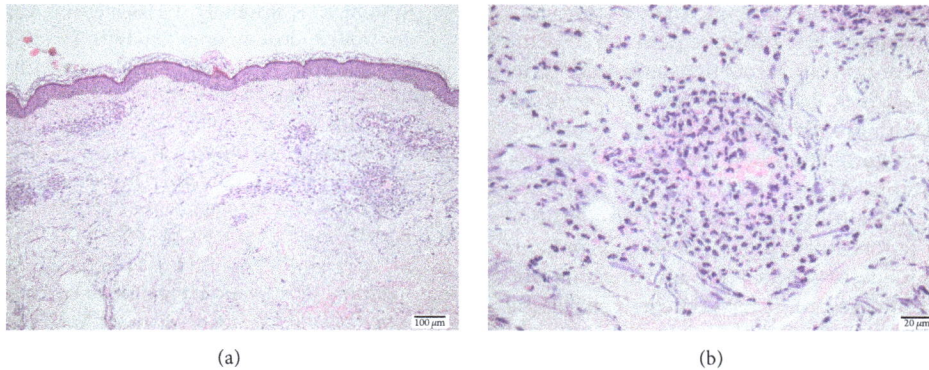

(a)   (b)

FIGURE 1: Histopathological sections of the patient showing leukocytoclastic vasculitis.

TABLE 1: Patients with urticarial vasculitis treated with omalizumab.

Author	Year	Case	Dose of omalizumab	Effect of omalizumab
Del Pozo et al. [3]	2012	Female, aged 51, with SLE and urticarial vasculitis. No improvement with oral corticosteroids, antihistamines, and azathioprine	Unknown: based on weight and IgE	Significant improvement Lesions disappeared. No hives or pain
Varricchi et al. [7]	2012	Female, aged 44, with asthma, Churg-Strauss syndrome, and urticarial vasculitis. No improvement with oral corticosteroids, antihistamines, azathioprine, and cyclosporine	300 mg s.c. every two weeks	Significant improvement of symptoms
Díez et al. [8]	2013	Three females with chronic spontaneous urticaria with autoimmune and pressure components plus vasculitis. No improvement with antihistamines, leukotriene receptor antagonists, and cyclosporine	150 mg s.c. every four weeks (two patients) and 300 mg s.c. every four weeks (one patient)	Remission of symptoms in all three patients
Sussman et al. [9]	2014	One patient, unknown gender and age, with urticarial vasculitis	150 mg s.c. every four weeks	Remission of symptoms. Details not given

2. Case Presentation

The patient was a 68-year-old man who unexpectedly developed severe, burning skin rashes clinically typical of urticarial vasculitis on his trunk, proximal upper extremities, and lower extremities during June 2014. The rashes consisted of erythematous and violaceous slightly ecchymotic infiltrated annular wheals lasting for more than 24 hours that resolved with slight postinflammatory hyperpigmentation. The patient had no angioedema and no extracutaneous manifestations such as fever, arthralgia, lymphadenopathy, uveitis, or serositis. Shortly before the onset of symptoms, he had a toe infection and received a short course of penicillin. The patient had a history of previous colon cancer for which he underwent surgery in 2008. Furthermore, he had total knee replacement surgery in 2012 due to arthritis, but he had no other previous history of rheumatic or collagen-vascular disease. He had basal cell carcinoma on the forehead in 2013. Routine blood tests including anti-cytoplasmic antibodies and anti-nuclear antibodies were normal, but he had slightly elevated secretion of protein in the urine. A skin biopsy revealed leukocytoclastic vasculitis with perivascular infiltrates primarily of neutrophils (Figure 1).

The patient was treated with oral prednisolone at a dose of 37.5 mg once daily for one week and an improvement was observed. The patient was then advised to reduce the dosage of prednisolone to 25 mg daily for three days and

then to 12.5 mg daily for one week and then slowly taper prednisolone altogether. After three months, the patient experienced relapse of skin rashes and was then treated with dapsone 50 mg twice daily for one month but without significant improvement. In December 2014, the patient was switched to omalizumab 300 mg s.c. once every four weeks, and already after one month a complete remission of the urticarial vasculitis and symptoms was observed. By July 2015, the patient is still being treated with omalizumab 300 mg s.c. every four weeks with sustained remission and no apparent adverse effects. The patient was not treated with oral antihistamines throughout the course of the disease.

3. Discussion

Clinical phase studies have shown that omalizumab is safe and reduces disease activity in patients with chronic urticaria [5, 6]. While there are no prospective clinical studies of omalizumab for urticarial vasculitis, a few case reports have shown that omalizumab might also be beneficial for this indication (Table 1). A case report by Del Pozo et al. described a female patient with systemic lupus erythematous and urticarial vasculitis. She was treated with oral antihistamines, oral corticosteroids, and azathioprine without improvement. She was then administered omalizumab based on weight and IgE levels, which showed great improvement as her lesions disappeared [3]. Another case by Varricchi et al. described a female patient with asthma, Churg-Strauss syndrome, and urticarial vasculitis. She also had no symptomatic improvement while being treated with oral antihistamines, oral corticosteroids, or other immunosuppressants such as azathioprine and cyclosporine. She was then treated with omalizumab 300 mg s.c. every two weeks as an add-on to antihistamines, oral corticosteroids, and immunosuppressants. After 6 months of treatment, the patient reported a significant improvement of her condition [7]. A Spanish case report involving three female patients with chronic spontaneous urticaria with autoimmune and pressure components and vasculitis also reported successful treatment with omalizumab [8]. Finally, an open-label study by Sussman et al. of patients with chronic urticaria involving also one patient with urticarial vasculitis noted that omalizumab was a sufficient treatment for the patients included in the study [9]. None of the patients included in these case studies experienced serious adverse effects during treatment.

Urticarial vasculitis with eruptive erythematous wheals resembles chronic urticaria, but the individual lesions usually last longer than in chronic urticaria. Symptoms are more frequently burning rather than itching and resolve with hyperpigmentation [1]. Several clinical studies have shown that omalizumab has great effect on chronic urticaria [5, 6] and while omalizumab is not the choice of treatment for urticarial vasculitis, it seems to have a beneficial effect on patients with urticarial vasculitis as reported herein and in the earlier published case reports. However, the mechanisms of action of omalizumab for urticarial vasculitis remain, in part, unresolved. Particularly, it is not known whether omalizumab is efficacious against both normocomplementaemic and hypocomplementaemic urticarial vasculitides. We did not measure levels of complement in blood in our patient.

4. Conclusion

Our report of successful treatment of urticarial vasculitis with omalizumab is important, as many patients with urticarial vasculitis cannot be treated successfully or experience significant side effects of the standard treatment. However, clinical trials with a greater number of patients with urticarial vasculitis that compare standard treatment with omalizumab are warranted.

Conflict of Interests

Simon Francis Thomsen is an advisory board member and speaker for Novartis.

References

[1] S. Chang and W. Carr, "Urticarial vasculitis," *Allergy and Asthma Proceedings*, vol. 28, no. 1, pp. 97–100, 2007.

[2] J. Venzor, W. L. Lee, and D. P. Huston, "Urticarial vasculitis," *Clinical Reviews in Allergy and Immunology*, vol. 23, no. 2, pp. 201–216, 2002.

[3] M. E. R. Del Pozo, N. P. M. Saenz, J. G. Vera, and J. L. Tiro, "Vasculitic urticaria treated with omalizumab. Case report," *World Allergy Organization Journal*, vol. 5, supplement 2, p. S106, 2012.

[4] S. Saini, K. E. Rosen, H.-J. Hsieh et al., "A randomized, placebo-controlled, dose-ranging study of single-dose omalizumab in patients with H $_1$-antihistamine-refractory chronic idiopathic urticaria," *Journal of Allergy and Clinical Immunology*, vol. 128, no. 3, pp. 567.e1–573.e1, 2011.

[5] T. Zuberbier, W. Aberer, R. Asero et al., "The EAACI/GA(2) LEN/EDF/WAO guideline for the definition, classification, diagnosis, and management of urticaria: the 2013 revision and update," *Allergy*, vol. 69, pp. 868–887, 2014.

[6] M. Maurer, K. Rosén, H. J. Hsieh et al., "Omalizumab for the treatment of chronic idiopathic or spontaneous urticaria," *The New England Journal of Medicine*, vol. 368, pp. 924–935, 2013.

[7] G. Varricchi, A. Detoraki, B. Liccardo et al., "Efficacy of omalizumab in the treatment of urticaria-vasculitis associated to Churg-Strauss syndrome: a case report," *World Allergy Organization Journal*, vol. 5, supplement 2, pp. S89–S90, 2012.

[8] L. S. Díez, L. M. Tamayo, and R. Cardona, "Omalizumab: therapeutic option in chronic spontaneous urticaria difficult to control with associated vasculitis, report of three cases," *Biomedica*, vol. 33, no. 4, pp. 503–512, 2013.

[9] G. Sussman, J. Hébert, C. Barron et al., "Real-life experiences with omalizumab for the treatment of chronic urticaria," *Annals of Allergy, Asthma and Immunology*, vol. 112, no. 2, pp. 170–174, 2014.

Lymphatic Malformation, Retinoblastoma, or Facial Cleft: Atypical Presentations of PHACE Syndrome

María Fernández-Ibieta[1] and Juan Carlos López-Gutiérrez[2]

[1]Pediatric Surgery Service, Hospital CU Virgen de la Arrixaca, El Palmar s/n, 30150 Murcia, Spain
[2]Vascular Anomalies Unit, Pediatric Surgery Department, Hospital La Paz, Madrid, Spain

Correspondence should be addressed to María Fernández-Ibieta; mfndezibieta@hotmail.com

Academic Editor: Masatoshi Jinnin

PHACE syndrome is a neurocutaneous disorder characterized by large cervicofacial infantile hemangiomas and associated anomalies: posterior fossa brain malformation, hemangioma, arterial cerebrovascular anomalies, coarctation of the aorta and cardiac defects, and eye/endocrine abnormalities of the brain. When ventral developmental defects (sternal clefting or supraumbilical raphe) are present the condition is termed PHACE. In this report, we describe three PHACE cases that presented unique features (affecting one of the organ systems described for this syndrome) that have not been described previously. In the first case, a definitive PHACE association, the patient presented with an ipsilateral mesenteric lymphatic malformation, at the age of 14 years. In the second case, an anomaly of the posterior segment of the eye, not mentioned before in PHACE literature, a retinoblastoma, has been described. Specific chemotherapy avoided enucleation. And, in the third case, the child presented with an unusual midline frontal bone cleft, corresponding to Tessier 14 cleft. Two patients' hemangiomas responded well to propranolol therapy. The first one was followed and treated in the pre-propranolol era and had a moderate response to corticoids and interferon.

1. Introduction

PHACE association affects 2.3% of all patients with infantile hemangioma (IH) and consists of a plaque-like IH in a "segmental" dermatomal distribution of the face with at least one of the following anomalies: posterior fossa brain malformation, hemangioma, arterial cerebrovascular anomalies, coarctation of the aorta and cardiac defects, and eye/endocrine abnormalities. When ventral developmental defects (sternal clefting or supraumbilical raphe) are present the condition is termed PHACES [1–3]. Cerebrovascular anomalies are the most common associated finding (72%) [1, 4]. Less than one-third of children have more than one extracutaneous feature. Because 8% of patients might have a stroke in infancy and 42% have a structural brain anomaly, patients with suspected PHACE association should have an MRI to evaluate brain structures and vasculature. Treatment is multidisciplinary and the angiomatous plaque usually responds well to propranolol [1–3].

2. Cases Presentation

2.1. Case 1. A 14-year-old girl with a history of PHACES association consisting in left angiomatous cervicofacial and thoracic plaque (Figure 1), left cerebellar hypoplasia, and moderate hypoplasia of ipsilateral internal carotid and ophthalmic artery presented with 6-month history of abdominal pain and distention. She had been treated with corticoids and interferon α2B for the hemangioma in the pre-propranolol era (with acceptable evolution, but she had neurologic sequelae consisting in fine movements incoordination). On abdominal examination, moderate ascites was found. In ultrasound, a well-defined liquid mass or cyst appeared, and a thoracoabdominal RM was performed. The final diagnose was a lymphatic mesenteric malformation, which surrounded stomach and spleen inferior pole, with a left caudal extension that compressed medially the bowel (Figure 1). A laparoscopy was performed, and the lymphatic malformation was enucleated from the mesentery, without recurrence.

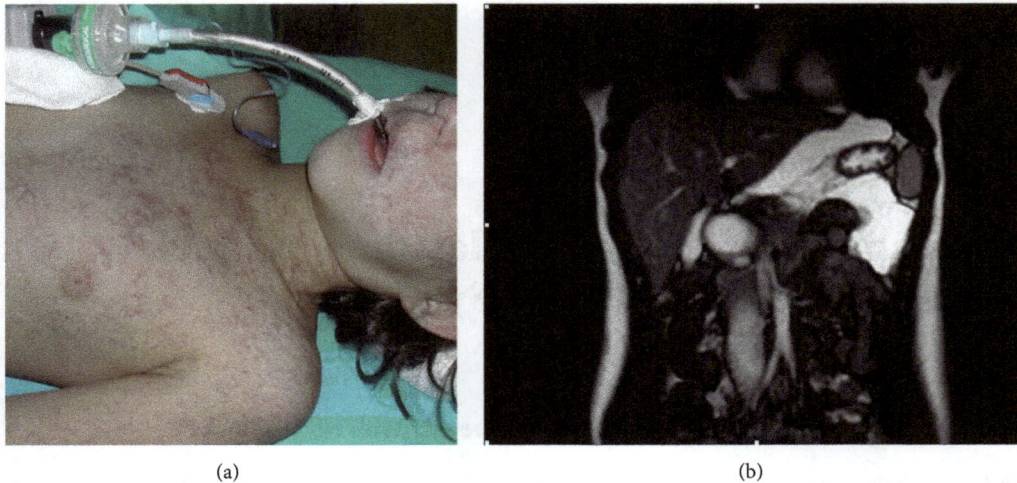

(a)   (b)

FIGURE 1: Left angiomatous cervicofacial and thoracic hemangioma plaque and lymphatic mesenteric malformation that surrounded stomach and spleen inferior pole.

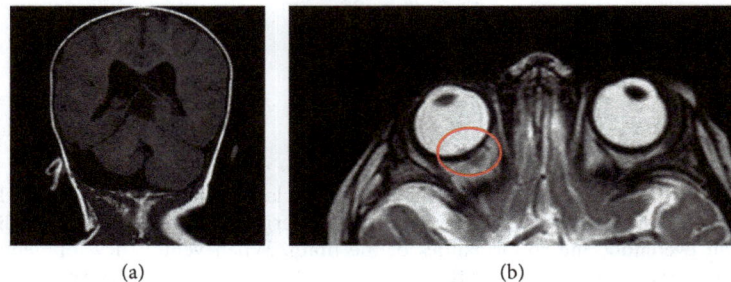

(a)   (b)

FIGURE 2: Right cerebellar and vermis hypoplasia plus a 2 mm length tumor of the retina (retinoblastoma).

2.2. Case 2. An 8-month-old male infant with well-defined PHACE association (right facial hemangiomatous plaque with right cerebellar and vermis hypoplasia plus a posterior fossa arachnoid cyst and pituitary cystic malformation, Figure 2) with good response to propranolol therapy presented with strabismus of the right eye. On ophthalmoscopic examination, a retinal papula was found. An ultrasound showed a 2 mm length tumor of the retina, and an eye RM was performed, where retinoblastoma was defined (Figure 2). Chemotherapy was then established, and enucleation was spared, with no relapse after one year follow-up.

2.3. Case 3. A one-month-old female presented in our office with facial and cranial angiomas. A cranial midline soft tissue protuberance was also observed. Magnetic resonance imaging of the brain showed a craniofacial cleft, corresponding to a Tessier 14 midline craniofacial cleft, between nose and facial bone (Figure 3). There were no intracranial lesions. A thyroglossal cyst was also found on the tongue base. The angiomatous plaques responded well to propranolol.

In this report, we describe three PHACE cases that are associated with unique features (affecting one of the organ systems described for this syndrome) that have not been described previously.

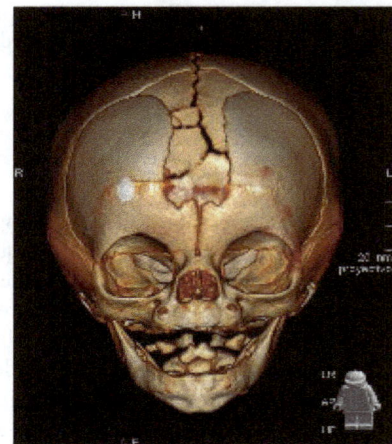

FIGURE 3: Craniofacial cleft, corresponding to a Tessier 14 midline craniofacial cleft, between nose and facial bone.

3. Discussion

The association between facial IH and cerebral anomalies was first described in 1978, and, since then, PHACES association has been recognized as the most frequent phacomatosis or neurocutaneous anomaly [5]. Its differential diagnosis comprises, among others, the Sturge-Weber syndrome, which is defined as capillary malformation (instead of a hemangioma) that is already present at birth, opposite to IH, which develops along the first weeks of life [5]. The hemangiomas in PHACES tend to be big (>5 cm) and evolve as a usual hemangioma in three phases, including development, arrest, and involution. Plus, it is seen in approximately 30% of those with >5 cm segmental hemangioma patients. They are segmental plaque-like hemangiomas, derived from embryological protuberances known as placodes, which contain neural crest cell migrated from the dorsal crest and develop into the mandibular, maxillar, and frontonasal processes [6, 7]. This may explain why patients with posterior fossa malformations have arterial and cutaneous anomalies in the same dermatome. A consensus statement on diagnostic criteria for PHACE syndrome has been reached recently [8], and the anomalies have been described as major or minor criteria. The most frequent structural brain anomalies are Dandy-Walker-type malformation and ipsilateral cerebellar hypoplasia. Cerebrovascular anomalies include hypoplasia or tortuosity of major vessels (internal carotid, anterior, middle or posterior cerebral arteries, or vertebrobasilar system) and persistence of embryonic vessels. These usually affect neurological development and most severe anomalies may present with stroke, global developmental delay, or seizures. The most cardiovascular malformations are coarctation of aorta, right-sided aortic arch, and ventricular septal defect. These are usually associated with sternal/umbilical/midline defects. Ophthalmological anomalies include posterior segment abnormalities (optic nerve hypoplasia and persistent fetal vasculature). Moreover, hypopituitarism and thyroid anomalies have been described [8–12]. According to the above-mentioned consensus, PHACE syndrome is defined in the presence of a plaque-like facial hemangioma and a major criterion (these are most prevalent features as posterior fossa anomalies, dysplasia of the large cerebral arteries, aortic arch anomaly, eye posterior segment anomaly, or sternal defect) or two minor criteria (callosal agenesis, pituitary malformation, ventricular septal defect, eye anterior segment anomaly, hypopituitarism, or ectopic thyroid, among others). The consensus defined the term "possible PHACE syndrome" when the patient presented with hemangioma/hemangiomatous plaque plus 1 minor criteria.

We have reported three PHACE cases, with unique features that have not been described before. In the first case, a definitive PHACE association, the patient presented with an ipsilateral mesenteric lymphatic malformation, at the age of 14 years. This finding might be more frequent as its clinical presentation is often symptomless for years until the cyst develops and causes pain or intestinal symptoms. The second case, again a definitive PHACE syndrome, an anomaly of the posterior segment of the eye, not mentioned before in PHACE literature, a retinoblastoma, has been described. And, in the third case, possible PHACE syndrome (facial hemangioma with an ectopic thyroid) presented with an unusual midline frontal bone cleft, corresponding to Tessier 14 cleft [13]. It is reasonable to speculate that if thoracic hemangiomas may associate midline sternal/umbilical clefts, facial ones could present cranial midline defects. Two patients' hemangiomas responded well to propranolol therapy [14–17]. The first one was followed and treated in the pre-propranolol era and had a moderate response to corticoids and interferon.

Conflict of Interests

The authors declare that there is no conflict of interests regarding the publication of this paper.

References

[1] A. K. Greene, "Management of hemangiomas and other vascular tumors," *Clinics in Plastic Surgery*, vol. 38, no. 1, pp. 45–63, 2011.

[2] C. J. Smithers and S. J. Fishman, "Vascular anomalies," in *Ashcraft's Pediatric Surgery*, pp. 982–996, Elsevier Saunders, Philadelphia, Pa, USA, 5th edition, 2010.

[3] A. M. Kulungowski and S. J. Fishman, "Vascular anomalies in Coran-Grosfeld's," in *Pediatric Surgery*, pp. 1610–1630, Saunders-Elsevier, Philadelphia, Pa, USA, 7th edition, 2012.

[4] A. N. Haggstrom, M. C. Garzon, E. Baselga et al., "Risk for PHACE syndrome in infants with large facial hemangiomas," *Pediatrics*, vol. 126, no. 2, pp. e418–e426, 2010.

[5] D. Metry, G. Heyer, C. Hess et al., "Consensus statement on diagnostic criteria for PHACE syndrome," *Pediatrics*, vol. 124, no. 5, pp. 1447–1456, 2009.

[6] M. Waner, P. E. North, K. A. Scherer, I. J. Frieden, A. Waner, and M. C. Mihm Jr., "The nonrandom distribution of facial hemangiomas," *Archives of Dermatology*, vol. 139, no. 7, pp. 869–875, 2003.

[7] M. Castillo, "PHACES syndrome: from the brain to the face via the neural crest cells," *American Journal of Neuroradiology*, vol. 29, no. 4, pp. 814–815, 2008.

[8] V. S. Oza, E. Wang, A. Berenstein et al., "PHACES association: a neuroradiologic review of 17 patients," *American Journal of Neuroradiology*, vol. 29, no. 4, pp. 807–813, 2008.

[9] D. W. Metry, C. F. Dowd, A. J. Barkovich, and I. J. Frieden, "The many faces of PHACE syndrome," *Journal of Pediatrics*, vol. 139, no. 1, pp. 117–123, 2001.

[10] A. M. Ruiz-de-Luzuriaga, D. Bardo, and S. L. Stein, "PHACES association," *Journal of the American Academy of Dermatology*, vol. 55, no. 6, pp. 1072–1074, 2006.

[11] G. L. Heyer, W. S. Millar, S. Ghatan, and M. C. Garzon, "The neurologic aspects of PHACE: case report and review of the literature," *Pediatric Neurology*, vol. 35, no. 6, pp. 419–424, 2006.

[12] G. L. Heyer, M. M. Dowling, D. J. Licht et al., "The cerebral vasculopathy of PHACES syndrome," *Stroke*, vol. 39, no. 2, pp. 308–316, 2008.

[13] J. P. Bradley and H. Kawamoto, *Craniofacial Clefts and Hypertelorbitism in Grabbs and Smith's Plastic Surgery*, Wolters Kluwer, Philadelphia, Pa, USA, 6th edition, 2007.

[14] B. A. Drolet, P. C. Frommelt, S. L. Chamlin et al., "Initiation and use of propranolol for infantile hemangioma: report of a consensus conference," *Pediatrics*, vol. 131, no. 1, pp. 128–140, 2013.

[15] G. Bronzetti, A. Patrizi, F. Giacomini et al., "A PHACES syndrome unmasked by propranolol interruption in a tetralogy of fallot patient: case report and extensive review on new

indications of β blockers," *Current Medicinal Chemistry*, vol. 21, no. 27, pp. 3153–3164, 2014.

[16] V. K. Sharma, F. O. G. Fraulin, D. O. Dumestre, L. Walker, and A. R. Harrop, "Beta-blockers for the treatment of problematic hemangiomas," *Canadian Journal of Plastic Surgery*, vol. 21, no. 1, pp. 23–28, 2013.

[17] M. Lynch, P. Lenane, and B. F. O'Donnell, "Propranolol for the treatment of infantile haemangiomas: our experience with 44 patients," *Clinical and Experimental Dermatology*, vol. 39, no. 2, pp. 142–145, 2014.

8

Reconstruction of a Large Anterior Ear Defect after Mohs Micrographic Surgery with a Cartilage Graft and Postauricular Revolving Door Flap

Stephanie Nemir,[1] **Lindsey Hunter-Ellul,**[2] **Vlad Codrea,**[3] **and Richard Wagner**[2]

[1]*Division of Plastic Surgery, Department of Surgery, University of Texas Medical Branch, Galveston, TX 77555, USA*
[2]*Department of Dermatology, University of Texas Medical Branch, Galveston, TX 77555, USA*
[3]*School of Medicine, University of Texas Medical Branch, Galveston, TX 77555, USA*

Correspondence should be addressed to Richard Wagner; rfwagner@utmb.edu

Academic Editor: Jacek Cezary Szepietowski

A novel postauricular revolving door island flap and cartilage graft combination was employed to correct a large defect on the anterior ear of an 84-year-old man who underwent Mohs micrographic surgery for an antihelical squamous cell carcinoma. The defect measured 4.6×2.4 cm and spanned the antihelix, scapha, a small portion of the helix, and a large segment of underlying cartilage, with loss of structural integrity and anterior folding of the ear. The repair involved harvesting 1.5 cm^2 of exposed cartilage from the scaphoid fossa and then sculpting and suturing it to the remnant of the antihelical cartilage in order to recreate the antihelical crura. The skin of the posterior auricle was then incised just below the helical rim and folded anteriorly to cover the cartilage graft. The flap remained attached by a central subcutaneous pedicle, and an island designed using the full-thickness defect as a stencil template was pulled through the cartilage window anteriorly to resurface the anterior ear. This case demonstrates the use of the revolving door flap for coverage of large central ear defects with loss of cartilaginous support and illustrates how cartilage grafts may be used in combination with the flap to improve ear contour after resection.

1. Introduction

The auricle is a very common site of skin cancers due to its projection from the head and subsequent actinic exposure [1]. This is particularly true in men, due to hairstyles that often do not protect the ear. Most auricular skin cancers are located on the helix, antihelix, and posterior ear, less frequently involving the lobule, tragus, or conchal bowl [2]. Large anterior auricular defects are a reconstructive challenge due to the complex topography of the ear, and second intention healing can lead to poor cosmetic outcomes, chondritis, or infection [3].

Repair is optimal for helical defects due to the high likelihood of cartilage desiccation and fibrosis that could result in notching [3]. One of the primary goals of ear reconstruction is to correct the shape of the auricle such that it does not attract attention when viewed by someone standing at a conversational distance [4]. Surgical options

include second intention healing, skin grafting, preauricular transposition flap, tubed pedicle flap, postauricular pull-through flap, and postauricular revolving door island flap [3]. We describe a patient with a large defect of the anterior ear resulting in compromised structural integrity. The defect was repaired with a cartilage graft that restored the antihelical contour, followed by a postauricular revolving door (also known as a trap door or flip-flop) island flap that restored the ear's structural integrity and provided skin coverage to the anterior ear and conchal bowl.

2. Case Report

An 84-year-old man underwent Mohs micrographic surgery for a primary squamous cell carcinoma on the left antihelix (Figure 1). At the time of the surgery, he was on anticoagulation therapy consisting of aspirin 81 mg po daily due to a

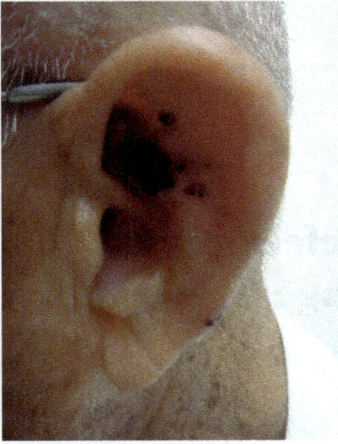

FIGURE 1: The preoperative photo of the left ear with squamous cell carcinoma on the antihelix.

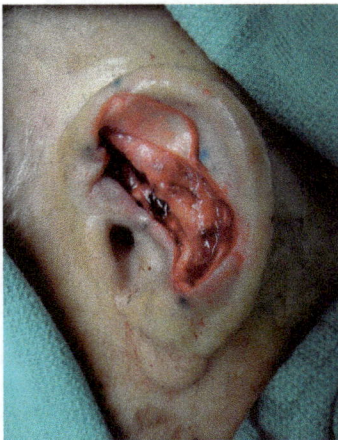

FIGURE 2: The final Mohs defect after two stages, measuring 4.6 × 2.4 cm.

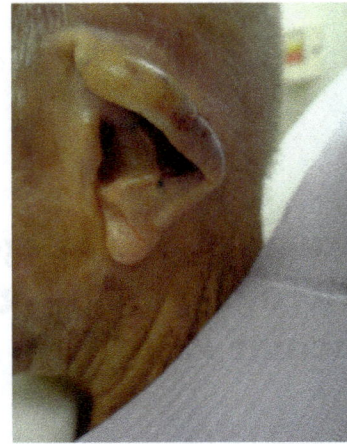

FIGURE 3: Lop-ear deformity.

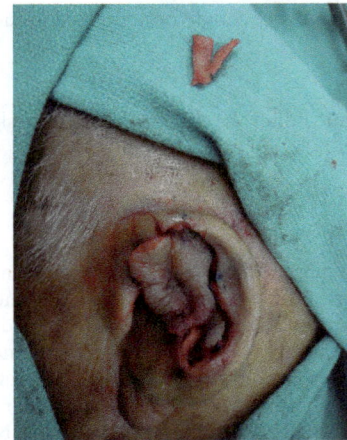

(a)

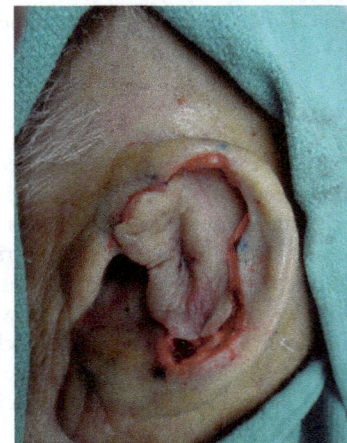

(b)

FIGURE 4: A 1.5 cm^2 cartilage graft was harvested from scaphoid fossa and attached to the antihelix region with quilting sutures. The postauricular skin was folded forward through the cartilage window to cover the cartilage graft.

history of myocardial infarction. He was given ciprofloxacin 500 mg by mouth twice daily starting two days preoperatively and continuing for a total of 14 days as surgical prophylaxis. Oncologic resection was complete after two stages, and the final defect measured 4.6 × 2.4 cm, involving the antihelix, scapha, underlying cartilage, and a small portion of the helix (Figure 2). The superior ear was structurally compromised due to the loss of cartilage, causing the ear to fold anteriorly (lop-ear deformity) (Figure 3). Retroauricular skin was intact, but there was exposed cartilage within the conchal bowl and at the scaphoid fossa.

Due to the size of the defect, limited laxity in surrounding tissues, and loss of structural integrity of the ear cartilage, primary closure and skin grafting were deemed to be sub-optimal wound management strategies. Instead, a 1.5 cm^2 cartilage graft was harvested from the exposed cartilage in the scaphoid fossa, sculpted, and sutured to the adjacent antihelix region with 4-0 poliglecaprone 25 suture, serving to recreate the crura of the antihelix (Figure 4(a)). The skin on the posterior auricle was then incised just below the helical

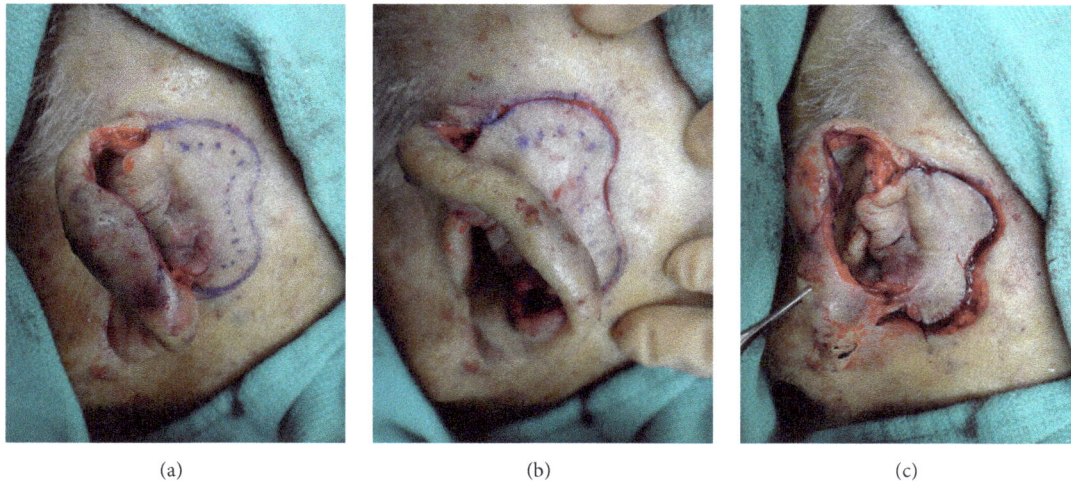

(a)   (b)   (c)

FIGURE 5: The defect served as a stencil on the postauricular skin to create the island, which was incised and undermined at the edges to allow for elevation.

rim, creating a full-thickness defect in the central ear. Skin elevation stopped at the auriculomastoid groove, leaving the skin based on a central subcutaneous pedicle, and the flap was folded anteriorly to cover the cartilage graft and then inset with 4-0 poliglecaprone 25 sutures tacking the flap dermis to the deeper tissues (Figure 4(b)). The full-thickness defect then served as the stencil template for the island portion of the revolving door flap (Figure 5(a)). The designed island was incised with 5 mm of undermining at the edges (Figure 5(b)) and then pulled through the cartilage window anteriorly (Figure 5(c)), thereby creating the revolving door. The flap was then inset into the ear defect anteriorly using 4-0 polypropylene suture. The wound edge on the posterior ear was similarly sutured to the incised skin edge on the postauricular skin, thereby pinning the helix to the mastoid region and correcting the lop-ear deformity. A tie-over bolster was made using fine mesh gauze impregnated with 3% bismuth tribromophenate in a petrolatum blend filled with sterile gauze fluffs and was affixed to the wound with 3-0 silk sutures. Patient was instructed to apply mupirocin 2% ointment to the postauricular suture line daily.

The bolster was taken down at 48 hours due to postoperative bleeding from the suture line and concerns for a possible hematoma. Upon inspection, the flap appeared well-perfused with no signs of underlying fluid collection and no active bleeding. A new bolster was placed at that time and was removed 8 days postoperatively. The immediate closure and 2-week and 3-month postoperative results are shown in Figures 6, 7, and 8.

3. Discussion

Though traditionally used for conchal bowl defects, postauricular revolving door (or trap door or flip-flop) island pedicle flaps can be used to repair large anterior ear defects that lack perichondrium and involve the helix, antihelix, and scapha [5, 6]. It was originally described by Masson

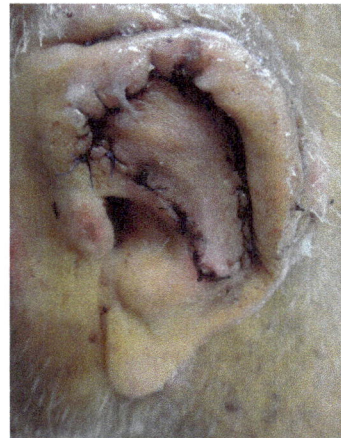

FIGURE 6: The flap was inset into the defect and sutured into place.

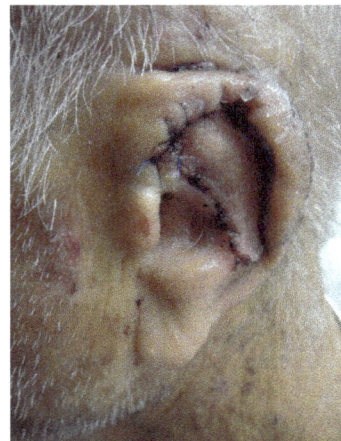

FIGURE 7: Two-week postoperative results.

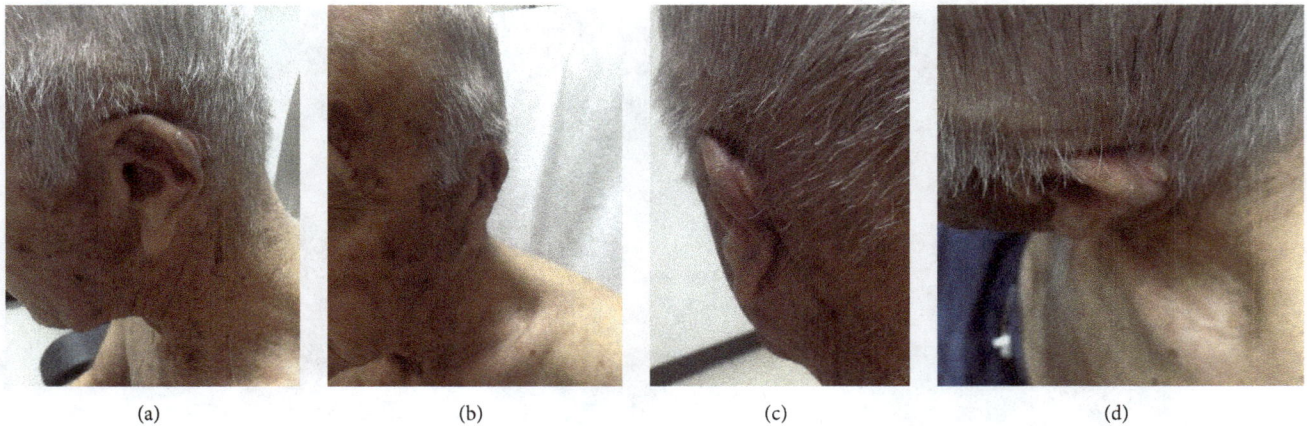

(a)   (b)   (c)   (d)

FIGURE 8: Three-month postoperative results.

in 1972 [7], with modifications by later authors serving to expand its indications to larger and more complex defects. While most commonly used for repair of Mohs defects after cancer resection, these flaps have also been successfully used in the repair of necrotic cartilage and antihelical skin caused by a second-degree burn [8]. This flap provides a varying amount of skin from the ipsilateral retroauricular and mastoid regions, depending on the size and position of the defect [4, 6], and has been described to cover defects as large as 6 × 6 cm [9]. The retroauricular skin has a rich blood supply, and island flaps utilizing this tissue minimize the risk of necrosis and hematoma formation [10]. The blood supply of this myocutaneous flap is the posterior auricular artery, which derives from the external carotid artery [9].

This flap has been described in previous literature as requiring more aggressive undermining of the postauricular skin, in order to prevent retroposition of the ear [3, 5]; up to 50% of the overall flap area may be undermined without affecting perfusion [11]. In this case, however, we felt that the patient would benefit from a superior cosmetic outcome if we used a modified, minimally elevated revolving door island flap in combination with a cartilage graft. This approach allowed us to simultaneously cover the exposed cartilage, recreate a portion of the normal contour, and correct the lop-ear deformity.

Advantages of this technique include color, texture, and thickness match, one-stage reconstruction, the ability to conceal the donor-site deformity, and results that are usually both functionally and aesthetically satisfactory for the patient [4, 6]. In addition to the postauricular area being relatively well concealed, adult patients typically have sufficient tissue to allow primary closure at the donor site [9]. Dessy et al. reported a superior cosmetic outcome with the revolving door flap compared to full-thickness skin grafts for wider skin tumor excisions of the auricular conchal defects among 40 skin cancer patients. Papadopoulos et al. describe a similar technique reconstructing the antihelix and concha with the postauricular island flap with excellent or adequate aesthetic outcomes in 74% and 24% of patients, respectively.

Disadvantages of this technique include pinning of the ear to the head, as with our patient, in addition to the surgical risks of necrosis, chondritis, infection, and the possible need for a postauricular drain (none of which occurred in this patient) [9]. Hematoma can also threaten the repair, and risk of hematoma is increased in patients on anticoagulation therapy, as in our patient. Meticulous hemostasis and flap immobilization with bolsters can minimize this risk. The degree to which pinning the ear to the head results in asymmetry and impacts the aesthetic outcome varies with how much an individual patient's ear naturally protrudes [3]. Other theoretical drawbacks include limited flap mobility due to the length of the pedicle and insufficient vascular supply in the event of parotid or mastoid surgery or external carotid artery ligation [9].

Additionally, we report an uncommon method of incorporating a cartilage graft underneath the flap to help recreate the ear's contour. Cartilage autografts such as the ones we used have been found to be superior to synthetic biomaterials or cadaveric grafts due to a lower risk of immunogenic rejections that cause inflammation and eventual graft failure. If available, as in this patient, the antihelix is the preferred harvest site for cartilage that will subsequently be used to enhance structural support of the auricle [12]. Use of a bolster or closed-suction drain after cartilage grafting, though cumbersome, is commonly used to maximize close adherence of flap to graft, minimize hematoma formation, and maximize aesthetic outcome. As with any reconstructive technique, proper planning and soft tissue management are imperative to minimize complications and further anatomical disfigurement.

Conflict of Interests

The authors declare that there is no conflict of interests regarding the publication of this paper.

References

[1] L. V. Reddy and M. F. Zide, "Reconstruction of skin cancer defects of the auricle," *Journal of Oral and Maxillofacial Surgery*, vol. 62, no. 12, pp. 1457–1471, 2004.

[2] H. Vuyk and T. Cook, "Auricular reconstruction after Mohs' surgery: a review," *FACE*, vol. 5, no. 1, pp. 9–21, 1997.

[3] T. R. Humphreys, L. H. Goldberg, and D. R. Wiemer, "The postauricular (revolving door) island pedicle flap revisited," *Dermatologic Surgery*, vol. 22, no. 2, pp. 148–150, 1996.

[4] L. A. Dessy, A. Figus, P. Fioramonti, M. Mazzocchi, and N. Scuderi, "Reconstruction of anterior auricular conchal defect after malignancy excision: revolving-door flap versus full-thickness skin graft," *Journal of Plastic, Reconstructive & Aesthetic Surgery*, vol. 63, no. 5, pp. 746–752, 2010.

[5] F. Schonauer, G. Vuppalapati, S. Marlino, A. Santorelli, L. Canta, and G. Molea, "Versatility of the posterior auricular flap in partial ear reconstruction," *Plastic and Reconstructive Surgery*, vol. 126, no. 4, pp. 1213–1221, 2010.

[6] I. T. Jackson, L. Milligan, and K. Agrawal, "The versatile revolving door flap in the reconstruction of ear defects," *European Journal of Plastic Surgery*, vol. 17, no. 3, pp. 131–133, 1994.

[7] J. K. Masson, "A simple island flap for reconstruction of concha-helix defects," *British Journal of Plastic Surgery*, vol. 25, pp. 399–403, 1972.

[8] M. Ruiz, O. Garcia, I. Hernán, J. Sancho, J. Serracanta, and J. P. Barret, "Revolving-door flap: an alternative for the coverage of acute burn defects of the auricle," *Burns*, vol. 37, no. 6, pp. e41–e43, 2011.

[9] Y. P. Krespi and B. R. Pate Jr., "Auricular reconstruction using postauricular myocutaneous flap," *Laryngoscope*, vol. 104, no. 6, part 1, pp. 778–780, 1994.

[10] O. N. Papadopoulos, D. K. Karypidis, C. I. Chrisostomidis, P. P. Konofaos, and M. B. Frangoulis, "One-stage reconstruction of the antihelix and concha using postauricular island flap," *Clinical and Experimental Dermatology*, vol. 33, no. 5, pp. 647–650, 2008.

[11] Y. P. Talmi, Z. Horowitz, L. Bedrin, and J. Kronenberg, "Technique of auricular reconstruction with a postauricular island flap 'flip-flop flap'," *Operative Techniques in Otolaryngology—Head and Neck Surgery*, vol. 11, no. 4, pp. 313–317, 2000.

[12] R. J. Sage, B. C. Leach, and J. Cook, "Antihelical cartilage grafts for reconstruction of mohs micrographic surgery defects," *Dermatologic Surgery*, vol. 38, no. 12, pp. 1930–1937, 2012.

9

Xanthoma Disseminatum with Tumor-Like Lesion on Face

Habib Ansarin,[1] Hoda Berenji Ardestani,[2] Seyed Mehdi Tabaie,[3] and Nasrin Shayanfar[4]

[1] Department of Dermatology, Hazrat-e Rasool University Hospital, Iran University of Medical Sciences, Tehran, Iran
[2] Skin and Stem Cell Research Center, Tehran University of Medical Sciences, Kamraniye Street, No. 4, Maryam Alley, Tehran 1937957511, Iran
[3] Iranian Center for Medical Laser, Academic Center for Education, Culture and Research, Tehran, Iran
[4] Department of Pathology, Iran University of Medical Sciences, Tehran, Iran

Correspondence should be addressed to Hoda Berenji Ardestani; hoda_b_a@yahoo.com

Academic Editors: H. Dobrev, B. Kumar, J. Y. Lee, A. Morita, and G. E. Piérard

Xanthoma disseminatum (XD) is a rare benign mucocutaneous xanthomatosis that is classified as a benign non-Langerhans cell histiocytosis. We report a 62-year-old man who presented with widespread yellow-brown papulonodular and tumoral lesions on face, flexors, and trunk. Histopathological features of the cutaneous lesions were typical of XD.

1. Introduction

Xanthoma disseminatum (XD) is a rare benign mucocutaneous xanthomatosis classified as a benign form of non-Langerhans cell histiocytosis [1–3]. Prominent flexural xanthomatous lesions and a frequent association with diabetes insipidus are characteristics of the disease. There is a high rate of mucosal lesions, as well as meningeal involvement leading to diabetes insipidus, but other viscera are rarely involved [3, 4]. We report a case of XD which had widespread yellow-brown papulonodular lesions on face, flexors, and trunk.

2. Case Report

A 62-year-old man was admitted to our department due to a gradually evolving disseminated papulonodular eruption on face, flexors, and trunk for 30 years ago. On examination, multiple, well-defined, yellowish brown papules and nodules and tumor-like lesions were seen symmetrically on upper and lower eyelids (Figure 1). Such papules also were observed on the cheeks and perioral region. On the anterior of the neck the lesions were confluent and formed a diffused plaque (Figure 2).

Hundreds of red to brown papules were distributed symmetrically on axilla, genitalia, poplitea, and trunk, some of which are confluent together and formed plaque or tumor-like lesions (Figures 3 and 4). There were also some papule and nodules on nasal mucosa (Figure 5).

He had no history of polyuria or any previous medical history.

Analysis at that point did not reveal any abnormalities in urine osmolality. Laboratory findings revealed a white blood cell count of 10,300 cells/mL containing 74% neutrophils. C-reactive protein was 7 mg/dL (normal values of 0.5 mg/dL).

Fasting cholesterol was 148 (normal values up to 200) and triglyceride was 141 (normal values up to 150).

Chest X-ray was normal.

Magnetic resonance imaging of the brain and pituitary revealed no abnormalities.

Histopathologic examination of skin biopsies showed a dense dermal diffuse histiocytic infiltration interspersed with mixed inflammatory cells and giant cells (Figures 6 and 7). Abundant foam cells were also seen (Figure 8). A neural infiltration was not present. Immunohistochemistry was positive for CD68 (KP1) (Figure 9) and negative for S-100 protein.

3. Discussion

Xanthoma disseminatum (XD) is a rare but distinct sporadic disorder, in which lipid deposition occurs secondary to

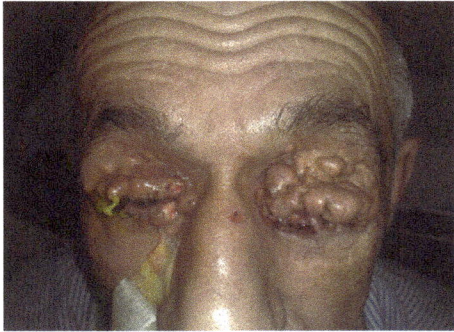

FIGURE 1: Tumor-like lesions on periorbital area, the ulceration like lesion do to biopsy's site.

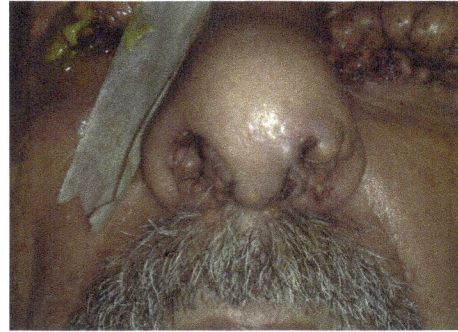

FIGURE 2: Involvement of flexural regions of neck with papule that confluent to plaque lesion.

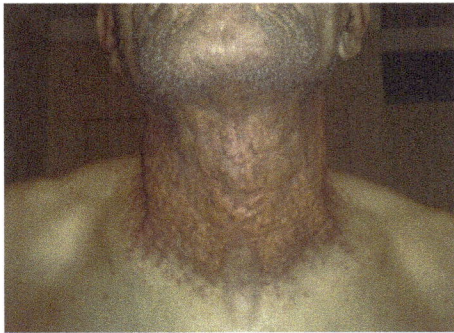

FIGURE 3: Involvement of red-brown papules.

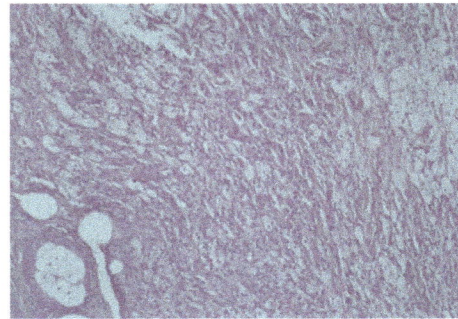

FIGURE 4: Papules, plaque, and tumor like lesions.

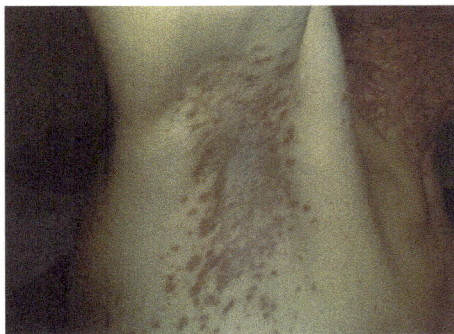

FIGURE 5: Involvement of nasal mucosa.

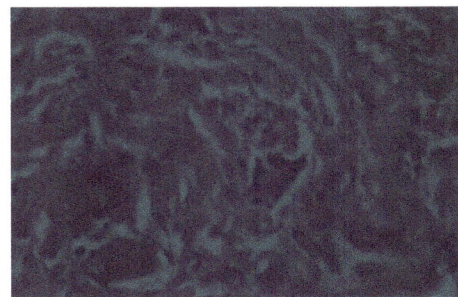

FIGURE 6: Dense dermal diffuse histiocytic infiltration.

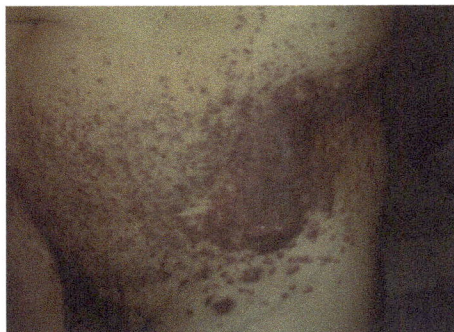

FIGURE 7: A dense dermal diffuse histiocytic infiltration interspersed with mixed inflammatory cells and giant cells.

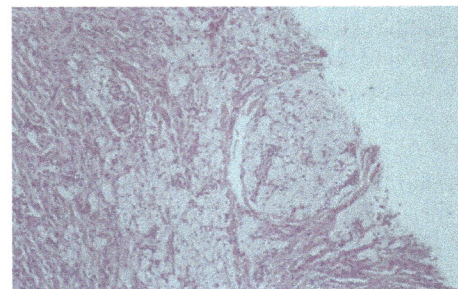

FIGURE 8: Foam cells were also seen.

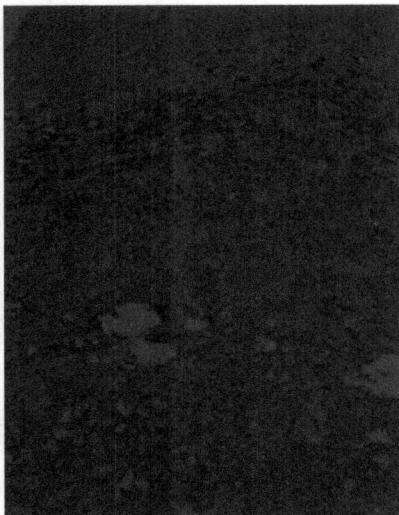

FIGURE 9: Immunohistochemistry was positive.

a proliferation of histiocytic cells. This is usually seen before 25 years, as rarely reported in the elderly [1]. XD is characterized by numerous features like widely disseminated but often closely set and even coalescing, round to oval, orange or yellow-brown papules, and nodules found mainly on the flexor surfaces, such as neck, axillae, antecubital fossae, groin, and perianal region. Often there are lesions around the eyes. The mucous membranes are affected in 40% to 60% of cases. In addition to oral lesions, there may be pharyngeal and laryngeal involvement.

The etiology of XD is unknown. It has been suggested that XD represents a reactive proliferation of histiocytes with secondary accumulation of lipid. But it is not associated with hyperlipidemia.

Three patterns have been identified; the most common pattern is the persistent form. Rarely, lesions may regress spontaneously, and even more infrequently in the progressive form there may be significant internal organ involvement [2]. XD consists of the triad of widespread normolipidemic xanthomata, mucous membrane involvement of the upper respiratory tract, and mild transient diabetes insipidus [1].

Mucous membrane involvements of XD have been reported in 40–60% of cases [4]. The most frequently affected mucosal areas are larynx, pharynx, mouth, trachea, and conjunctiva, although in postmortem studies involvement of the esophagus and stomach was reported as well [5]. Our patient had multiple xanthomatous papules and nodules in his nasal mucosa, but investigation for involvement of other mucosal regions was not carried out.

Meningeal involvement is common, leading to diabetes insipidus when infiltration at the base of the brain is present. This condition is encountered in about 40% of cases but usually is less severe than that associated with Langerhans cell disease. Characteristically, internal lesions other than diabetes insipidus are absent. Our patient did not have any sign or symptom of diabetes insipidus [6].

In a few instances multiple osteolytic lesions have been found, especially in the long bones, as well as lung and central nervous system infiltrates.

Histopathologically, in early lesions, scalloped macrophages dominate the histologic picture, with few foamy cells. Well-developed lesions may still show scalloped cells, but xanthomatization occurs in most cases. Most well-developed lesions contain a mixture of scalloped cells, foamy cells, and inflammatory cells, as well as Touton and foreign-body giant cells. XD histiocytes stain for lysozyme and aI-antitrypsin and also express CD68, CDllb, CD14, CDllc, and factor XIIIa [7].

The main differential diagnosis of XD is generalized eruptive histiocytosis (GEH) and progressive nodular histiocytosis (PNH). Multiple skin lesions occurring in adolescence or young adulthood with prominent involvement of flexural areas, as well as viscera and mucosa, and comprising mainly xanthomatous cells are XD; multiple lesions appearing in crops, generally sparing the flexures, and occurring in normolipemic patients are GEH, while multiple lesions arising in skin of an older patient and progressing to form large nodules, with no evidence of spontaneous regression and comprising mainly spindle-shaped histiocytes, are PNH [8].

We report this case for its unusual large tumor-like lesions around the eyes. In the literature, some authors have previously described cases of XD with eyelid or periocular accentuation of lesions [9, 10].

There are various treatment modalities, like vasopressin, corticosteroids, antiblastic chemotherapy, radiotherapy, cryotherapy, CO_2 LASER therapy, and surgical resection, used alone or in combination [3, 8]. Oral prednisolone (2 mg/kg/day) and azathioprine (2 mg/kg/day) did not show significant efficacy; a combination of lipid-lowering agents or azathioprine and cyclophosphamide was reportedly useful [3]; combination of systemic steroids, clofibrate, and chemotherapy was effective in some studies [3]. Bone marrow transplantation has been used successfully in life-threatening XD [11]. 2-Chlorodeoxyadenosine therapy was found useful in maintaining remission and long-term control of cutaneous lesions [12].

Conflict of Interests

The authors declare that there is no conflict of interests regarding the publication of this paper.

References

[1] J. Altman and R. K. Winkelman, "Xanthoma disseminatum," Archives of Dermatology, vol. 86, pp. 582–596, 1962.

[2] R. Caputo, S. Veraldi, R. Grimalt et al., "The various clinical patterns of Xanthoma disseminatum. Considerations on seven cases and review of the literature," Dermatology, vol. 190, no. 1, pp. 19–24, 1995.

[3] T. W. Kang and S. C. Kim, "A case of xanthoma disseminatum presenting as pedunculating nodules and plaques," Korean Journal of Dermatology, vol. 45, no. 3, pp. 290–293, 2007.

[4] V. K. Mahajan, A. L. Sharma, and P. S. Chauhan, "Xanthoma disseminatum: a red herring xanthomatosis," Indian Journal of

Dermatology, Venereology and Leprology, vol. 79, pp. 253–254, 2013.

[5] J. J. Powell, P. Marren, F. Wojnarowska, and C. Davies, "Xanthoma disseminatum with multi-system involvement and fatal outcome," *Journal of the European Academy of Dermatology and Venereology*, vol. 12, no. 3, pp. 276–278, 1999.

[6] I. T. Zak, D. Altinok, S. S. F. Neilsen, and K. K. Kish, "Xanthoma disseminatum of the central nervous system and cranium," *American Journal of Neuroradiology*, vol. 27, no. 4, pp. 919–921, 2006.

[7] B. Zelger, R. Cerio, G. Orchard, P. Fritsch, and E. Wilson-Jones, "Histologic and immunohistochemical study comparing xanthoma disseminatum and histiocytosis X," *Archives of Dermatology*, vol. 128, no. 9, pp. 1207–1212, 1992.

[8] K. Eisendle, D. Linder, G. Ratzinger et al., "Inflammation and lipid accumulation in xanthoma disseminatum: therapeutic considerations," *Journal of the American Academy of Dermatology*, vol. 58, pp. S47–S49, 2008.

[9] J. Y. Kim, H. Daejung, Y. S. Choe et al., "A case of xanthoma disseminatum accentuating over the eyelids," *Annals of Dermatology*, vol. 22, no. 3, pp. 353–357, 2010.

[10] C. Papagoras, G. Kitsos, P. V. Voulgari et al., "Periocular xanthogranuloma: a forgotten entity?" *Clinical Ophthalmology*, vol. 4, no. 1, pp. 105–110, 2010.

[11] S. Savaşan, L. Smith, C. Scheer, R. Dansey, and E. Abella, "Successful bone marrow transplantation for life threatening xanthogranuloma disseminatum in neurofibromatosis type-1," *Pediatric Transplantation*, vol. 9, no. 4, pp. 534–536, 2005.

[12] F. Khezri, L. E. Gibson, and A. Tefferi, "Xanthoma disseminatum: effective therapy with 2-chlorodeoxyadenosine in a case series," *Archives of Dermatology*, vol. 147, no. 4, pp. 459–464, 2011.

10

Angioedema due to Systemic Isotretinoin Therapy

Pelin Üstüner

Dermatology Clinic, Rize State Hospital, Eminettin Mahallesi, 53100 Rize, Turkey

Correspondence should be addressed to Pelin Üstüner; pelindogaustuner@gmail.com

Academic Editor: Christos C. Zouboulis

Angioedema is the swelling of the mucosal membranes as a variant of urticaria induced by hereditary C1 esterase inhibitor enzyme deficiency, certain foods, or drugs. Herein, we report the case of a 23-year-old woman, with mild-moderate acne presenting with widespread facial angioedema on the 2nd day of systemic isotretinoin treatment. The patient had taken no drugs other than isotretinoin in the preceding days and had no known food allergy. Her angioedema was resolved after the isotretinoin was discontinued. We want to draw the attention of dermatologists to this rare adverse allergic effect of isotretinoin which is frequently used in the treatment of acne vulgaris.

1. Introduction

Retinoids are widely used to treat many conditions; in particular, isotretinoin is known as the first choice treatment for nodulocystic acne vulgaris that is unresponsive to conventional therapies [1]. While cheilitis, mucositis, xerophthalmia, xerosis, retinoid dermatitis, dyslipidemia, photosensitivity, pyogenic granuloma, onycholysis, and paronychia are the well-known, frequent adverse effects of isotretinoin [2], angioedema due to the use of isotretinoin has only been reported in 3 cases to date [3–5].

Angioedema is the swelling of mucosal membranes as a variant of urticaria which can be induced by hereditary C1 esterase inhibitor enzyme deficiency, certain foods, or drugs [6]. Angioedema may have many causes such as nonsteroidal anti-inflammatory drugs, angiotensin-converting enzyme inhibitors, radiocontrast media, antibiotics, or sea food. Angioedema consists of an allergic (IgE-mediated) or nonallergic hypersensitivity reaction, such as pseudoallergy or idiosyncrasy [6]. Skin tests and determination of specific IgE antibodies with standardized allergens are available, but the pathogenesis of drug-induced urticaria and angioedema is rarely clear. It can involve an allergic (IgE-mediated) or non-allergic hypersensitivity reaction, both with a similar clinical presentation.

2. Case Report

A 23-year-old white woman with mild-moderate acne was referred to our dermatology department with facial recalcitrant acne of 2 years duration. She was unresponsive to previous tetracycline treatment (1000 mg daily) for 1 year and was started on oral isotretinoin. After taking just two doses of 30 mg/day isotretinoin, the patient presented the next day with widespread facial swelling predominant in the periorbital areas. She had no previous history of urticaria or angioedema and no known food allergy. She was on a normal diet and had taken no drugs other than isotretinoin in the preceding days. Her medical history and systemic medication were unremarkable. She had no other symptoms. The results of the blood tests including C1 esterase inhibitor, ASO, hepatitis markers, HIV, and parasitological tests were normal. She stated that she had no prior infectious diseases, contact allergic reactions, or food allergies. Dermatological examination revealed bilateral periorbital oedema, widespread facial erythema, and mild desquamation (Figure 1). No other parts of the body were involved. We diagnosed angioedema due to isotretinoin use, and a systemic steroid 40 mg prednol IM for 3 sequential days and oral levocetirizine 5 mg were initiated. Before the occurrence of the angioedema the patient also had mild seborrhoeic dermatitis. The angioedema disappeared

TABLE 1: Brief summary of the cases of angioedema due to the treatment of isotretinoin.

Cases	Age	Sex	Clinical features
Saray and Seçkin [5].	18	F	First episode: oedema of the lips, eyelids, and periorbital region. Second episode: erythematous and oedematous plaques on the dorsum of hands and knees
Filho et al. [3].	24	F	Lip oedema
	48	M	Bilateral periorbital oedema*
Scheinfeld and Bangalore [4].	32	M	Facial swelling
The presented case.	23	F	Widespread facial swelling, periorbital oedema, facial erythema, and mild desquamation. Oral provocation test: facial oedema and periorbital swelling

*The case treated with acitretin.

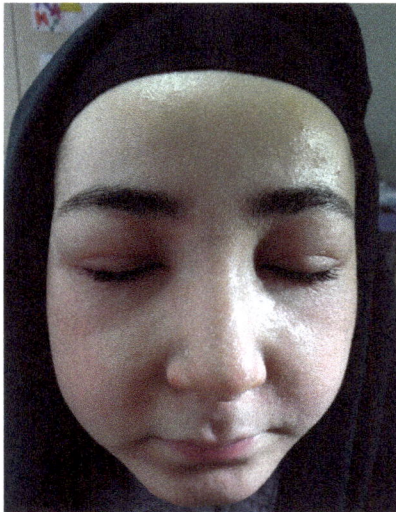

FIGURE 1: Bilateral periorbital edema, facial widespread erythema, and mild desquamation.

completely in a few days, and the treatment was discontinued.

The patient was rehospitalized for the oral provocation test with 30 mg/day isotretinoin treatment. Vasoactive drugs for cardiopulmonary resuscitation (adrenaline and atropine), methylprednisolone, pheniramine maleate ampules, and tracheal intubation were all prepared before the drug administration in case of an angioedema attack and anaphylactic shock. After reexamination of the similar facial oedema and periorbital swelling that appeared in a few hours, systemic steroid treatment was restarted and angioedema was finally reameliorated. In the following 12 months she had no relapses.

3. Discussion

We considered that certain drugs might have been recently started before the occurrence of the angioedema; however, the patient was receiving no drugs apart from isotretinoin. Due to the lack of treatment alternatives and the tendency for the patient to develop scars, an oral provocation test was administered ten days after she was rehospitalized and restarted on isotretinoin therapy. We verified that isotretinoin caused angioedema in this case. Similar facial oedema and

periorbital swelling were reinduced on the first day of the second cure. Systemic steroid treatment was restarted and angioedema was finally reameliorated. In the following 12 months she had no relapses.

The possible reasons for this patient's facial swelling include some type of retinoid induced angioedema, exacerbation of inflammation by isotretinoin, and isotretinoin induced capillary leak syndrome [4]. In this case, the etiology of angioedema was evaluated and other common causes, such as food and drug allergies, were eliminated since there was no history of suspicious food intake at the time the lesions developed and the patient was taking no other medications. Furthermore, the facial angioedema appeared shortly after the isotretinoin intake, disappeared after the drug was discontinued, and recurred after it was restarted. In addition, there were no later recurrences of angioedema. Therefore, we were able to confirm the exact etiology of the angioedema as isotretinoin. The desquamation was also attributed to the fact that she also had mild seborrhoeic dermatitis before the occurrence of angioedema, since there was no suspicious contact history and the desquamation was predominantly common in seborrheic areas.

Angioedema has only been reported in 3 cases due to the use of isotretinoin and in 1 case due to the use of acitretin to date [3–5] (Table 1). In one of these cases, both urticaria and angioedema were reported due to systemic isotretinoin treatment in an 18-year-old female referred with facial nodulocystic acne of two years duration [5]. Oedema of the lips and periorbital region and urticarial plaques on the patient's knees 1 day after isotretinoin reintake were revealed. Upon questioning, the patient admitted that she had restarted the isotretinoin treatment on her own the day before [5]. Lip swelling due to the intake of systemic isotretinoin has also been reported in a 15-year-old boy presenting with a severe lip abscess requiring incision and drainage and hospital admission for the application of an intravenous antibiotic [7]. Although rare, lip abscesses related to isotretinoin therapy present with substantial morbidity and should be promptly recognized. Misdiagnosis of mucositis and angioedema may delay the administration of appropriate therapy. Furthermore, perioral abscess formation in patients taking isotretinoin may also masquerade as angioedema or severe mucositis [8]. However, to date only one case of a 48-year-old man with bilateral periorbital oedema related to acitretin 25 mg/day use has been reported [3].

Isotretinoin capsules contain several additives, such as butylated hydroxyanisole, parabens, vegetable oils, and dyes. It is possible that one of these additives might have been the cause of the angioedema [5]. Gelatine capsules contain glycerine and parabens (methyl and propyl), with the following dye systems: 10 mg iron oxide (red) and titanium dioxide; 20 mg FD&C Red No. 3, FD&C Blue No. 1, and titanium dioxide; 40 mg FD&C Yellow No. 6, D&C Yellow No. 10, and La Roche-type titanium dioxide [3]. However, these additives in drugs and foods have not been found to produce angioedema [3]. We were also able to exclude the possible diagnosis of soybean, peanut, titanium dioxide, or iron oxide dermatitis after the application of the allergy prick test with these ingredients, as they are known to be also included in the isotretinoin capsules.

We think that some angioedema cases might have been misdiagnosed, since isotretinoin is not known to have any allergic side effects. Since isotretinoin is frequently used, we believe that dermatologists should be aware of this rare adverse effect of this drug. Furthermore, more clinical and experimental studies should be undertaken to determine the exact association between isotretinoin and angioedema.

Conflict of Interests

The author declares that there is no conflict of interests regarding the publication of this paper.

References

[1] D. K. Wysowski, J. Swann, and A. Vega, "Use of isotretinoin (Accutane) in the United States: rapid increase from 1992 through 2000," *Journal of the American Academy of Dermatology*, vol. 46, no. 4, pp. 505–509, 2002.

[2] P. K. Rao, R. M. Bhat, B. Nandakishore, S. Dandakeri, J. Martis, and G. H. Kamath, "Safety and efficacy of low-dose isotretinoin in the treatment of moderate to severe acne vulgaris," *Indian Journal of Dermatology*, vol. 59, no. 3, p. 316, 2014.

[3] R. R. D. C. Filho, H. L. de Almeida Jr., and J. D. A. Breunig, "Angioedema due to oral acitretin and isotretinoin," *Anais Brasileiros de Dermatologia*, vol. 86, no. 4, pp. 28–30, 2011.

[4] N. Scheinfeld and S. Bangalore, "Facial edema induced by isotretinoin use: a case and a review of the side effects of isotretinoin," *Journal of Drugs in Dermatology*, vol. 5, no. 5, pp. 467–468, 2006.

[5] Y. Saray and D. Seçkin, "Angioedema and urticaria due to isotretinoin therapy," *Journal of the European Academy of Dermatology and Venereology*, vol. 20, no. 1, pp. 118–120, 2006.

[6] A. J. Bircher, "Drug-induced urticaria and angioedema caused by non-IgE mediated pathomechanisms," *European Journal of Dermatology*, vol. 9, no. 8, pp. 657–663, 1999.

[7] K. C. Huoh and K. W. Chang, "Lip abscess associated with isotretinoin treatment of acne vulgaris," *JAMA Dermatology*, vol. 149, no. 8, pp. 960–961, 2013.

[8] K. Beer, H. Oakley, and J. Waibel, "Perioral abscess associated with isotretinoin," *Journal of Drugs in Dermatology*, vol. 8, no. 11, pp. 1034–1036, 2009.

11

Acquired Brachial Cutaneous Dyschromatosis in a 60-Year-Old Male: A Case Report and Review of the Literature

Nadia Abidi, Kristen Foering, and Joya Sahu

Department of Dermatology, Jefferson Medical College, Thomas Jefferson University, 833 Chestnut Street, Suite 740, Philadelphia, PA 19107, USA

Correspondence should be addressed to Joya Sahu; joya.sahu@jefferson.edu

Academic Editor: Alireza Firooz

Acquired brachial cutaneous dyschromatosis is an acquired pigmentary disorder that has been described in only 20 patients but likely affects many more. This case of a man with acquired brachial cutaneous dyschromatosis is unique as most reports are in women. We report the case of a 60-year-old male who presents with an asymptomatic eruption characterized by hyperpigmented and telangiectatic macules coalescing into patches on the bilateral extensor aspects of the forearms which is consistent clinically and histopathologically with acquired brachial cutaneous dyschromatosis. Given its presence in patients with clinical evidence of chronic sun exposure and its histopathological finding of solar elastosis, acquired brachial cutaneous dyschromatosis is likely a disorder caused by cumulative UV damage. However, a possible association between angiotensin-converting enzyme inhibitors and acquired brachial cutaneous dyschromatosis exists. Further investigation is needed to elucidate both the pathogenesis of the disorder and forms of effective management. Treatment of the disorder should begin with current established treatments for disorders of dyspigmentation.

1. Case Report

A 60-year-old male presented for an annual skin examination. Physical exam incidentally revealed two large, well-delineated patches on the bilateral forearms comprised of hyperpigmented, hypopigmented, telangiectatic, and slightly atrophic macules (Figures 1 and 2). Superficial telangiectasias were also present on the neck and anterior chest. The patient was unsure as to when the forearm lesions first appeared but reported a gradual onset and progressive course over several years. On further questioning he denied any associated symptoms. The patient reported a 25-year history of chronic sun exposure secondary to his profession as a fleet service agent handling aircraft cargo transport outdoors. He denied using any consistent form of photoprotection in the form of sunscreen or physical barriers.

The patient is Fitzpatrick skin type III. Past medical history included hypertension, hyperlipidemia, type 2 diabetes mellitus, asthma, and a history of basal cell carcinoma. Current medications include amlodipine/benazepril, which the patient had been taking since his diagnosis of hypertension six years earlier, chlorthalidone, rosuvastatin, metformin, and inhaled mometasone.

Potassium hydroxide (KOH) preparation on lesion scrapings, performed to rule out underlying fungal infection, was negative. A punch biopsy was obtained from a representative patch on the forearm. Biopsy of the lesion revealed epidermal atrophy with blunting of the rete ridges. There was increased pigmentation of the basal layer without melanin incontinence. There were prominent superficial blood vessels (Figure 3).

2. Discussion

Acquired brachial cutaneous dyschromatosis (ABCD) is an acquired disorder of pigmentation of the skin that presents as asymptomatic, gray-brown patches with an irregular geographical border, interspersed with hypopigmented macules on the dorsal aspect of the forearms [1]. It is usually bilateral and distally distributed. On histology, ABCD is characterized by a poikilodermatous-like tissue pattern with epidermal atrophy, increased basal layer pigmentation, solar elastosis,

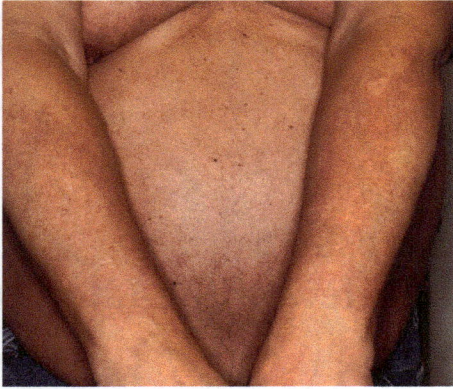

FIGURE 1: Clinical presentation of acquired brachial cutaneous dyschromatosis. There are irregular hyper- and hypopigmented macules coalescing into large patches on the bilateral dorsal forearms.

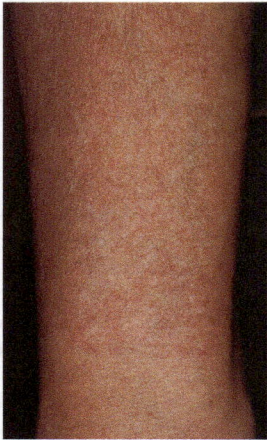

FIGURE 2: Clinical presentation of acquired brachial cutaneous dyschromatosis. Closer inspection of the left forearm reveals hyperpigmented patches and hypopigmented, slightly depressed, atrophic plaques with prominent telangiectasia. Note the relative sharp demarcation at the distal forearm/wrist.

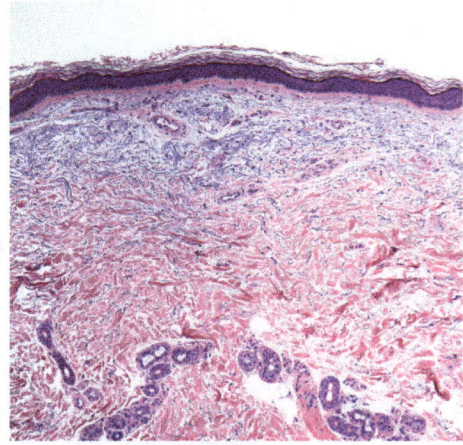

FIGURE 3: Histopathological examination of acquired brachial cutaneous dyschromatosis. Note the pronounced atrophy of the viable epidermis and papillary dermis, increased telangiectasias, abundant solar elastosis, and scattered melanophages, consistent with ABCD 100x magnification, H&E.

and superficial telangiectases [1–3]. However, unlike poikiloderma, no pigmentary incontinence is seen [1–3]. It has been reported most frequently in middle-aged, postmenopausal women with Fitzpatrick skin types III-IV [1]. Additionally, an association with poikiloderma of Civatte has been found in 45% of cases [1].

The differential diagnosis includes melasma, tinea versicolor, and other disorders of pigmentation. Melasma is comprised of sharply delineated, hyperpigmented macules and patches found primarily on the malar eminences, forehead, upper lip, and mandible of women. It is similar to ABCD histologically in that there is increased basal layer pigmentation, but there is no epidermal atrophy or telangiectasia. Tinea versicolor is characterized by hyper- and hypopigmented macules and patches with fine scale and is commonly found on the neck and trunk in a seborrheic distribution. It is easily diagnosed by microscopic examination of KOH-dissolved scale.

Other pigmentary disorders could look similar clinically but they are discernable by histologic examination. Lichen planus pigmentosus (LPP) is characterized by grey to dark brown macules in sun exposed areas such as the face, neck, trunk, and limbs and in sun-protected sites such as the flexural folds [4]. Erythema dyschromicum perstans (EDP) is characterized by asymptomatic, grayish macules involving the trunk and proximal extremities [5]. For both entities, the color is distinctive and different from ABCD and histologically these conditions show interface dermatitis, melanophages, and variability in epidermal change and inflammatory infiltrate [4, 6].

Finally, drugs are known to cause pigmentary disorders and they include nonsteroidal anti-inflammatory drugs, antimalarials, amiodarone, cytotoxic drugs, tetracyclines, heavy metals, and psychotropic drugs [7]. Thorough history distinguished drug-induced hyperpigmentation from ABCD in our patient.

Currently, two hypotheses on the etiopathogenesis of ABCD exist. In its first description in the literature by Rongioletti and Rebora, authors observed a large proportion of their cohort (65%) suffered from hypertension and had been taking antihypertensive drugs for years prior to the onset of the pigmentation—with angiotensin-converting enzyme inhibitors (ACEIs) being the most commonly used [1]. These findings led to the hypothesis of a direct association of ABCD with hypertension and/or with antihypertensive—specifically ACEI—use [1]. Later, Hu et al. disputed over this conclusion, suggesting the association between ABCD and hypertension or antihypertensives as more likely a consequence of the commonality of hypertension and its treatment regimens [2]. Instead, due to its histopathological resemblance to poikiloderma of Civatte, in which epidermal atrophy, hyperpigmentation, and telangiectasias are also seen, Hu et al. suggest the disorder is a manifestation of chronic sun damage—either due to cumulative UV exposure or a pattern produced by drug-induced (possibly ACE-I induced) photosensitivity [2].

Although drug induced pigmentation represents 10–20% of all acquired hyperpigmentation [8], there is currently no data associating ACEIs and cutaneous dyschromia. However, one study reports photosensitivity as an adverse cutaneous reaction to ACEI use [9], therefore potentially backing Hu et al.'s two-hit drug-induced photosensitivity hypothesis. In this case, our patient's long-standing hypertension, use of an ACEI, and chronic sun exposure lend support to either proposed hypothesis.

Though not uncommon according to Rebora and Rongioletti, ABCD is subtle and asymptomatic and thus likely underreported; as such, there is little known about successful treatments. Established treatments for other acquired forms of dyspigmentation, including topical depigmenting agents, chemical peels, and laser treatments, may be considered [10]. To obtain satisfactory cosmetic results, treatment of cutaneous hyperpigmentation often requires the combination of multiple modalities of treatment as well as strict photoprotection. In a 2010 review, authors reported significantly greater improvements in skin pigmentation disorders with treatment using nonablative and ablative fractional photothermolysis (NAFP and AFP) in comparison to treatment with other resurfacing devices [11]. One study utilizing AFP for treatment of poikiloderma of Civatte observed a 65.0% improvement in erythema/telangiectasia and a 66.7% improvement in dyschromia with the average number of 1.4 treatments required for improvement. Due to the histopathological similarities seen in ABCD and poikiloderma of Civatte, we expect that a series of AFP treatments for our patient would result in similar improvement.

In summary, we describe a case of acquired brachial cutaneous dyschromatosis in a 60-year-old male with a history of hypertension, ACEI use, and chronic sun exposure. In most reported cases thus far, individuals have had some evidence of chronic sun exposure either histologically with the presence of solar elastosis or clinically with the presence of poikiloderma of Civatte. Although this most likely indicates a primary sun-exposure component to the etiology of ABCD, pathogenesis via ACEI-induced photosensitivity remains to be investigated. To determine appropriate treatments for ABCD, trials in its management are needed and should be guided by current forms of treatment used for other pigmentation disorders, including topical depigmenting agents, chemical peels, laser treatments, and strict photoprotection.

Conflict of Interests

J. Sahu served as a consultant to Celgene. The authors declare that there is no other conflict of interests regarding the publication of this paper.

References

[1] F. Rongioletti and A. Rebora, "Acquired brachial cutaneous dyschromatosis: a common pigmentary disorder of the arm in middle-aged women," *Journal of the American Academy of Dermatology*, vol. 42, no. 4, pp. 680–684, 2000.

[2] S. W. Hu, J. Chu, S. Meehan, H. Kamino, and M. K. Pomeranz, "Acquired brachial cutaneous dyschromatosis," *Dermatology Online Journal*, vol. 17, no. 10, article 16, 2011, http://escholarship.org/uc/item/09r7454f.

[3] D. Lipsker, "What is poikiloderma?" *Dermatology*, vol. 207, no. 3, pp. 243–245, 2003.

[4] M. E. Vega, L. Waxtein, R. Arenas, M. T. Hojyo, and L. Dominguez-Soto, "Ashy dermatosis versus lichen planus pigmentosus: a controversial matter," *International Journal of Dermatology*, vol. 31, no. 2, pp. 87–88, 1992.

[5] T. F. Cestari, L. P. Dantas, and J. C. Boza, "Acquired hyperpigmentations," *Anais Brasileiros de Dermatologia*, vol. 89, no. 1, pp. 11–25, 2014.

[6] L. D. Soto, M. E. V. Memije, R. Arenas, and L. W. Morgenstein, "Dermatosis cinecienta. A clinico-pathological study of 20 patients (1989–1990)," *Gaceta Médica de México*, vol. 128, no. 6, pp. 623–628, 1992.

[7] D. Dereure, "Drug-induced skin pigmentation," *American Journal of Clinical Dermatology*, vol. 2, no. 4, pp. 253–262, 2001.

[8] O. Dereure, "Drug-induced skin pigmentation epidemiology, diagnosis and treatment," *The American Journal of Clinical Dermatology*, vol. 2, no. 4, pp. 253–262, 2001.

[9] U. M. Steckelings, M. Artuc, T. Wollschläger, S. Wiehstutz, and B. M. Henz, "Angiotensin-converting enzyme inhibitors as inducers of adverse cutaneous reactions," *Acta Dermato-Venereologica*, vol. 81, no. 5, pp. 321–325, 2001.

[10] M. Picardo and M. Carrera, "New and experimental treatments of cloasma and other hypermelanoses," *Dermatologic Clinics*, vol. 25, no. 3, pp. 353–362, 2007.

[11] E. P. Tierney and C. W. Hanke, "Review of the literature: treatment of dyspigmentation with fractionated resurfacing," *Dermatologic Surgery*, vol. 36, no. 10, pp. 1499–1508, 2010.

12

Cutaneous Metastasis of Medullary Carcinoma Thyroid Masquerading as Subcutaneous Nodules Anterior Chest and Mandibular Region

Rahul Mannan,[1] **Jasmine Kaur,**[2] **Jasleen Kaur,**[3] **Sanjay Piplani,**[1] **Harjot Kaur,**[1] **and Harleen Kaur**[1]

[1] Department of Pathology, SGRDIMSR, Amritsar, Punjab 143001, India
[2] Department of Oral and Maxillofacial Surgery, SGRDIMSR, Amritsar, Punjab, India
[3] Department of Dermatology, SGRDIMSR, Amritsar, Punjab, India

Correspondence should be addressed to Rahul Mannan; rahulmannan@gmail.com

Academic Editor: Gérald E. Piérard

Cutaneous metastasis of underlying primary malignancies can present to dermatologist with chief complaints of cutaneous lesions. The underlying malignancy is generally diagnosed much later after a complete assessment of the concerned case. Medullary carcinoma thyroid (MCT) is a relatively uncommon primary neoplasia of the thyroid. Very few cases presenting as cutaneous metastases of MCT have been reported in the literature. Most of the cases which have been reported are of the papillary and the follicular types. We here report a case of a patient who presented in the dermatology clinic with the primary complaint of multiple subcutaneous nodules in anterior chest wall and left side of body of mandible. By systematic application of clinical and diagnostic skills these nodules were diagnosed as cutaneous metastasis of MCT bringing to the forefront a history of previously operated thyroid neoplasm. So clinically, the investigation of a flesh coloured subcutaneous nodule, presenting with a short duration, particularly in scalp, jaw, or anterior chest wall should include possibility of metastatic deposits. A dermatologist should keep a possibility of an internal organ malignancy in patients while investigating a case of flesh coloured subcutaneous nodules, presenting with short duration. A systematic application of clinical and diagnostic skills will eventually lead to such a diagnosis even when not suspected clinically at its primary presentation. A prompt and an emphatic diagnosis and treatment will have its bearing on the eventual outcome in all these patients.

1. Introduction

Organ specific malignancies rarely present clinically as cutaneous metastasis. Such patients often report to a dermatologist with the chief complaint of cutaneous lesions. The underlying malignancy is generally diagnosed after a complete assessment of the concerned case [1]. Medullary carcinoma thyroid (MCT) is a relatively uncommon primary neoplasia of the thyroid. Very few cases presenting as cutaneous metastases of MCT have been reported in the literature. Most of the cases which have been reported are of the papillary and the follicular types with the most frequent site of presentation being scalp [2].

We report a case of a patient who presented in the dermatology clinic with the primary complaint of multiple subcutaneous nodules in anterior chest wall and left side of body of mandible. These nodules were diagnosed as cutaneous metastasis of MCT on cytology bringing to the forefront a history of previously operated thyroid neoplasm.

2. Case Report

A 43-year-old female patient presented in the dermatology clinic of a tertiary care teaching hospital with primary complaint of gradually increasing multiple painless swellings on the anterior chest wall and in the jaw for the past 3 months. On examination, subcutaneous nodules were observed and their size ranged from the smallest being 1.0 cm (left side mandible) to the largest which measured 3.0 cm (below the right breast) with the overlying skin being normal in colour

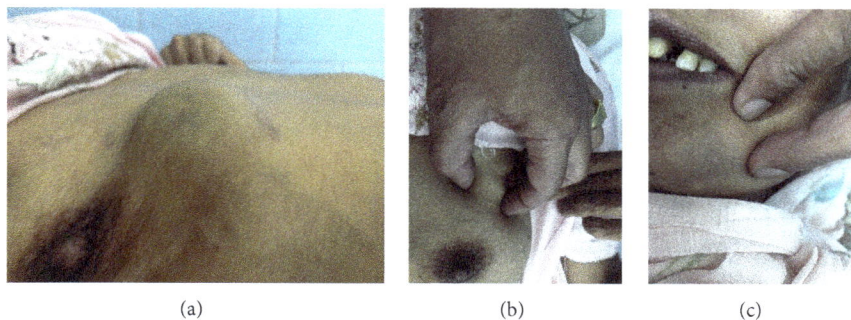

FIGURE 1: (a) Subcutaneous nodule seen in the anterior chest wall below the right breast. (b) Another subcutaneous nodule seen in the anterior chest wall just near the left breast. (c) Subcutaneous nodule in the mandible.

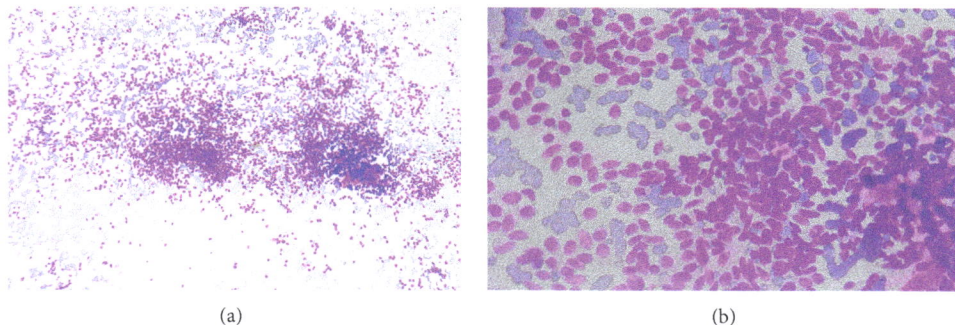

FIGURE 2: (a) Singly scattered cellular aspirate with cells of variable sizes and shapes on fine needle aspiration [MGG ×100]. (b) Higher magnification exhibiting predominantly oval and spindloid to plasmacytoid cells on fine needle aspiration [H & E 400x].

(Figures 1(a), 1(b), and 1(c)). On palpation these nodules were nontender with no temperature elevation, nonitchy, soft to firm in consistency, freely mobile, and not fixed to the underlying tissues.

General clinical examination of the patient was non-significant. The various routine haematological parameters were within normal limits with no eosinophilia or atypical cell noted in peripheral smear examination. Her biochemical tests were within range and serological investigations noncontributory (nonreactive viral markers including negative VDRL serology). On the basis of clinical picture, lab investigations and symptomatology the clinical differentials of lipomatous lesion, benign neural sheath tumour, fibroblastic/fibrohistiocytic lesion, adnexal tumour, and amelanotic melanoma were made.

To ascertain the etiology of the nodules, fine needle aspiration cytology (FNAC) was planned under the guidance of dermatologist in order to aspirate the material from correct representative site. The procedure was done from multiple sites with the help of 23 G needles and 2-3 passes were given. Material aspirated was serosanguinous. Smears prepared were air dried and alcohol fixed. May grunwald giemsa (MGG) and hematoxylin and eosin (H & E) stains were done, respectively. Extra blood admixed material was taken and cell block was made which was sent to histopathology unit for tissue processing.

The smears prepared showed dispersed cellular aspirate with cells of variable sizes and shapes. The cells were predominantly oval and spindloid to plasmacytoid. The nuclei of these cells exhibited mild anisokaryosis, presence of small inconspicuous nucleoli, and speckled (salt and pepper) chromatin (Figures 2(a) and 2(b)). The cytoplasm of these cells was eosinophilic and demonstrated fine, pinkish cytoplasmic granularity. Focally, presence of small quantity of amorphous pinkish material (amyloid like material) was also observed.

The cytological opinion was thus in favour of subcutaneous deposits of a "neuroendocrinal" lesion. In context of the cytological findings the patient was reevaluated at the dermatological clinic for the same. During reevaluation the patient concurred with the symptoms associated with neuroendocrinal lesions of intermittent episodes of flushing. Based on these findings a provisional diagnosis of a neuroendocrinal lesion arising from the gastrointestinal tract, lungs or thyroid was made. The patient was asked about history of any previous surgery in relation to the abovementioned sites. The patient subsequently provided a history of thyroid surgery 5 years back at another centre. On examination a fine scar was noted in one of the neck creases. The previous treatment records and reports were not available with the patient which is quite the norm in many instances in resource challenged countries. Based on these findings, a working diagnosis of cutaneous metastatic deposits of MTC was suggested with histopathology report of cell block awaited.

Patient was advised radiological examination (CT scan and ultrasonography). CT scan revealed destruction of the

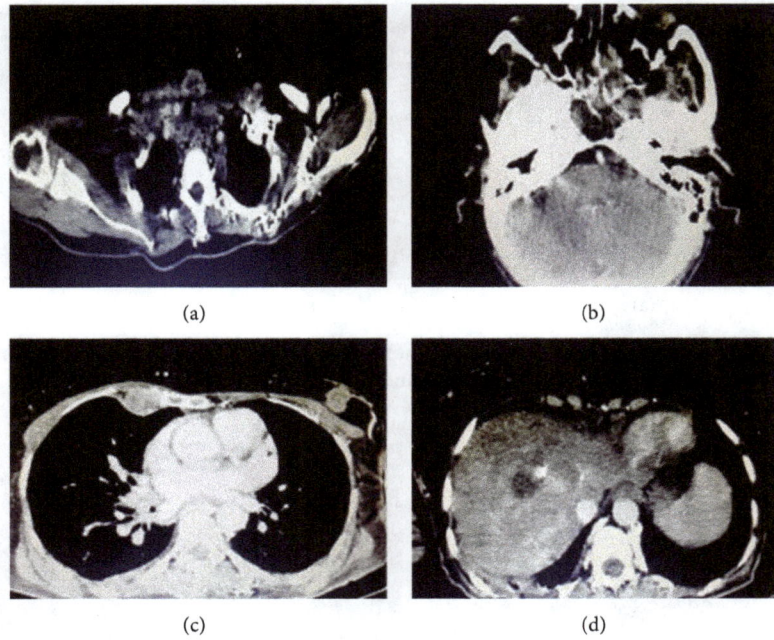

(a)

(b)

(c)

(d)

FIGURE 3: (a) Destruction of the right 4th rib along with erosion of the spinous processes of the thoracic vertebra and sclerotic lesions in the body of the vertebrae. (b) Destruction of the floor of middle cranial fossa, posterior ethmoidal air cells and sphenoid sinus. (c) Lesions in the mediastinum. (d) In liver multiple variable sized heterogeneous lesions containing foci of calcification were observed.

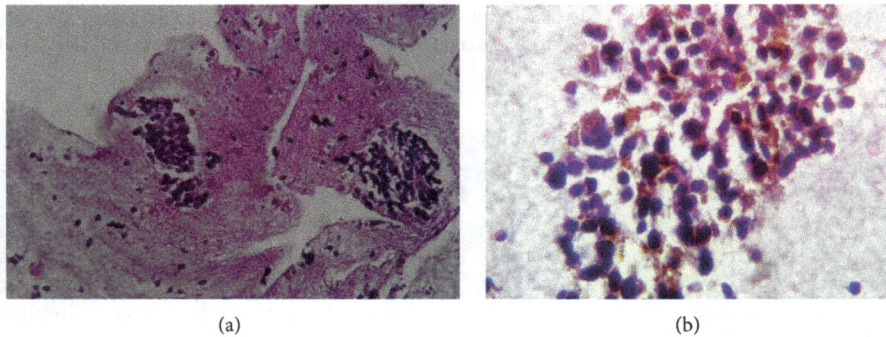

(a)

(b)

FIGURE 4: (a) Small nests of cohesive malignant cells within areas of hemorrhage [H & E 100x]. (b) Higher magnification detailing the cell morphology of spindle to oval shaped cells [H & E 400x].

floor of middle cranial fossa, posterior ethmoidal air cells, and sphenoid sinus. In the maxillofacial region there was destruction of the left condylar process of mandible with soft tissue mass extending into the infratemporal fossa. Destruction of the left alveolar margin of the mandible was also present. CT scan of the neck region showed a heterogeneously enhanced nodular mass in the residual thyroid gland with retrosternal extension. Multiple lymph nodes were seen at level II, III, and supraclavicular region bilaterally. In the thoracic region, three irregular nodular spiculated masses with central necrosis were seen in the right breast parenchyma. Destruction of the right 4th rib along with erosion of the spinous processes of the thoracic vertebra and sclerotic lesions in the body of the vertebrae were noted. In liver multiple variable sized heterogeneous lesions containing foci of calcification were observed. These were also noted as multiple hyperechoic

lesions in both lobes of liver on USG (suggestive of metastatic deposits) (Figure 3).

The histopathology report of the cell block showed a lesion composed of nests of cohesive malignant cells within areas of hemorrhage (Figure 4(a)). The individual cells were predominantly spindle shaped to epithelioid in morphology. They contained a moderate amount of amphophilic cytoplasm with irregular, hyperchromatic nuclei containing prominent nucleoli exhibiting characteristic "salt and pepper" chromatin. The cytoplasm was minimal but showed fine eosinophilic granules (Figure 4(b)).

On immunohistochemical studies (IHC), tumor cells were positive for calcitonin, TTF-1, and thyroglobulin thus confirming the primary site to be thyroid and the tumor. Hence a final diagnosis of cutaneous metastasis of MTC was rendered. Patient was advised whole body scan, calcitonin and CEA serum assays for further evaluation and also offered chemotherapy and palliative radiotherapy which the patient refused due to economic constraints. Patient and her attendants were advised and encouraged to undergo a full clinical/radiological examination and screening for germ line mutation. Patient was also unable to give a proper family history or presence of any relative with such manifestations/thyroid swelling.

For treatment purposes she was referred to a higher centrally funded apex centre where she could receive adequate subsidized therapy for the same.

3. Discussion

Subcutaneous nodules can cause a dilemma to both the treating physician (in this case dermatologist) and the cytopathologist to reach a conclusive diagnosis. This is more so pronounced in reaching a cytodiagnosis of cutaneous metastasis in the absence of history of primary tumour as in the present case. In cutaneous metastasis of MCT, the cytology and the clinical opinion can be biased towards a diagnosis of adnexal tumour/fibrous lesion (due to presence of spindloid cells of MCT). So a caution has to be exercised.

Skin metastasis of thyroid cancer has been rarely reported and of which most of the cases documented are of papillary and follicular type [3] with MCT being the least common with around 10 cases reported worldwide. The most common site of cutaneous metastasis of thyroid neoplasia reported in the literature is scalp [4].

In the present case report, a point of difference from the other case reports detailing the cutaneous metastasis of MCT was localization (absence of scalp lesions and presence of nodule in mandible region) and presentation (as the nodules were skin coloured, nonitching, and nonulcerative) and associated with no granulation tissue and hyperkeratinization.

MCT is a variant of thyroid carcinoma which originates from the parafollicular cell (C cells), which produce calcitonin and has a neuroendocrine histogenesis [5]. An overview of MCT is discussed under Table 1.

Two different forms of MCT are recognized: the sporadic form, which accounts for about 75% of cases, and the hereditary or familial form accounting for the remaining 25%. RET (REarranged during Transfection) proto-oncogene mutation is identified on hot spots in most of the hereditary cases of MTC and less than half the cases of sporadic forms. RET tyrosine kinase receptor like other tyrosine kinases is involved in the regulation of differentiation, proliferation, survival, and cell motility processes through several intracellular signalling and hence plays a major role in histogenesis and evolution of MCT [6].

In recent years there has been gradual advancement of identification of more mutations like RAS in the so called RET negative cases. There is newer stress on reclassifying cases of MCT on the basis of molecular biology (Table 2). These along with a novel mutated form M918T are associated with more aggressive disseminated forms and presence of MCT in children including those seen in the present case of dermatological metastases (which are thought to carry some additional mutations) and carry poor prognosis [7, 8].

TABLE 1: Medullary carcinoma thyroid: an overview.

Clinical examination

(i) Incidence

3.0% of all thyroid cancers

(ii) Age at presentation

5th and 6th decade

(iii) Clinical presentation at diagnosis

    (a) Cervical swelling (cervical lymphadenopathy) with midline neck swelling

    (b) Hoarseness, dysphagia, and stridor

    (c) Paraneoplastic syndromes (uncommon)

    (d) Diarrhoea

(iv) Propensity for regional and distant metastasis

    (a) Cervical Lymphadenopathy present in 50% cases at the time of diagnosis

    (b) Liver, lung, and bone metastasis by hematogenous route in 5–10% cases at the time of diagnosis

Diagnostic options

(i) Cytology

(ii) Histopathology followed by immunohistochemical stains

(iii) Serum calcitonin and CEA levels

(iv) 24 hours urinalysis for catecholamine metabolites to rule out asso MEN 2 syndrome

(v) Radiological assessment

    (a) Whole body CT scan

    (b) Ultrasonography of neck and abdomen

(vi) Screening for missense mutation in RET in leucocytes

Management options

(i) Surgery

    (a) Total thyroidectomy with or without neck dissection

    (b) Prophylactic thyroidectomy in carriers

(ii) Radiotherapy (adjuvant)

(iii) Chemotherapy (palliative in advanced cases)

(iv) Newer modalities (tyrosine kinase inhibitors)

    (a) Vandetanib

    (b) Cabozantinib

The newer research queers the pitch further by finding of an additional RAS mutations in all so called RET negative patients. One of the study has calculated the prevalence of RAS positivity in the range of 68% in RET negative MCT and only 2.8% in RET positive MCT [9] suggesting that RAS mutations could represent alternative genetic events in sporadic MCT tumorigenesis.

Thus a dermatologist/treating physician and pathologists should be aware of genetic classification of MTC (Table 2) in setting of dermatological metastases or other multicentric metastases in sporadic cases of young as various investigations and tools for genetic screening of patients and their relatives are now available which can identify germ line RET as well as other non-RET mutations. This in turn has helped treating physicians worldwide to understand the disease pathology, to tailor make the therapeutic response, and to

TABLE 2: Molecular classification of MCT (Modified from 2012 Europen thyroid cancer association guidelines and with work done by Boichard et al. [8]).

Hereditary MTC (25% Cases): Associated with almost all cases with germline RET mutation (Exon 5, 8, 10, 11, 13, 14, 15 & 16).
- MEN 2A: 85% cases mutation at Exon 11, codon 634
Other mutations Exon 10 and 11, codon 609, 611, 618, 620
- MEN 2B: Exon 16, codon 918 (Most common)
- Disseminated and aggressive variant (commonly in children and young): M918T
Sporadic MTC (75% of all cases):
- RET positive group: 35% cases with somatic RET mutations
- RET negative group:
(1) Criteria: Negative for common germline mutations in Exon 5, 8, 10, 11, 13, 14, 15 & 16
(2) Other Mutations to be identified:
(i) RAS mutation—(Almost 80% of remaining RET negative cases)
(ii) H-RAS (>50%): Exon 2, codon 13; Exon 3, codon 61; Exon 4, codon 63
(iii) K-RAS (<30%): Exon 3, codon 61; Exon 2, codon 13; Exon 4, codon 117

frame recommendations in setting of MCT which can have a direct impact on disease free survival and can lessen the associated morbidity as well.

According to the latest recommendations it is encouraged that once an RET mutation has been confirmed in a patient, all first degree relatives should be screened to identify 50% who must have inherited the mutation (especially children) and are therefore at risk for development of MCT. All such patients can undergo prophylactic thyroidectomy [10] (Table 1). The newer research goes a step further with investigation a patient of non-RET mutation to investigate for other mutations such as RAS [11]. This approach has led to availability of newer therapeutic strategies involving newer tyrosine kinase inhibitors such as vandetanib and cabozantinib which are the drugs currently approved by US food and drug administration (FDA) for treatment of metastatic MCT. Till date no case has been documented which has utilized above two drugs to treat cutaneous metastasis [12, 13] for all such cases which are more complicated, undergone wide metastases (including dermatological), and patients having novel mutations. It is imperative to note though that till date no Ras-targeted therapies have been successful in these cases but have met with a little success in setting of aggressive mutation M918T [8] (Table 2). However, the documentation of such mutations in MCT may lead to designing of drug particularly targeting these mutations in near future.

A conclusive diagnosis of cutaneous metastasis of MCT usually requires a high index of suspicion and histopathological backing with immunohistochemical analysis. Apart from the characteristic "neuroendocrine" morphology noted on cytology and histology, MCT is immunopositive for markers such as calcitonin (most specific tumour marker), synaptophysin, chromogranin, and CD56.

These arrays of IHC markers which are positive for neuroendocrine tumours can be seen in other tumours such as small cell (SC) carcinoma lung, carcinoid tumours (of thoracic, abdominal, and head-neck region), and even merkel cell carcinoma. All these can also present as subcutaneous chest and scalp swellings. Here a unique and novel IHC marker, thyroid transcription factor (TTF-1), can be a very effective tool in distinguishing the type of malignancy [11]. TTF-1 is expressed in thyroid follicular cells, thyroid C cells, and pneumocytes. So it can effectively rule out carcinoid tumors/other neuroendocrine tumors of extra-thyroid sites and hence narrowing the differentials to MCT and SC carcinoma lung.

The differentiation between MCT and SC carcinoma lung (as both express TTF-1 and neuroendocrine markers) can be easily done on the basis of expression of thyroglobulin which is negative in the latter [14].

The tumour cells in the present case were immunoreactive to calcitonin, TTF-1, and thyroglobulin. It was immunonegative for S-100 which ruled out the possibility of subcutaneous amelanotic melanoma. Hence a final diagnosis of cutaneous metastasis of MCT was reported.

The cutaneous metastasis of thyroid carcinoma is a sign of dissemination and reflects a very poor prognosis (mean survival rate of 7–19 months) [4]. The residual tumour tissue metastasis can be measured by PET-CT scan by identifying the hypermetabolic foci in the skin lesions. Conventionally as illustrated in Table 1, the management of MCT includes surgery (alone, when condition detected early) and if high risk of regional metastasis is suspected then surgery is supplanted with radiotherapy. Unlike the other variants of thyroid malignancy, there is no role of radioiodine treatment in cases of MCT because of difference in histogenesis. Due to small number of MCT cases with skin metastasis the biological behaviour of tumour to various modalities has not been studied in detail. Till date, combination of radiotherapy (RT) and chemotherapy (CT) or CT alone have been tried with 50% success rate [4, 15]. The response to CT is predicted by estimating serum calcitonin and CEA levels. Another proposed clinical indicator, calcitonin doubling time (CDT), has been proposed which better predicts MCT survival and prognosis [13, 16].

As described above the newer modalities which are targeting the tyrosine kinase proteins (involved in growth of medullary cancer cells) have opened a new vista in the treatment of MCT. These have utilized the principle of molecular genetics involved in tumorogenesis of MCT.

The present case report is worth reporting as it not only presents a rare presentation of secondary cutaneous metastasis of MCT but also illustrates instance of careful clinical assessment while evaluating a case of skin nodule showing spindloid/plasmacytoid cytology. So clinically, the investigation of a flesh coloured subcutaneous nodule, presenting with a short duration, particularly in scalp, jaw, or anterior chest wall, should include possibility of metastatic deposits.

A dermatologist should be clinically aware of the possibility of an internal organ malignancy in patients with such presentation and ready to think "out of box" and get all the necessary investigations including utilizing the technologies such as FNAC, IHC, and molecular studies to identify gene mutations for proper evaluation. These principles were employed in the present case report to reach a diagnosis as diagnosis of MCT was not suspected clinically at its primary presentation.

A prompt and an emphatic diagnosis and treatment will have its bearing on the eventual outcome in all these patients.

Disclosure

All authors take full responsibility and have full knowledge of the details described in the observation.

Conflict of Interests

There is no conflict of interests amongst the authors.

Authors' Contribution

Rahul Mannan worked as the principal author and diagnosed the case. Harjot Kaur and Sanjay Piplani collected the materials. Harleen Kaur handled the photography and Jasmine Kaur and Jasleen Kaur were the clinical supervisors and did the proof reading of the manuscript.

References

[1] A. Pushkar, L. Khan, P. Singh, and A. Agarwal, "Cutaneous metastasis from visceral malignancy: a rare presentation," Journal of Cytology, vol. 26, no. 3, pp. 109–110, 2009.

[2] P. R. Dahl, D. G. Brodland, J. R. Goellner, and I. D. Hay, "Thyroid carcinoma metastatic to the skin: a cutaneous manifestation of a widely disseminated malignancy," Journal of the American Academy of Dermatology, vol. 36, no. 4, pp. 531–537, 1997.

[3] W. J. Choi, Y. Y. Lee, S. Kim et al., "A case of medullary Ca thyroid in which the skin metastasis was concurrently present and response occured to chemotherapy," Cancer Research and Treatment, vol. 40, no. 4, pp. 202–206, 2008.

[4] S. Alwaheeb, D. Ghazarian, S. L. Boerner, and S. L. Asa, "Cutaneous manifestations of thyroid cancer: a report of four cases and review of the literature," Journal of Clinical Pathology, vol. 57, no. 4, pp. 435–438, 2004.

[5] E. D. Williams, "Histogenesis of medullary carcinoma of the thyroid.," Journal of Clinical Pathology, vol. 19, no. 2, pp. 114–118, 1966.

[6] C. Nashed, S. V. Sakpal, S. Cherneykin, and R. S. Chamberlain, "Medullary thyroid carcinoma metastatic to skin," Journal of Cutaneous Pathology, vol. 37, no. 12, pp. 1237–1240, 2010.

[7] R. Elisei, M. Alevizaki, B. Conte-Devolx, K. Frank-Raue, V. Leite, and G. R. Williams, "2012 European thyroid association guidelines for genetic testing and its clinical consequences in medullary thyroid cancer," European Thyroid Journal, vol. 1, no. 4, pp. 216–231, 2013.

[8] A. Boichard, L. Croux, A. Al Ghuzlan et al., "Somatic RAS mutations occur in a large proportion of sporadic RET-negative medullary thyroid carcinomas and extend to a previously unidentified exon," Journal of Clinical Endocrinology and Metabolism, vol. 97, no. 10, pp. E2031–E2035, 2012.

[9] M. M. Moura, B. M. Cavaco, A. E. Pinto, and V. Leite, "High prevalence of RAS mutations in RET-negative sporadic medullary thyroid carcinomas," The Journal of Clinical Endocrinology and Metabolism, vol. 96, no. 5, pp. E863–E868, 2011.

[10] Thyroid carcinoma, "NCCN guidelines," July 2014, http://www.nccn.org/prefii/physician-df/throid.pdf.

[11] N. G. Ordonez and N. A. Samaan, "Medullary carcinoma of the thyroid metastatic to the skin: report of two cases," Journal of Cutaneous Pathology, vol. 14, no. 4, pp. 251–254, 1987.

[12] S. A. Wells Jr., B. G. Robinson, R. F. Gagel et al., "Vandetanib in patients with locally advanced or metastatic medullary thyroid cancer: a randomized, double-blind phase III trial," Journal of Clinical Oncology, vol. 30, no. 2, pp. 134–141, 2012.

[13] C. D. Hart and R. H. De Boer, "Profile of cabozantinib and its potential in the treatment of advanced medullary thyroid cancer," OncoTargets and Therapy, vol. 6, pp. 1–7, 2013.

[14] P. A. Bejarano, Y. E. Nikiforov, E. S. Swenson, and P. W. Biddinger, "Thyroid transcription factor-1, thyroglobulin, cytokeratin 7, and cytokeratin 20 in thyroid neoplasms," Applied Immunohistochemistry and Molecular Morphology, vol. 8, no. 3, pp. 189–194, 2000.

[15] S. A. Wells Jr., B. G. Robinson, R. F. Gagel et al., "Vandetanib in patients with locally advanced or metastatic medullary thyroid cancer: a randomized, double-blind phase III trial," Journal of Clinical Oncology, vol. 30, no. 2, pp. 134–141, 2012.

[16] B. Niederle, F. Sebag, and M. Brauckhoff, "Timing and extent of thyroid surgery for gene carriers of hereditary C cell disease—a consensus statement of the European Society of Endocrine Surgeons (ESES)," Langenbeck's Archives of Surgery, vol. 399, no. 2, pp. 185–197, 2014.

Iatrogenic Anetoderma of Prematurity: A Case Report and Review of the Literature

Laura Maffeis,[1] **Lorenza Pugni,**[1] **Carlo Pietrasanta,**[1] **Andrea Ronchi,**[1] **Monica Fumagalli,**[1] **Carlo Gelmetti,**[2] **and Fabio Mosca**[1]

[1] *NICU, Department of Clinical Sciences and Community Health, Fondazione IRCCS Ca' Granda Ospedale Maggiore Policlinico, University of Milan, Via della Commenda 12, 20122 Milan, Italy*
[2] *Pediatric Dermatology Unit, Fondazione IRCCS Ca' Granda Ospedale Maggiore Policlinico, University of Milan, Via Pace 9, 20122 Milan, Italy*

Correspondence should be addressed to Lorenza Pugni; lorenza.pugni@mangiagalli.it

Academic Editor: Gérald E. Piérard

Anetoderma is a skin disorder characterized by focal loss of elastic tissue in the mid dermis, resulting in localized areas of macular depressions or pouchlike herniations of skin. An iatrogenic form of anetoderma has been rarely described in extremely premature infants and has been related to the placement of monitoring devices on the patient skin. Because of the increasing survival of extremely premature infants, it is easy to foresee that the prevalence of anetoderma of prematurity will increase in the next future. Although it is a benign lesion, it persists over time and can lead to significant aesthetic damage with need for surgical correction. Sometimes the diagnosis can be difficult, especially when the atrophic lesions become evident after discharge. Here, we report on a premature infant born at 24 weeks of gestation, who developed multiple anetodermic patches of skin on the trunk at the sites where electrocardiographic electrodes were previously applied. The knowledge of the disease can encourage a more careful management of the skin of extremely premature babies and aid the physicians to diagnose the disease when anetoderma patches are first encountered later in childhood.

1. Introduction

Anetoderma is a rare benign dermatosis characterized by focal loss of mid dermal elastic tissue, resulting in well-circumscribed areas of macular depressions or pouchlike herniations of skin [1–4]. The term *anetoderma* is derived from the Greek words *anetos* (relaxed) and *derma* (skin). Histological examination of the lesion typically reveals not only normal skin findings on hematoxylin-eosin staining, but also a significant reduction in elastic fibers within the dermis on Verhoeff-Van Gieson staining. The loss of elastic tissue could be caused by either decreased production or increased destruction of elastic fibers [5, 6].

Anetoderma may occur as a primary idiopathic phenomenon or secondary to many autoimmune, infectious, inflammatory, tumor, or drug-induced diseases (Table 1) [5, 6]. Historically, primary anetoderma was subclassified into two types, the Jadassohn-Pellizzari type and the Schweninger-Buzzi type, depending, respectively, on the presence or absence of prior inflammation at the site of the lesion. However, this classification is of historical interest because histologic features and prognosis are the same in both conditions [5, 6]. Among the primary forms of anetoderma, familial forms have been described [2, 7].

Anetoderma has rarely been reported in newborns. Both congenital and acquired iatrogenic forms have been described in preterm infants. The congenital form has been reported in babies born between 24 and 25 weeks of gestation and its origin is still unclear, even if a congenital defect in the production of elastic fibers in the dermis has been hypothesized [5, 6]. The acquired iatrogenic form has been reported in infants born between 24 and 32 weeks of gestation, who spent a long time in neonatal intensive care unit (NICU). Its origin has been related to the placement of monitoring devices (transcutaneous oxygen monitoring, electrocardiographic electrodes, temperature probes, adhesives, etc.) on the patient

(a) Primary anetoderma (idiopathic)

Jadassohn-Pellizzari type (precedent clinical inflammation)

Schweninger-Buzzi type (no precedent clinical inflammation)

Familial

Congenital

(b) Secondary anetoderma (diseases associated with anetoderma)

(1) Autoimmune conditions	(i) Addison disease (ii) Antiphospholipid syndrome (iii) Discoid lupus (iv) Graves disease (v) Haemolytic anemia (vi) Sjögren syndrome (vii) Systemic lupus erythematosus (viii) Takayasu arteritis
(2) Infectious conditions	(i) Chicken pox (ii) HIV infection (iii) Leprosy (iv) Lyme disease (v) Molluscum contagiosum (vi) Syphilis (vii) Tuberculosis
(3) Inflammatory conditions	(i) Acne vulgaris (ii) Granuloma annulare (iii) Insect bites (iv) Mastocytosis (v) Prurigo nodularis
(4) Tumor/deposition conditions (benign and malignant)	(i) Cutaneous plasmacytoma (ii) Lymphocytoma cutis (iii) Melanocytic naevi (iv) Myxofibrosarcoma (v) Nodular amyloidosis (vi) Pilomatricomas (vii) Schwannomas (viii) Xanthomas
(5) Drug induced	(i) Penicillamine (ii) Hepatitis B vaccination
(6) Iatrogenic	Anetoderma of prematurity

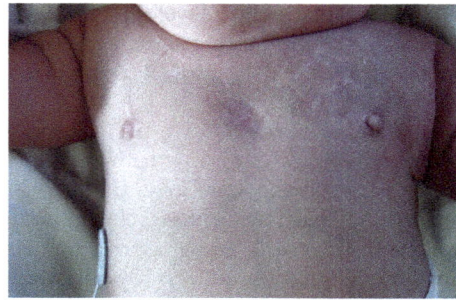

FIGURE 1: Ovalar, light-violaceous patches in the middle of upper chest. Translucent, coalescing, and bilateral lesions in subclavicular regions.

and the 10th centile for weight. Her Apgar score was 3 at 1 minute. She was intubated at 1 minute and transferred to the NICU, where she was treated for respiratory distress and a patent ductus arteriosus which failed to close with medical treatment and required a surgical intervention. She developed a severe bronchopulmonary dysplasia requiring prolonged noninvasive ventilatory support.

Numerous, localized, round-flat, and atrophic patches of skin on her upper chest were first noticed between the 4th and the 5th month of age while in NICU. All lesions were ventrally located and were between 5 and 15 mm in diameter. The largest lesions were localized in the middle of the chest and were ovalar, well-demarcated with a light-violaceous hue, without herniation (Figure 1). In the subclavicular areas, the lesions were less demarcated and more coalescing. Her skin was otherwise normal. None of the lesions was present at birth. Some bruise-like and ecchymotic lesions on the chest without necrosis or atrophy were described on medical records during the second week of extrauterine life. The location of the skin lesions corresponded to the sites of electrocardiographic electrodes placement.

The baby is now 7 months old and is still in NICU because of severe bronchopulmonary dysplasia, which is still requiring ventilatory support. Since their onset, the anetodermic lesions showed no changes and they are not yet evolved into the herniated anetoderma. Histological examination was not performed because of the very typical clinical presentation of the disease.

3. Discussion

Iatrogenic anetoderma of prematurity is clinically characterized by atrophic, round-flat or ovalar, skin-colored to violaceous, and brown or gray depressions or outpouchings of the skin, ranging from several millimeters to several centimeters in diameter. They are localized on the ventral surface of the chest, abdomen, upper arms, and proximal thighs, where monitoring leads or other medical devices are usually placed [3, 8–10]. Sometimes the atrophic lesions are preceded by erosive or ecchymotic patches, but in most cases previous skin lesions are absent or not diagnosed.

Iatrogenic anetoderma of prematurity was firstly described by Golden [9] in 1981. They reported on

skin [3, 8–10]. Although it is a benign lesion, it persists over time and can lead to disfigurement with need for surgical correction.

Here, we report on a premature infant born at 24 weeks of gestation, who developed multiple anetodermic patches of skin on the trunk at the sites where electrocardiographic electrodes were previously applied.

2. Case Report

Our patient was born at 24 weeks of gestation by caesarean section. She was the second-born infant in a monochorionic diamniotic twin pregnancy. The twins' mother was well throughout the pregnancy. No history of infections in pregnancy was reported. Her twin sister died at one week of age because of a severe intraventricular haemorrhage. Her birth weight was 470 g, placing her between the 3rd two premature infants, who developed anetoderma at transcutaneous oxygen monitoring sites. It was hypothesized that the intense heat under the probes could have caused a first-degree burn.

Subsequently, only 25 cases have been reported in the medical literature. Prizant et al. [3] reported on 9 cases of anetoderma in patients who were born between 24 and 29 weeks of gestation. The newborns developed anetodermic patches of skin on the trunk and the proximal extremities during their stay in NICU. The authors hypothesized that this acquired form of anetoderma could be due to the monitoring leads or adhesives tapes which were placed on the skin of the newborns.

Colditz et al. [8] described two infants born at 27 weeks of gestation who presented multiple lesions of anetoderma on the forehead at 3 months of age. The lesions appeared at the sides of gel electrocardiographic electrodes placement for electrical impedance tomography. Local hypoxemia due to pressure from the electrodes on immature skin was thought to be the cause of the disorder. The infants reported by Colditz were both growth-retarded (birth weight: 630 and 520 g). Reduced growth and thickness of the epidermis associated with intrauterine growth retardation may contribute to the formation of anetoderma.

This observation agrees with that of Todd [4] who reported an anetoderma associated with a monitoring lead in a severely growth-retarded twin (gestational age at birth: 32 weeks; birth weight: 794 g).

Ben-Amitai et al. [1] described two identical twins born at 26 weeks of gestation (birth weight: 1200 and 1050 g) who presented with a similar atrophic patch on the abdomen just lateral to the umbilicus at age 3 months. The authors suggested the possible role of genetic factors in the onset of the disease. However, since only two pairs of monozygotic twins concordant for anetoderma have been reported [1, 6], genetic factors probably are not pivotal.

The highest number of case series was reported by Goujon et al. [10] in 2010. Anetoderma was diagnosed clinically between the age of 6 weeks and 5 months in 11 preterm infants (gestational age at birth: 25–30 weeks; birth weight: 725–1250 g). Previous placement of monitoring leads was reported in most cases. Local hypoxemia due to pressure on immature skin or excessive traction on the skin when adhesive electrodes or tapes are removed was assumed to be the cause of the lesions. The thinness of the skin, the immaturity of its structure, an altered elastin metabolism, or an easier activation of elastolytic enzymes, such as metalloproteases, may give reason for the premature skin predisposition to anetoderma formation.

In our case, the correspondence between the site of involvement and placement of electrocardiographic leads was evident, since some lesions had the size and the shape of electrodes. Furthermore, the anetoderma was noticed when the patient was still in NICU and the electrocardiographic leads were still located on the lesional skin. No lesions were present at birth, so a congenital anetoderma was excluded. Our patient was growth-retarded and had an extremely low birth weight. Some authors believe that intrauterine and postnatal growth retardation may be more related to the onset

of anetoderma than a low gestational age [4, 8]. The skin lesions were extensive and should be monitored over time to assess the severity of the aesthetic damage.

We believe that neonatologists, pediatricians, and dermatologists should be aware of iatrogenic anetoderma of prematurity. Firstly, the disease, although benign, persists over time and can lead to a significant aesthetic damage with psychological disorders of the patient and need for surgical correction. Secondly, the frequency of the disease, probably underestimated, is likely to increase given the increased survival of extremely premature infants.

The knowledge of iatrogenic anetoderma of prematurity can help neonatologists to prevent it, paying particular attention to the use of medical devices such as electrodes, adhesive tapes, and other medical stuff in order not to stress such an immature and predisposed skin, and can help pediatricians and dermatologists in a correct diagnosis when lesions become evident after discharge. In this case, a prolonged hospitalization in NICU and a thorough history regarding the presence or absence of skin lesions at birth may facilitate the differential diagnosis with congenital anetoderma and other dermatoses present at birth, such as Goltz syndrome (focal dermal hypoplasia), aplasia cutis congenita, and congenital erosive and vesicular dermatosis. Technological improvement has significantly increased neonatal survival, but it should match a higher "refinement of care," that is, attention to detail, which can improve the quality of life.

Consent

Patient's parents gave their informed consent for the inclusion in the study. This paper is a case report containing no identifying patient information, and examinations and treatment of the patient fall in clinical practice. All procedures followed were in accordance with the Helsinki Declaration of 1975, as revised in 2008.

Conflict of Interests

The authors declare that there is no conflict of interests regarding the publication of this paper.

Authors' Contribution

Laura Maffeis, Lorenza Pugni, Carlo Pietrasanta, Andrea Ronchi, and Monica Fumagalli designed the study, reviewed the literature, and wrote the paper. Fabio Mosca revised the final draft. All authors contributed to the intellectual contents and approved the final version.

Acknowledgments

The authors would like to thank the patient and her family for their participation.

References

[1] D. Ben-Amitai, M. Feinmesser, E. Wielunsky, P. Merlob, and M. Lapidoth, "Simultaneous occurrence of anetoderma in premature identical twins," *Israel Medical Association Journal*, vol. 10, no. 6, pp. 431–432, 2008.

[2] A. Patrizi, I. Neri, A. Virdi, C. Misciali, and C. D'acunto, "Familial anetoderma: a report of two families," *European Journal of Dermatology*, vol. 21, no. 5, pp. 680–685, 2011.

[3] T. L. Prizant, A. W. Lucky, I. J. Frieden, P. S. Burton, and S. M. Suarez, "Spontaneous atrophic patches in extremely premature infants: anetoderma of prematurity," *Archives of Dermatology*, vol. 132, no. 6, pp. 671–674, 1996.

[4] D. J. Todd, "Anetoderma of prematurity," *Archives of Dermatology*, vol. 133, no. 6, p. 789, 1997.

[5] E. M. Wain, J. E. Mellerio, A. Robson, and D. J. Atherton, "Congenital anetoderma in a preterm infant," *Pediatric Dermatology*, vol. 25, no. 6, pp. 626–629, 2008.

[6] G. L. Zellman and M. L. Levy, "Congenital anetoderma in twins," *Journal of the American Academy of Dermatology*, vol. 36, no. 3, pp. 483–485, 1997.

[7] S. J. Friedman, P. Y. Venencie, R. R. Bradley, and R. K. Winkelman, "Familial anetoderma," *Journal of the American Academy of Dermatology*, vol. 16, no. 2, pp. 341–345, 1987.

[8] P. B. Colditz, K. R. Dunster, G. J. Joy, and I. M. Robertson, "Anetoderma of prematurity in association with electrocardiographic electrodes," *Journal of the American Academy of Dermatology*, vol. 41, no. 3, pp. 479–481, 1999.

[9] S. M. Golden, "Skin craters—a complication of transcutaneous oxygen monitoring," *Pediatrics*, vol. 67, no. 4, pp. 514–516, 1981.

[10] E. Goujon, F. Beer, S. Gay, D. Sandre, J.-B. Gouyon, and P. Vabres, "Anetoderma of prematurity: an iatrogenic consequence of neonatal intensive care," *Archives of Dermatology*, vol. 146, no. 5, pp. 565–567, 2010.

14

Ulcerated Radiodermatitis Induced after Fluoroscopically Guided Stent Implantation Angioplasty

Maira Elizabeth Herz-Ruelas,[1] **Minerva Gómez-Flores,**[1]
Joaquín Moxica-del Angel,[2] **Ivett Miranda-Maldonado,**[3] **Ilse Marilú Gutiérrez-Villarreal,**[4]
Guillermo Antonio Guerrero-González,[1] **and Adriana Orelia Villarreal-Rodríguez**[2]

[1] *Dermatology Department, Hospital Universitario "Dr. José Eleuterio González," Universidad Autónoma de Nuevo León,*
   Monterrey, Mexico
[2] *Christus Mugerza Sur Hospital, Monterrey, Mexico*
[3] *Pathology Department, Hospital Universitario "Dr. José Eleuterio González," Universidad Autónoma de Nuevo León,*
   Monterrey, Mexico
[4] *School of Medicine, Universidad Autónoma de Nuevo León, Monterrey, Mexico*

Correspondence should be addressed to Maira Elizabeth Herz-Ruelas; mairaherz@yahoo.com

Academic Editor: Julia Y. Lee

Cases of radiation-induced skin injury after fluoroscopically guided procedures have been reported since 1996, though the majority of them have been published in Radiology and Cardiology literature, less frequently in Dermatology journals. Chronic radiation dermatitis induced by fluoroscopy can be difficult to diagnose; a high grade of suspicion is required. We report a case of an obese 46-year-old man with hypertension, dyslipidemia, and severe coronary artery disease. He developed a pruritic and painful atrophic ulcerated skin plaque over his left scapula, six months after fluoroscopically guided stent implantation angioplasty. The diagnosis of radiodermatitis was confirmed histologically. We report this case to emphasize the importance of recognizing fluoroscopy as a cause of radiation dermatitis. A good clinical follow-up at regular intervals is important after long and complicated procedures, since the most prevalent factor for injury is long exposure time.

1. Introduction

Cases of radiation-induced skin injury after fluoroscopically guided procedures have been reported since 1996; however, diagnosis and treatment of such lesions remain difficult [1]. Fluoroscopy-induced chronic radiation dermatitis often requires a high clinical suspicion to establish a correct diagnosis [2]. Ionizing radiation during interventional procedures is often underestimated. The risk of developing this reaction is directly related to the radiation dose, which depends on the type of procedure, technique, time of exposure, and the patient's body constitution [3]. The period between radiation exposure and manifestation of skin injuries varies, from 15 days up to months or years.

The incidence of radiodermatitis after percutaneous coronary interventions by X-ray fluoroscopic procedures is rising; case reports have been increasingly documented. The skin lesions encompass a wide spectrum, such as erythema, telangiectasias, atrophy, hyperpigmentation and hypopigmentation, necrosis, chronic ulceration, and squamous cell carcinoma [4].

Chronic radiation dermatitis induced by fluoroscopy can be difficult to diagnose. There are some histopathology features such as ulceration, prominent telangiectasia, and atypical stellate fibroblasts. Absence of lymphocytic infiltrate, inflammation, and presence of hyperkeratosis are helpful diagnosing this entity from others such as morphea and lichen sclerosus [5].

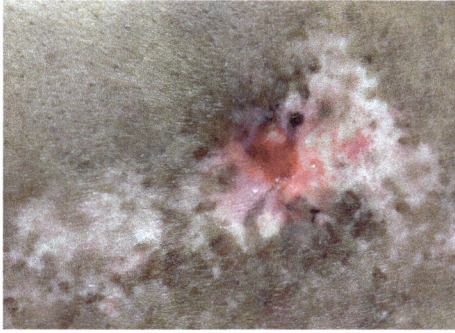

FIGURE 1: Ulcered, atrophic plaque with hypopigmentation and hyperpigmentation, as well as superficial telangiectasia.

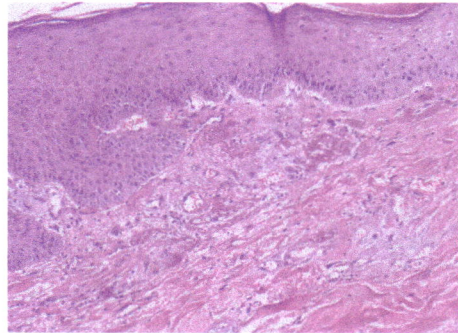

FIGURE 3: Hematoxylin and eosin, 10X. Epidermis with acanthosis and superficial prominent telangiectasia, with fibrin and fibrosis.

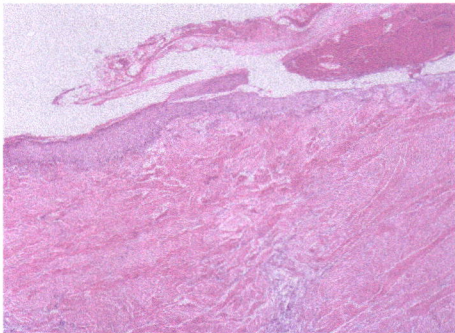

FIGURE 2: Hematoxylin and eosin. 5X. Atrophic epidermis with necrosis and central ulceration. Dermal sclerosis, loss of dermal appendages.

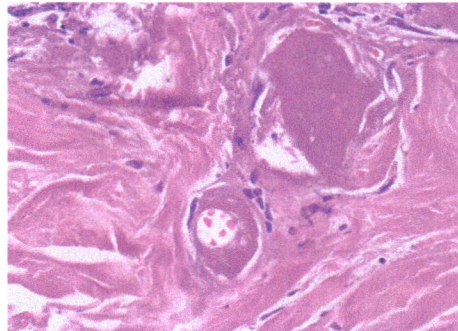

FIGURE 4: Hematoxylin and eosin. 40X. Superficial dermal telangiectasia with fibrin thrombi and fibrosis.

2. Case Presentation

An obese 46-year-old man with hypertension, dyslipidemia, and severe coronary artery disease referred a history of fluoroscopically guided stent implantation angioplasty six months before his Dermatology consultation. His medications included nebivolol, cilostazol, clopidogrel, and rosuvastatin. He referred an erythematous patch over his left scapula when discharged from the hospital.

The lesion evolved in 3 months into an atrophic plaque that was pruritic, tender, and painful. Over the following 3 months, the lesion became indurated, ulcerated, developing hypopigmentation and hyperpigmentation, as well as superficial telangiectasia. The lesion was well demarcated, 8 × 5 cms (Figure 1). A skin biopsy specimen demonstrated changes consistent with chronic radiation dermatitis (Figures 2, 3, and 4). The histological findings, along with the location over the left scapula and the history of fluoroscopic exposure during cardiac catheterization, led to the clinical diagnosis of fluoroscopy-induced chronic radiation dermatitis.

The ulcer was treated with bismuth subgallate powder, applied every four days and left under occlusion. The ulcer resolved after thirty days of treatment. A hydrophilic ointment was indicated on the rest of the plaque.

3. Discussion

This case emphasizes the importance of fluoroscopic procedures as a cause of radiation dermatitis. The diagnosis of fluoroscopy-induced chronic radiation dermatitis should be considered in patients with a recent vascular lesion or morphea-like lesion, or an unexplained ulcer localized over previously radiated sites [6].

Follow-up is important after procedures that include radiation exposure [4]. Radiodermatitis has been described during many other vascular procedures like radiofrequency catheter ablation, renal angioplasty, interventional neuroradiology, implantation of cardiac resynchronization devices, and implantable cardioverter defibrillator pacemaker systems.

Radiation dermatitis' treatment outcome is limited. Simple skin grafting often fails because of poor vascularity.

With the increase of minimally invasive procedures involving fluoroscopy, radiation dermatitis is becoming more prevalent. Though rare, radiation dermatitis must always be considered as a complication of fluoroscopic procedures. Physicians involved in this type of interventions should be aware of side effects and implement measures to minimize exposure time in order to prevent development of radiation skin injuries [7].

Conflict of Interests

The authors declare that there is no conflict of interests regarding the publication of this paper.

References

[1] I. Hashimoto, H. Sedo, K. Inatsugi, H. Nakanishi, and S. Arase, "Severe radiation-induced injury after cardiac catheter ablation: a case requiring free anterolateral thigh flap and vastus lateralis muscle flap reconstruction on the upper arm," *Journal of Plastic, Reconstructive and Aesthetic Surgery*, vol. 61, no. 6, pp. 704–708, 2008.

[2] A. Jeskowiak, M. Hubmer, G. Prenner, and H. Maechler, "Radiation induced cutaneous ulcer on the back in a patient with congenital anomaly of the upper cava system," *Interactive Cardiovascular and Thoracic Surgery*, vol. 12, no. 2, pp. 290–292, 2011.

[3] A. K. Schecter, M. D. Lewis, L. Robinson-Bostom, and T. D. Pan, "Cardiac catheterization-induced acute radiation dermatitis presenting as a fixed drug eruption," *Journal of Drugs in Dermatology*, vol. 2, no. 4, pp. 425–427, 2003.

[4] A. Aerts, T. Decraene, J. J. van den Oord et al., "Chronic radiodermatitis following percutaneous coronary interventions: a report of two cases," *Journal of the European Academy of Dermatology and Venereology*, vol. 17, no. 3, pp. 340–343, 2003.

[5] J. Boncher and W. F. Bergfeld, "Fluoroscopy-induced chronic radiation dermatitis: a report of two additional cases and a brief review of the literature," *Journal of Cutaneous Pathology*, vol. 39, no. 1, pp. 63–67, 2012.

[6] T. H. Frazier, J. B. Richardson, V. C. Fabré, and J. P. Callen, "Fluoroscopy-induced chronic radiation skin injury: a disease perhaps often overlooked," *Archives of Dermatology*, vol. 143, no. 5, pp. 637–640, 2007.

[7] M. Dandurand, P. Huet, and B. Guillot, "Secondary radiodermatitis caused by endovascular explorations: 5 cases," *Annales de Dermatologie et de Vénéréologie*, vol. 126, no. 5, pp. 413–417, 1999.

15

Relapsing Polychondritis

Beata Sosada, Katarzyna Loza, and Ewelina Bialo-Wojcicka

Department of Dermatology, Miedzyleski Specialist Hospital in Warsaw, ul. Bursztynowa 2, 04-479 Warsaw, Poland

Correspondence should be addressed to Beata Sosada; beatasosada@wp.pl

Academic Editor: Alexander A. Navarini

Relapsing polychondritis (RP) is a rare systemic disease characterized by recurrent, widespread chondritis of the auricular, nasal, and tracheal cartilages. Additional clinical features include audiovestibular dysfunction, ocular inflammation, vasculitis, myocarditis, and nonerosive arthritis. Although the cause remains unknown, the etiology is suspected to be autoimmune. We describe a case of a 31-year-old woman with a four-month history of bilateral auricular and nasal chondritis. Infectious and neoplastic diseases were excluded by imaging and laboratory examinations. RP was diagnosed based on three McAdam's criteria. The patient was medicated with oral prednisolone and methotrexate with positive clinical response. In this case clinical history and detailed physical examination were fundamental in concluding the correct diagnosis and administrating the appropriate medication.

1. Introduction

Relapsing polychondritis (RP) is a rare inflammatory disease primarily affecting the cartilaginous structures of the ear, nose, joints, tracheobronchial tree, and cardiovascular system. Cardiovascular and respiratory complications of RP are associated with high morbidity and mortality. The first case of RP was described in 1923 by Jaksch-Wartenhorst [1]. The term "relapsing polychondritis" was first used by Pearson et al. in 1960 in their review of 12 cases [2]. RP was usually observed in the fourth and fifth decade of life with no sex predilection [3–5].

The McAdam's criteria were the initial diagnostic criteria of RP [3] and required meeting three out of six of the following: bilateral auricular chondritis, nonerosive seronegative inflammatory arthritis, nasal chondritis, ocular inflammation, respiratory tract chondritis, and audiovestibular damage. Modified criteria have been proposed by Damiani and Levine [4] which include meeting one McAdam's criterion plus histopathological confirmation or two McAdam's criteria plus response to corticosteroids or dapsone. Currently, the diagnosis of RP relies mostly on the criteria established by Michet et al. [5] which require the presence of a proven inflammation in at least two of three of the auricular, nasal, or laryngotracheal cartilages or the proven inflammation in one of these cartilages plus two other signs, including ocular inflammation, vestibular dysfunction, seronegative inflammatory arthritis, or hearing loss (Table 1).

The exact cause of RP is still unknown but the disease is mostly seen as an immune-mediated disease, as there is a well-documented overlap of RP with other rheumatic and autoimmune diseases [3, 6]. Although a large number of cases have been reported recently and the knowledge on the clinical spectrum, pathogenesis, and management in RP has grown considerably, only limited microscopic data is available in the literature [4, 7]. The histologic features of the chondritis include loss of basophilic staining of the cartilage matrix followed by cartilage destruction with replacement by fibrous tissue and cellular infiltration with plasma cells and lymphocytes. A rare disease RP is described occurring extremely rarely in young women.

2. Case Report

A 31-year-old Caucasian woman was consulted in our department for recurrent swellings of both pinnae which had been present for approximately 4 months. About two weeks before coming to hospital she suffered from pain and tenderness of both auricles, the nose as well as the left elbow. Her personal and family history was unremarkable. She was a smoker (10 pack-years). During physical examination both

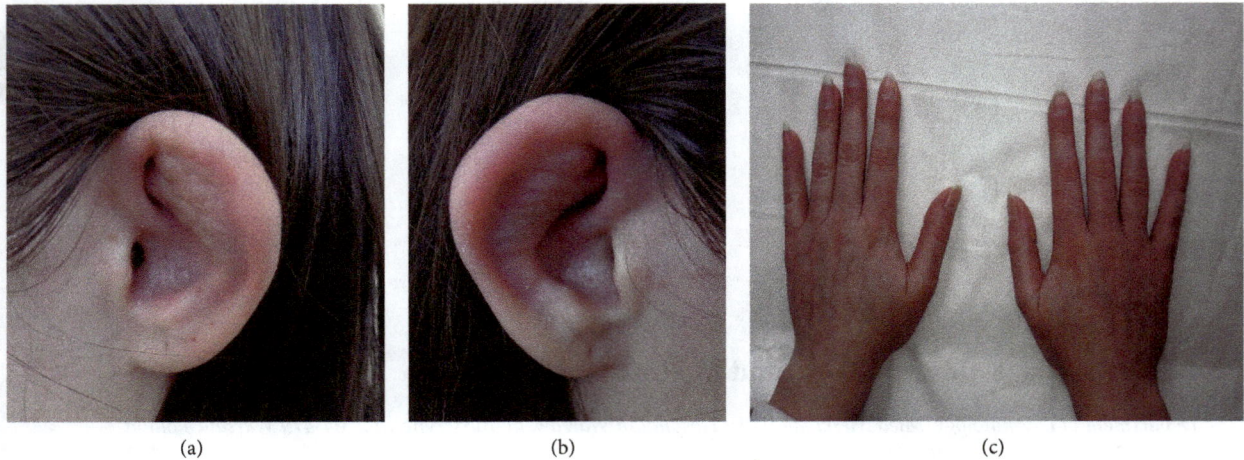

(a) (b) (c)

FIGURE 1: (a, b) Cauliflower ears. Swelling and erythema of the cartilaginous part of the ear, sparing the lobule which lacks cartilage. (c) The Raynaud's phenomenon.

TABLE 1: Diagnostic criteria for RP.

McAdam et al. [3]	(1) Recurrent chondritis of both auricles (2) Nonerosive inflammatory polyarthritis (3) Chondritis of nasal cartilages (4) Inflammation of ocular structures (5) Chondritis of respiratory tract (6) Cochlear and/or vestibular damage (requirement—three out of six criteria)
Damiani and Levine [4]	(1) Three out of six McAdam et al.'s [3] criteria (2) One out of six McAdam et al.'s [3] criteria and a positive histologic confirmation (3) Two out of six McAdam et al.'s criteria and response to corticosteroid or dapsone (requirement—any of these)
Michet et al. [5]	(1) Proven inflammation in two out of three cartilages: auricular, nasal, and laryngotracheal (2) Proven inflammation in one of the above and meeting two other signs from ocular inflammation, hearing loss, vestibular dysfunction, or seronegative inflammatory arthritis (requirement—any of these)

pinnae lost their firmness, became soft and floppy, and had a cauliflower-like appearance (Figures 1(a) and 1(b)). In addition Raynaud's phenomenon was found (Figure 1(c)) and evidenced by nailfold capillaroscopy.

Routine blood investigations revealed normocytic normochromic anemia, elevated erythrocyte sedimentation rate. The rheumatoid factor was within normal limits. Other clinical parameters (urinalysis, thyroid tests, and liver function tests) resulted within normal range. Antinuclear antibodies (ANA) titer was 1 : 320. Antiphospholipid antibodies, antineutrophil cytoplasmic antibodies (ANCAs), anti-Borrelia burgdorferi antibodies IgG/IgM, rheumatoid factor, anti-HIV-1, anti-HIV-2, and VDRL tests were negative. Two biopsy specimens were taken, one from the skin and another from the cartilage of the pinna for histopathological study. Histologic pictures show cellular infiltrates by lymphocytes, neutrophils, and plasma cells, most evident in the cartilage-skin interface, as well as the reduced number of chondrocytes seen in areas of cartilage destruction (Figures 2(a), 2(b), and 2(c)).

The skin tissue was also processed for direct immunofluorescence (DIF) studies where isolated IgG staining at the BMZ was observed. Spirometry, computer tomography, and radiography of the chest did not reveal any laryngotracheobronchial symptoms. No ocular disorders in ophthalmologic consultations were found. Doppler echocardiography and electrocardiography did not reveal any abnormalities. The patient started on prednisolone 30 mg daily with improvement in symptoms. Approximately 8 weeks following discharge, while tapering prednisolone to 15 mg daily, she had recurrence of nasal pain and auricular swelling. Prednisolone dose was increased to 30 mg daily and a combination therapy with methotrexate 15 mg weekly was recommended. After 6 months, corticosteroids were reduced to 5 mg daily and methotrexate was increased to 17,5 mg weekly. The patient is still on followup with no progression during this period. Moreover, ANA titer decreased to 1 : 160.

3. Discussion

RP is an autoimmune disease in which target antigens are still unknown. Both circulating antibodies and immune complex deposits in the affected cartilaginous tissue could be present. Studies [8, 9] have shown that 33% of patients with RP had circulating antibodies of type II collagen in

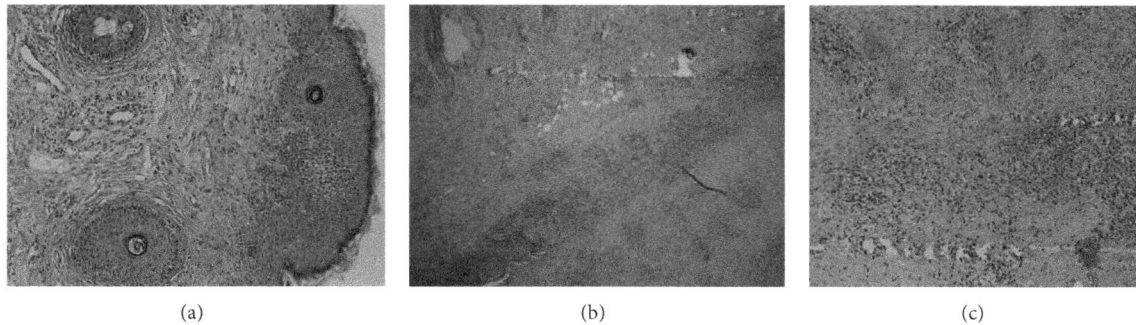

(a)   (b)   (c)

FIGURE 2: (a) The dermis contains a mild focal lymphohistiocytic infiltrate. H&E, ×100. (b) Degenerative and inflammatory changes affecting the marginal chondrocytes with loss of basophilia and poor alcian blue staining of the cartilaginous tissue. H&E, ×40. (c) The inflammatory cells infiltrate, including lymphocytes, plasma cells, and histiocytes, infiltrate the degenerative cartilage. H&E, ×100.

the active phase of the disease and their titres also corresponded to the disease activity. Autoimmunity to collagen type II has also been described in systemic lupus erythematosus (SLE) and rheumatoid arthritis. Other studies [10, 11] showed that the antibodies are generated against not only native and denatured collagen type II but also collagen types IX and XI, which form the major extracellular scaffold in the cartilage. Matrilin-1 is a cartilage-specific protein and is highly expressed in tracheal and nasal but not in normal adult articular cartilage [12]. Saxne and Heinegard in their studies [12, 13] revealed that an increased serum level of matrilin-1 could be found in patients with RP in the active phase, suggesting that the release of matrilin-1 resulted from the destruction of the involved cartilage. However, neither anti-collagen type II nor anti-matrilin-1 antibodies are sensitive and specific enough and consequently cannot be used for diagnostic purposes. The diagnosis of RP is largely based on the clinical features and the role of laboratory and imaging investigations is purely supportive to rule out other related or associated systemic diseases. Clinical, histopathological, and DIF features together or in combination are helpful in the final diagnosis. The treatment of RP is symptomatic and should be tailored to each individual patient based on disease activity and severity.

Glucocorticoid therapy is fundamental in the treatment of RP and is used chronically in most patients. Less severe symptoms are generally treated with nonsteroid anti-inflammatory drugs. Dapsone may also be used as an initial therapy but results in many adverse reactions. Severe symptoms of disease, including ocular or laryngotracheal involvement, systemic vasculitis, and severe polychondritis require systemic corticosteroids. In patients intolerant to, rarely unresponsive to, steroid therapy or in whom a steroid sparing therapy is required, immunosuppressants play a role. Immunosuppressive agents like methotrexate, azathioprine, and cyclosporine may be given to patients with severe respiratory or vascular involvement and to those with steroid-resistant or steroid-dependent disease. Trentham and Le [14] observed that methotrexate in dose of 17,5 mg/week was the most effective nonsteroid drug in causing symptomatic benefit and reducing the steroid requirement. Intravenous cyclophosphamide and plasmapheresis could be used in patients with organ-threatening and life-threatening diseases, including glomerulonephritis or acute airways obstruction. The autoimmune theory of pathogenesis of RP makes immunomodulatory agents (biologics) an important treatment alternative to other medical therapies. However, data from clinical trials is scarce; there are many case reports of satisfactory response to biologic therapy in RP. Standard management cannot be established due to its rarity.

Conflict of Interests

The authors declare that there is no conflict of interests regarding the publication.

Acknowledgment

The authors would like to thank Dr. Kazimierz Kalbarczyk, who unfortunately passed away this year. He was a great dermatopathologist in Department of Dermatology at the Miedzyleski Specialist Hospital in Warsaw and gave opportunity to all young dermatologists to discover the fascinating world of dermatopathology.

References

[1] R. Jaksch-Wartenhorst, "Polychondropathia," *Wiener Archiv für Innere Medizin*, vol. 6, pp. 93–100, 1923.

[2] C. M. Pearson, H. M. Kline, and V. D. Newcomer, "Relapsing polychondritis," *The New England Journal of Medicine*, vol. 263, pp. 51–58, 1960.

[3] L. P. McAdam, M. A. O'Hanlan, and R. C. M. Pearson, "Relapsing polychondritis: prospective study of 23 patients and a review of the literature," *Medicine*, vol. 55, no. 3, pp. 193–215, 1976.

[4] J. M. Damiani and H. L. Levine, "Relapsing polychondritis. Report of ten cases," *The Laryngoscope*, vol. 89, no. 6, pp. 929–946, 1979.

[5] C. J. Michet Jr., C. H. McKenna, H. S. Luthra, and W. M. O'Fallon, "Relapsing polychondritis: survival and predictive role of early disease manifestations," *Annals of Internal Medicine*, vol. 104, no. 1, pp. 74–78, 1986.

[6] J.-C. Piette, R. El-Rassi, and Z. Amoura, "Antinuclear antibodies in relapsing polychondritis," *Annals of the Rheumatic Diseases*, vol. 58, no. 10, pp. 656–657, 1999.

[7] S. Frisenda, C. Perricone, and G. Valesini, "Cartilage as a target of autoimmunity: a thin layer," *Autoimmunity Reviews*, vol. 12, no. 5, pp. 591–598, 2013.

[8] J. M. Foidart, S. Abe, G. R. Martin et al., "Antibodies to type II collagen in relapsing polychondritis," *The New England Journal of Medicine*, vol. 299, no. 22, pp. 1203–1207, 1978.

[9] L. Giroux, F. Paquin, M. J. Guerard Desjardins, and A. Lefaivre, "Relapsing polychondritis: an autoimmune disease," *Seminars in Arthritis and Rheumatism*, vol. 13, no. 2, pp. 182–187, 1983.

[10] C. L. Yang, J. Brinckmann, H. F. Rui et al., "Autoantibodies to cartilage collagens in relapsing polychondritis," *Archives of Dermatological Research*, vol. 285, no. 5, pp. 245–249, 1993.

[11] S. Alsalameh, J. Mollenhauer, F. Scheuplein et al., "Preferential cellular and humoral immune reactivities to native and denatured collagen types IX and XI in a patient with fatal relapsing polychondritis," *Journal of Rheumatology*, vol. 20, no. 8, pp. 1419–1424, 1993.

[12] T. Saxne and D. Heinegard, "Involvement of nonarticular cartilage, as demonstrated by release of a cartilage-specific protein, in rheumatoid arthritis," *Arthritis and Rheumatism*, vol. 32, no. 9, pp. 1080–1086, 1989.

[13] T. Saxne and D. Heinegard, "Serum concentrations of two cartilage matrix proteins reflecting different aspects of cartilage turnover in relapsing polychondritis," *Arthritis and Rheumatism*, vol. 38, no. 2, pp. 294–296, 1995.

[14] D. E. Trentham and C. H. Le, "Relapsing polychondritis," *Annals of Internal Medicine*, vol. 129, no. 2, pp. 114–122, 1998.

16

A Life Threatening Rash, an Unexpected Cause

Dhiraj Jain,[1] Stalin Viswanathan,[1] and Chandramohan Ramasamy[2]

[1] Department of General Medicine, Indira Gandhi Medical College & RI, Pondicherry 605009, India
[2] Department of Cardiology, Jawaharlal Institute of Postgraduate Medical Education and Research, Pondicherry 605006, India

Correspondence should be addressed to Stalin Viswanathan; stalinviswanathan@ymail.com

Academic Editor: Thomas Berger

We describe a 74-year-old man with purpura fulminans and altered sensorium following an acute febrile illness. Intensive sepsis management was to no avail, until institution of doxycycline therapy following confirmation of scrub typhus. Empirical doxycycline needs to be considered in endemic areas for patients presenting with purpura fulminans.

1. Introduction

Skin manifestations of rickettsial infections include eschars (single or multiple due to *Orientia tsutsugamushi* and *Rickettsia africae*, resp.) and eruptions which may be either macular, maculopapular, vesicular, or purpuric [1]. Scrub typhus is a ubiquitous infection in the tropics but is usually not considered in the differential diagnosis of life-threatening dermatoses. Rickettsial infections have been, on occasions, reported to cause purpura fulminans. Herein we describe an elderly man with scrub typhus-related purpura fulminans who was cured of his illness, following administration of doxycycline.

2. Case

This 74-year-old man presented with continuous fever of five days' duration. Headache, myalgia, and productive cough were also present. There was altered sensorium in the form of decreased speech and irritable behavior one day prior to admission, without vomiting, seizures, or limb weakness. There were no cardiorespiratory, gastrointestinal, or renal complaints. The patient did not have history of diabetes, hypertension, or addiction to either alcohol or tobacco.

On examination, the patient was irritable and disoriented, with a temperature of 38.8°C, pulse of 104 beats/minute, blood pressure of 90/60 mm Hg, and respiratory rate of 24/min. He had pedal edema and an otherwise normal systemic examination. Pending results, ceftriaxone and amikacin were administered for probable sepsis. His investigations were as follows: hemoglobin 12 g%, total leukocyte count 21×10^9/L, associated with left shift and toxic granulations, platelet count 18×10^9/L, blood urea 160 mg/dL, serum creatinine 2.6 mg/dL, INR 1.6, aPTT prolongation 10 seconds, D-dimer 400 ng/mL, total/direct bilirubin 3/2.8 mg/dL, and SGOT/SGPT 73/64 U/L. His blood and urine cultures were noncontributory. Lumbar puncture was deferred in view of severe thrombocytopenia. Computed tomography of head was normal. Following investigations, he was switched to renal-modified doses of ceftazidime. On the second day, he developed a symmetrical purpuric rash involving the palms, soles, arms, and legs which later became bullous, confluent, black, and necrotic over the next 48 hours (Figures 1(a) and 1(b)). Peripheral smear on 3rd day showed features of microangiopathic hemolytic anemia. Serological testing for hepatitis B, hepatitis C, HIV, leptospirosis, scrub typhus, and systemic lupus was ordered. Echocardiography and ultrasonography were noncontributory. Meropenem was substituted for ceftazidime on day 3. On the fourth day, scrub IgM (PanBio, Brisbane, Australia; Scrub Typhus IgM and IgG Rapid Immunochromatographic test) returned positive. Doxycycline was initiated, with which his fever, altered sensorium, and hepatorenal dysfunction improved. His skin lesions resolved without sequelae and he was discharged from hospital on the 7th day of admission.

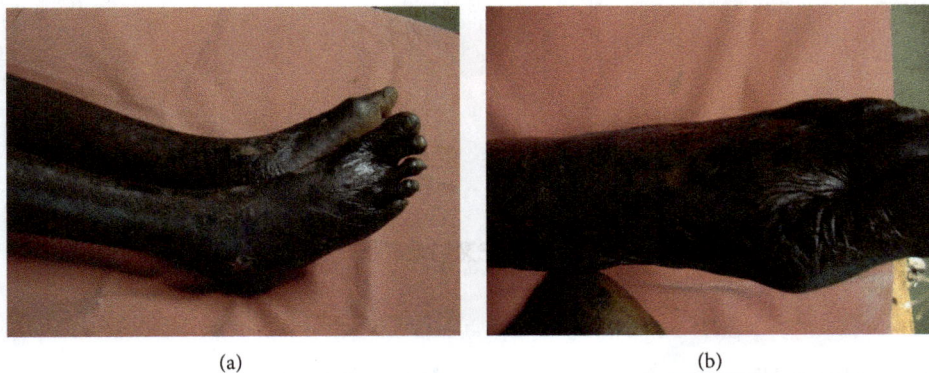

(a)   (b)

FIGURE 1: (a) Blotchy purpuric rash over both lower limbs mainly in the extremities, with some healed areas 48 hours after doxycycline therapy. (b) Closer view of left foot showing involvement of all toes and dorsum of foot, with some healed lesions showing hypopigmentation.

3. Discussion

Purpura fulminans (PF) is a triad of skin ecchymoses, infarction/necrosis, and hemorrhagic bullae which occurs due to both infectious and noninfectious causes [2]. According to one large case series, skin discoloration, disseminated intravascular coagulation, and septic shock were the commonest features of PF [3]. Gangrene occurs distally and is usually symmetrical. This condition is more common in pediatric age groups [4]. Abnormalities can ensue in either the fibrinolytic or coagulation system [4]. Infectious causes of PF include meningococcal (classical) and pneumococcal sepsis and infections due to varicella, influenza, and *Candida albicans* [4]. Congenital and acquired protein C/S deficiencies, antiphospholipid syndrome, paroxysmal nocturnal hemoglobinuria [5], vasculitides, animal/insect toxins, and drugs such as phenytoin, ketorolac, quinidine, and diclofenac contribute to noninfectious PF [2, 4]. Leptospirosis [6], malaria [7], and dengue [8] are some tropical infections reported to have caused PF. Among the rickettsiae, *R. conorii*, *R. rickettsii*, and *R. australis* have produced fatal PF [9, 10]. Antibodies to *R. conorii* were not tested due to its unavailability in our hospital. Indian tick typhus has been described as an etiological factor for PF from various parts of India [11–13]. But scrub typhus has not been previously reported to cause PF. Infectious PF usually develops 1–3 weeks after the infective episode [4].

Management of PF requires a multidepartment effort that involves physicians/pediatricians, surgeons, radiologists, nurses, and physiotherapists. Interventions such as debridement, fasciotomy, amputations, and thrombolysis may be sometimes necessary [3, 14]. For compartment syndromes arising due to PF, relief should be provided within six hours. Medical therapy comprises antibiotics, steroids, and protein C infusion [15] along with routine sepsis care. Our patient did not require any surgical intervention and improved with doxycycline alone.

In conclusion, PF is a potentially fatal dermatological emergency that requires intensive and multidisciplinary care. Purpura fulminans may be treated more appropriately by familiarizing oneself with prevalence of illnesses in the locality, which could reduce morbidity, mortality, and

hospitalization stay. Although scrub typhus has been widely reported from many states in India, the exact prevalence is not known. Though Indian tick typhus much more commonly causes rickettsia-related purpuric eruptions, scrub typhus, by virtue of its prevalence in the tsutsugamushi triangle, should not be forgotten in the Indian subcontinent.

Conflict of Interests

The authors declare that there is no conflict of interests regarding the publication of this paper.

References

[1] P. Parola and D. Raoult, "Tropical rickettsioses," *Clinics in Dermatology*, vol. 24, no. 3, pp. 191–200, 2006.

[2] N. Kosaraju, V. Korrapati, A. Thomas, and B. R. James, "Adult purpura fulminans associated with non-steroidal antiinflammatory drug use," *Journal of Postgraduate Medicine*, vol. 57, no. 2, pp. 145–146, 2011.

[3] B. J. Childers and B. Cobanov, "Acute infectious purpura fulminans: a 15-year retrospective review of 28 consecutive cases," *The American Surgeon*, vol. 69, no. 1, pp. 86–90, 2003.

[4] S. N. Faust and S. Nadel, "Purpura fulminans," in *Life-Threatening Dermatoses and Emergencies in Dermatology*, J. Revuz, J.-C. Roujeau, F. Kerdel, and L. Valeyrie-Allanore, Eds., pp. 45–55, Springer, Berlin, Germany, 2009.

[5] C. May, K. O'Rourke, K. Jackson, L. Francis, and G. A. Kennedy, "Purpura fulminans in a patient with paroxysmal nocturnal haemoglobinuria," *Internal Medicine Journal*, vol. 43, no. 1, p. 102, 2013.

[6] A. Talwar, S. Kumar, M. Gopal, and A. Nandini, "Spectrum of purpura fulminans: report of three classical prototypes and review of management strategies," *Indian Journal of Dermatology, Venereology and Leprology*, vol. 78, no. 2, p. 228, 2012.

[7] P. Corne, F. Bruneel, C. Biron-Andreani, and O. Jonquet, "Purpura fulminans due to imported falciparum malaria," *Intensive Care Medicine*, vol. 34, no. 11, pp. 2123–2124, 2008.

[8] D. H. Karunatilaka, J. R. de Silva, P. K. Ranatunga, T. M. Gunasekara, M. A. Faizal, and G. N. Malavige, "Idiopathic purpura fulminans in dengue hemorrhagic fever," *Indian Journal of Medical Sciences*, vol. 61, no. 8, pp. 471–473, 2007.

[9] M. Weinberger, A. Keysary, J. Sandbank et al., "Fatal Rickettsia conorii subsp. israelensis infection, Israel," *Emerging Infectious Diseases*, vol. 14, no. 5, pp. 821–824, 2008.

[10] W. J. McBride, J. P. Hanson, R. Miller, and D. Wenck, "Severe spotted fever group rickettsiosis, Australia," *Emerging Infectious Diseases*, vol. 13, no. 11, pp. 1742–1744, 2007.

[11] S. Tirumala, B. Behera, S. Jawalkar et al., "Indian tick typhus presenting as purpura fulminans," *Indian Journal of Critical Care Medicine*, vol. 18, pp. 476–478, 2014.

[12] E. Jayseelan, S. C. Rajendran, S. Shariff, D. Fishbein, and J. S. Keystone, "Cutaneous eruptions in Indian tick typhus," *International Journal of Dermatology*, vol. 30, no. 11, pp. 790–794, 1991.

[13] A. Kundavaram, N. R. Francis, A. P. J. Jude, G. M. Varghese, and K. P. P. Abhilash, "Acute infectious purpura fulminans due to probable spotted fever," *Journal of Postgraduate Medicine*, vol. 60, no. 2, pp. 198–199, 2014.

[14] R. G. Jones, G. P. Gardner, and M. E. Morris, "Catheter-directed thrombolysis in a patient with purpura fulminans," *American Surgeon*, vol. 78, no. 11, pp. E448–E449, 2012.

[15] P. Schellongowski, T. Staudinger, W. R. Sperr, and C. Scheibenpflug, "Treatment of infection-associated purpura fulminans with protein C zymogen is associated with a high survival rate," *Blood*, vol. 122, article 3606, 2013.

17

Paget Disease of the Vulva: Diagnosis by Immunohistochemistry

Andressa Gonçalves Amorim,[1] **Brunelle Batista Fraga Mendes,**[1]
Rodrigo Neves Ferreira,[2] **and Antônio Chambô Filho**[1]

[1]*Department of Obstetrics and Gynecology, Santa Casa de Misericórdia Hospital, 29025-023 Vitória, ES, Brazil*
[2]*Pathology Department, Santa Casa de Misericórdia Hospital, Dr. João dos Santos Neves Street 143, 29025-023 Vitória, ES, Brazil*

Correspondence should be addressed to Andressa Gonçalves Amorim; andressaamorim88@hotmail.com

Academic Editor: Jaime A. Tschen

The objective of this paper is to report a case of extramammary Paget disease of the vulva, to describe its diagnosis, surgical treatment, and outcome, and to discuss the general characteristics of this pathology. This is a rare neoplasm, found principally in areas in which apocrine and eccrine glands are numerous. This case report is relevant to the literature since the differential diagnosis of extramammary Paget disease is difficult to be done only with the macroscopic appearance of the lesion and even with the microscopic characteristics, requiring further studies, immunohistochemistry, as to differentiate pathologies. The present report describes the case of a 63-year-old patient at the Santa Casa de Misericórdia Hospital in Vitória, Espírito Santo, Brazil, who presented with a hardened, ulcerated, and purplish lesion with hyperchromic and hypochromic spots, measuring 4 cm in diameter, located on the lower third of right labium majus, close to the vaginal fourchette. A right hemivulvectomy was performed, leaving wide margins all around. The patient progressed satisfactorily following surgery. Although extramammary Paget disease is rare, its incidence increases as a function of the patient's age. Patients should be followed up closely because of the risk of persistence and/or recurrence of the disease.

1. Introduction

James Paget was the first to describe Paget disease (PD) in 1874, while extramammary Paget disease (EMPD) was first described by Crocker in 1888 [1]. The condition consists of an intraepithelial adenocarcinoma.

In general, EMPD lesions are found in areas such as the vulva, anus, perianal region, and axillae in which the density of apocrine glands is high. In women, the most common site of EMPD is the vulva; however, EMPD is responsible for less than 1% of all vulvar neoplasms [2]. Diagnosis of EMPD usually occurs between 50 and 80 years of age, with the disease being more common in Caucasian women [3]. The most common clinical symptom is pruritus. The lesion may be erythematous or eczematous, with islands of hyperkeratosis [4].

Surgical resection with wide margins is considered the standard treatment; however, successful surgical excision of the disease is a challenge and recurrences are common. Alternative treatments such as photodynamic therapy, laser therapy, radiotherapy, topical treatments such as 5% imiquimod cream, or even chemotherapy have been the subjects of debate and it is important to evaluate the available evidence [5].

The present paper reports a case with histopathological findings of extramammary Paget disease in a patient receiving care at the Department of Obstetrics and Gynecology, Santa Casa de Misericórdia Hospital, Vitória, Espírito Santo, Brazil. Prior to publication, the paper was submitted to and approved by the internal review board, reference number 35177714.70000.5065. The patient gave her written consent for the publication of this report and the accompanying images.

2. Case Presentation

The patient in question is a 63-year-old, married, black female patient, who became menopausal at 48 years of age. She had controlled hypertension, was not in use of hormone therapy, had no family history of gynecological cancer, and reported being a nonsmoker. She was seen at the Gynecology

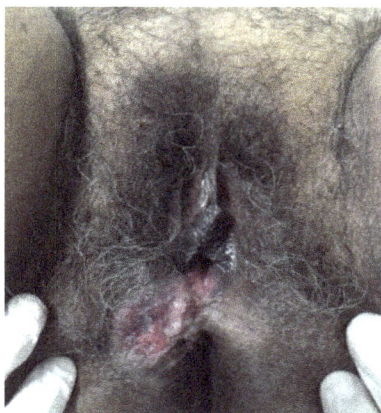

FIGURE 1: Photograph of the lesion prior to surgery.

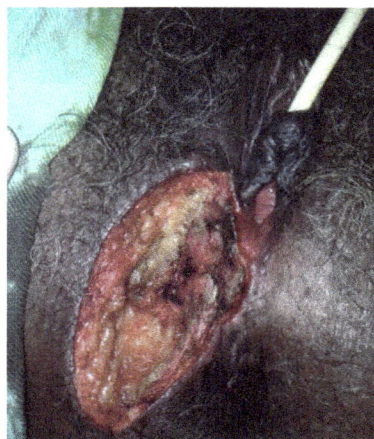

FIGURE 2: Photograph taken during surgery showing resection margins.

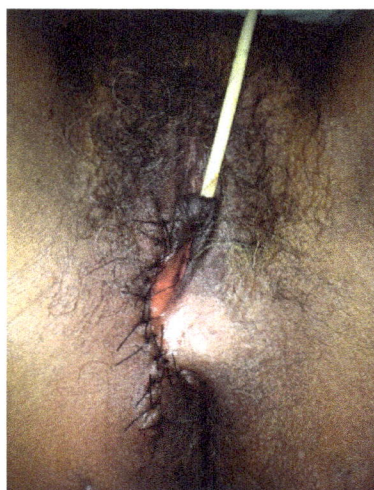

FIGURE 3: View of the completed surgical procedure.

Department's Vulva Clinic with a complaint of intense vulvar pruritus over a prolonged period of time, associated with the appearance of a purplish lesion with white striae three months previously. She reported no other signs or symptoms.

Physical examination revealed that the patient was in a good general state of health, well hydrated, and afebrile, with no signs of anemia, jaundice, or cyanosis. Physical examination of the cardiovascular and respiratory systems and of the abdomen showed no abnormalities. Breasts were voluminous and pendulous, with no nodulations or retractions. Examination of the vulva revealed normal hair distribution for age, a hypertrophic vulva, and the presence of a hardened, ulcerated, purplish lesion measuring 4 cm in diameter, with hyperchromic and hypochromic spots, situated on the lower third of the right labium majus, close to the vaginal fourchette (Figure 1). Speculum examination revealed a cervix with an apparently normal epithelium and external os with no pathological discharge. Manual examination revealed a closed, mobile, and painless cervix with fibroelastic consistency. Bimanual palpation showed a pelvic uterus. The inguinal lymph nodes were nonpalpable.

Colposcopy and cytology were performed, revealing an intense inflammatory process and no neoplastic cells. No abnormalities were found at bilateral mammography or on transvaginal or transabdominal ultrasonography.

An incisional biopsy was proposed. Histopathology revealed malignant intraepidermal neoplasia with large cells, karyomegaly, visible nucleolus, and clear cytoplasm. The cells were focally positive for periodic acid Schiff (PAS) staining. Blackened pigment was present in some cells from the basal layer and there was a focus of ulceration. Histopathology findings were compatible with malignant intraepithelial neoplasia. An immunohistochemical study was then carried out to differentiate between melanoma and extramammary Paget disease.

2.1. Immunohistochemistry. Immunohistochemistry revealed positivity for cytokeratins (CK7 and CK8/18) and negativity for S100 protein and Melan A. Taken together with the morphological features, these findings permitted a diagnosis

of Paget disease to be made. Consequently, surgery (right hemivulvectomy) was proposed to remove the lesion.

2.2. Surgery. Right hemivulvectomy was performed with wide margins all around (Figures 2 and 3). Following surgery, the patient progressed satisfactorily with no complications and was discharged from hospital.

2.2.1. Histopathology of the Surgical Specimen

Macroscopy. There was elliptical segment of light brown, wrinkled skin measuring 5.7 × 4.5 × 3.0 cm, with a hypochromic area measuring 3.5 × 2.2 cm. Sectioned tissue appeared yellowish and elastic.

Microscopy. Presence of vacuolized cytoplasm in the epidermis was detected. These cells were surrounded by a clear

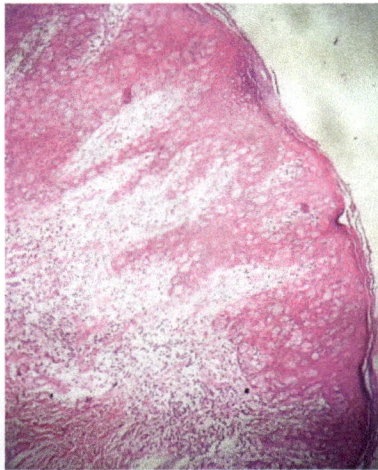

FIGURE 4: HE, 100x, Paget cells with clear cytoplasm inside the epidermis.

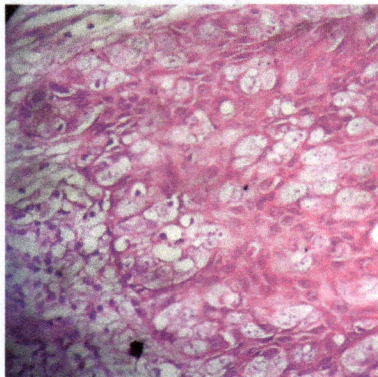

FIGURE 5: HE, 400x, Paget cells in the basal layer, some with melanic pigment.

halo and had granular cytoplasm containing mucopolysaccharides. The nucleus was very large with a visible nucleolus. There were foci of blackened pigment compatible with melanin in the basal cells. The dermis was unaffected by the lesion. The surgical margins were free (Figures 4 and 5).

Immunohistochemistry. Table 1 shows the differences in the immunohistochemical profile commonly found in skin melanomas and in Paget disease as compared to the findings in the present case, thus confirming the diagnosis.

The patient was referred to the Vulva Clinic of the Gynecology Department, Santa Casa de Misericórdia Hospital in Vitória, for follow-up.

3. Discussion

Extramammary Paget disease consists of a rare intraepithelial adenocarcinoma that has been described as an apocrine gland tumor. It may be benign or malignant with the potential to metastasize [6]. Nothing at all from the patient's family, social, or environmental history suggests the etiology of the development of EMPD or any predisposition towards the disease [7]. The symptoms are nonspecific. Clinical presentation is generally characterized by vulvar and perianal pruritus [8].

The clinical appearance is of an erythematous plaque with squamous or crusted areas. The size of the plaque may vary from less than 1 cm to lesions taking up the entire anogenital region. The margins of the affected region are generally clearly outlined, raised, and erythematous, resembling contact dermatitis, eczema, or even a bacterial infection. The symptoms may have been present for a long period of time. There is generally a history of various unsuccessful attempts at treating the lesion dermatologically [9].

The presence of these characteristics should raise several different suspicions, and therefore a biopsy is recommended to enable a differential diagnosis to be made with other dermatological/oncological pathologies such as melanoma, squamous cell carcinoma, hidradenitis suppurativa, psoriasis, fungal infections, contact dermatitis, and lichen sclerosus, among others [8].

Paget disease is characterized microscopically by the presence of atypical cells in the epidermis, and these cells have a large nucleus, visible nucleolus, and vacuolized cytoplasm. With their high mucin content, Paget cells stain positively for acid and neutral mucopolysaccharides, with periodic acid Schiff (PAS) stain being commonly used to clarify diagnosis. In some cases, the cells may contain granules of melanin [10]. There are theories to explain the presence of this pigment in Paget disease cells: (1) production of chemotactic factor by the neoplastic cells, generating a proliferation of dendritic melanocytes, and (2) Paget cells that may phagocyte the melanin from the melanocytes. Nevertheless, the actual physiopathology remains unknown [11].

Although finding melanin in Paget disease is rare, this fact may potentially serve as a trap when trying to reach a diagnosis, since it may mimic melanoma both at clinical examination and histologically. One architectural characteristic is that in EMPD the atypical cells with pigments of melanin are situated in the suprabasal layer, whereas, in melanomas, the malignant cells usually also surround the dermoepidermal junction [12].

If necessary, diagnosis can be confirmed using immunohistochemistry. In Paget disease, the positive epithelial markers are CK7, EMA, CEA, and mucin, whereas Melan A, HMB45, and S100 are negative in Paget disease but positive in cases of melanoma. Paget cells express HER2/neu receptors and c-erb-2 oncogene, indicating a biological origin similar to that of breast carcinoma [13].

Surgical resection is the standard treatment for EMPD and most often involves local resection and reconstruction by various means [14]. Nevertheless, because of the multifocal nature of EMPD, surgery is limited as far as prognosis is concerned and is sometimes associated with severe morbidity and functional disability. Therefore, radiotherapy has been used in certain circumstances such as in elderly patients who are clinically incapacitated for surgery or as an alternative treatment in the case of patients with a recurrence of EMPD after various surgical attempts and in those who refuse to undergo surgery [15].

TABLE 1: Differentiation between the immunohistochemical profile commonly found in skin melanomas and that found in Paget disease in comparison to the present case.

Antigen investigated	Melanoma in situ	Paget disease	Present case
Melan A	+	−	−
S100 protein	+	−	−
Cytokeratins	−	+	+
Carcinoembryonic antigen (CEA)	−	+	+
Epithelial membrane antigen (EMA)	−	+	+

In one-third of cases, there may be a recurrence of EMPD irrespective of the surgical margins. The disease may also recur in skin grafts removed from another part of the body and for as long as fifteen years after treatment as a consequence of the retrograde dissemination of Paget cells through the lymph vessels from a previously occult site of metastasis. The lesion that appears as a recidivist is almost always in situ. When affecting the perianal region, the five-year recurrence rate of Paget disease is 61% [2]. Since Paget disease does not regress spontaneously and is progressive in nature, constant follow-up is required to ensure early diagnosis of recurrences. In view of the limited experience with this disease, further studies are necessary to enable a consensus to be reached in relation to the optimal treatment for EMPD.

4. Conclusion

EMPD is rare; however, its incidence increases as a function of the patient's age. Clinical diagnosis is difficult, since the characteristics of the disease are nonspecific and variable; therefore, histopathology and immunohistochemical studies are required to enable a differential diagnosis to be made with melanoma, hidradenitis suppurativa, psoriasis, and contact dermatitis, among other conditions. Patients should be followed up closely because of the risk of persistence and/or recurrence of the disease. This is an original case report of interest to gynecology.

Consent

Written informed consent was obtained from the patient for publication of this case report and accompanying images. A copy of the written consent is available for review.

Conflict of Interests

The authors declare that they have no competing interests.

Authors' Contribution

Antônio Chambô Filho performed the biopsy and wide surgical excision and followed up the patient. Andressa Gonçalves Amorim designed the study and wrote the first draft of this paper. Brunelle Batista Fraga Mendes collected pertinent data and Rodrigo Neves Ferreira performed the histopathological

evaluation. All authors reviewed and approved the final version of the paper.

References

[1] D. Barmon, L. Imchen, A. Kataki, and J. Sharma, "Extra mammary Paget's disease of the vulva," *Journal of Mid-life Health*, vol. 3, no. 2, pp. 100–102, 2012.

[2] E. S. Trindade, P. A. Polcheira, D. B. Basílio, Z. N. Rocha, J. L. Rocha Júnior, and G. R. Primo, "Invasive Paget's disease of the vulva and perianal region: a case report," *Revista Brasileira de Ginecologia e Obstetrícia*, vol. 26, pp. 329–335, 2004.

[3] C. O. Onaiwu, P. T. Ramirez, A. Kamat, L. C. Pagliaro, E. E. Euscher, and K. M. Schmeler, "Invasive extramammary Paget's disease of the bladder diagnosed 18 years after noninvasive extramammary Paget's disease of the vulva," *Gynecologic Oncology Case Reports*, vol. 8, pp. 27–29, 2014.

[4] S. K. Simon, I. K. Bolanča, K. Šentija, V. Kukura, J. Valetić, and A. Škrtić, "Vulvar Paget's disease a case report," *Collegium Antropologicum*, vol. 34, no. 2, pp. 649–652, 2010.

[5] K. A. Edey, E. Allan, J. B. Murdoch, S. Cooper, and A. Bryant, "Interventions for the treatment of Paget's disease of the vulva," *The Cochrane Database of Systematic Reviews*, vol. 10, Article ID CD009245, 2013.

[6] Y. Merot, G. Mazoujian, G. Pinkus, K. Momtaz-T, and G. F. Murphy, "Extramammary Paget's disease of the perianal and perineal regions: evidence of apocrine derivation," *Archives of Dermatology*, vol. 121, no. 6, pp. 750–752, 1985.

[7] C. W. Helm, "Rare tumours of the vulva," in *Cancer and Pre-Cancer of the Vulva*, D. M. Luesley, Ed., pp. 151–154, Arnold, London, UK, 1st edition, 2000.

[8] G. Márquez-Acosta, EJ. Olaya-Guzmán, J. Jiménez-López, D. Gómez-Pue, and M. Pérez-Quintanilla, "Extensive Paget's disease of the vulva: case report and a conservative management proposal," *Perinatología y Reproducción Humana*, vol. 27, pp. 44–50, 2013.

[9] J. Mann, A. Lavaf, A. Tejwani, P. Ross, and H. Ashamalla, "Perianal Paget disease treated definitively with radiotherapy," *Current Oncology*, vol. 19, no. 6, pp. e496–e500, 2012.

[10] R. Amin, "Perianal Paget's disease," *British Journal of Radiology*, vol. 72, pp. 610–612, 1999.

[11] T. V. B. Gabbi, N. Y. S. Valente, and L. G. M. Castro, "Pigmented Paget's disease of the nipple mimicking cutaneous melanoma: importance of the immunohistochemical profile to differentiate between these diseases," *Anais Brasileiros de Dermatologia*, vol. 81, no. 5, pp. 457–460, 2006.

[12] J. Vincent and J. M. Taube, "Pigmented extramammary Paget disease of the abdomen: a potential mimicker of melanoma," *Dermatology Online Journal*, vol. 17, article 13, 2011.

[13] B. R. Vani, M. U. Thejaswini, V. Srinivasamurthy, and M. S. Rao, "Pigmented Paget's disease of nipple: a diagnostic challenge on cytology," *Journal of Cytology*, vol. 30, no. 1, pp. 68–70, 2013.

[14] B. Berman, J. Spencer, A. Villa, V. Poochareon, and G. Elgart, "Successful treatment of extramammary Paget's disease of the scrotum with imiquimod 5% cream," *Clinical and Experimental Dermatology, Supplement*, vol. 28, no. 1, pp. 36–38, 2003.

[15] S. H. Son, J. S. Lee, Y. S. Kim et al., "The role of radiation therapy for the extramammary paget's disease of the vulva; experience of 3 cases," *Cancer Research and Treatment*, vol. 37, pp. 365–369, 2005.

18

Unilateral Oral Mucous Membrane Pemphigoid: Refractory Atypical Presentation Successfully Treated with Intravenous Immunoglobulins

André Laureano and Jorge Cardoso

Department of Dermatology and Venereology, Hospital de Curry Cabral, Centro Hospitalar de Lisboa Central, 1069-166 Lisboa, Portugal

Correspondence should be addressed to André Laureano; andre.oliveira@sapo.pt

Academic Editor: Gérald E. Piérard

A 57-year-old male presented with a 6-month history of blisters and painful erosions on the right buccal mucosa. No skin or other mucosal involvement was seen. The findings of histopathological and direct immunofluorescence examinations were sufficient for the diagnosis of oral mucous membrane pemphigoid in the context of adequate clinical correlation. No response was seen after topical therapies and oral corticosteroids or dapsone. Intravenous immunoglobulin was started and repeated every three weeks. Complete remission was achieved after three cycles and no recurrence was seen after two years of follow-up. The authors report a rare unilateral presentation of oral mucous membrane pemphigoid on the right buccal and hard palate mucosa, without additional involvement during a period of five years. Local trauma or autoimmune factors are possible etiologic factors for this rare disorder, here with unique presentation.

1. Introduction

Mucous membrane pemphigoid (MMP) describes a heterogeneous group of chronic autoimmune subepithelial blistering diseases, primarily affecting mucous membranes, with or without skin involvement [1]. Although scarring is the clinical hallmark, it may not be obvious in the oral mucosa, which is the most commonly affected site. Lesions typically consist of desquamative gingivitis, erythematous patches, blisters, and erosions covered by pseudomembranes [2]. Autoantibodies binding to the epithelial basement membrane zone (BMZ) have been demonstrated in this subset, targeting bullous antigens 1 and 2, laminin 332 and laminin 311, type VII collagen, β4-integrin subunit, and some nonidentified basal membrane zone antigens [3, 4]. Any oral cavity location can be involved and patients usually have a good prognosis.

2. Case Presentation

A 57-year-old male presented with a 6-month history of blisters and painful erosions on the right buccal mucosa. His medical history was relevant for hypertension and hypothyroidism. He had been taking valsartan and levothyroxine for years and denied the use of topical drugs and previous dental procedures. On physical examination, the patient was found to have few bullae, erosions, and pseudomembrane-covered erosions on the right buccal mucosa (Figure 1).

No skin or other mucosal involvement was seen. He had fragmented teeth with sharp edges adjacent to the lesions. Laboratory evaluation was unremarkable. Histopathological examination of bullous lesion revealed a subepithelial blister with a mostly lymphocytic infiltrate in the upper corion (Figure 2).

Direct immunofluorescence of peribullous mucosa showed a linear band of IgG, IgA, and complement component 3 (C3) at the epithelial BMZ (Figure 3).

ELISA was negative for antibodies against bullous pemphigoid antigens 180 and 230 and desmogleins 1 and 3. Correlation between these features allowed the diagnosis of MMP. Application of dipropionate betamethasone cream, twice daily, was started. After one year the patient had

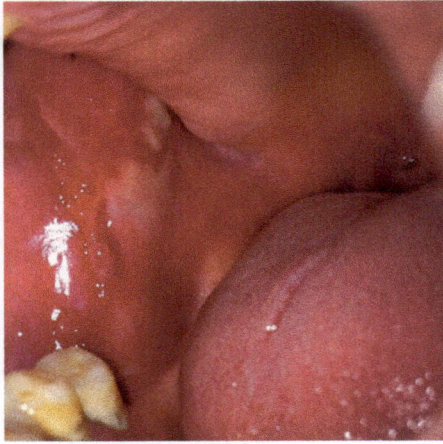

FIGURE 1: At presentation multiple painful erosions and pseudomembrane-covered erosions on the right buccal mucosa were seen.

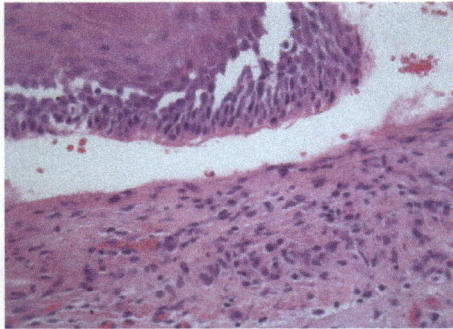

FIGURE 2: Histopathological examination of a bullous lesion revealed a subepithelial blister with a mostly lymphocytic and neutrophilic dense inflammatory infiltrate in the upper corion (hematoxylin and eosin, original magnification ×100).

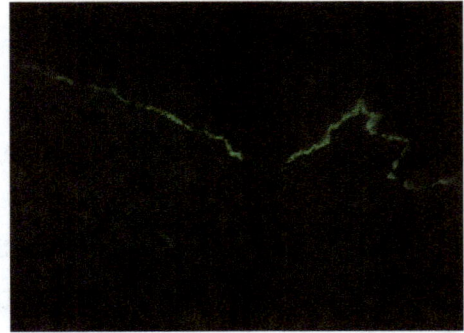

FIGURE 3: Direct immunofluorescence showed a linear band of IgG, IgA, and C3 at the epithelial BMZ (original magnification ×40).

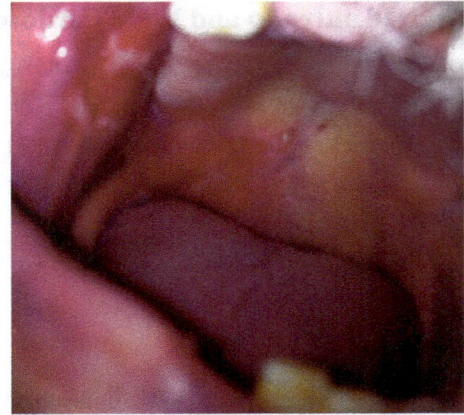

FIGURE 4: No response after topical and systemic treatment with corticosteroids and dapsone, with further involvement of the right hard palate mucosa.

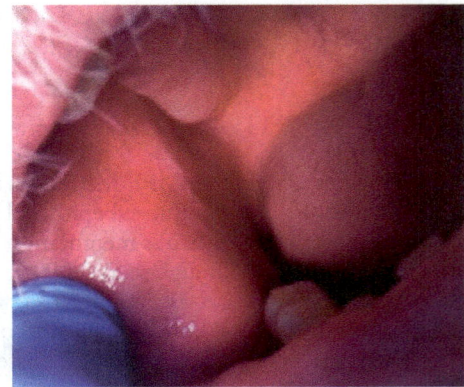

FIGURE 5: Complete response after IVIg therapy and only a delicate white pattern of reticulated scarring on the buccal mucosa had been seen after 3 years of follow-up.

persistent bullae and erosions on the right buccal mucosa that healed without scarring. Oral prednisolone (0.5 mg/kg/d) was started for six months, and as no response was achieved, treatment with dapsone (100 mg/d) was administered during one year. Further involvement of the right hard palate mucosa occurred, erosions were extremely painful, and the patient had difficulty in eating and depression (Figure 4).

Intravenous immunoglobulin (IVIg) at a dose of 2 g/kg/cycle was started and repeated every three weeks. Complete remission was achieved after three cycles. IVIg therapy was maintained for six additional months. No recurrence was seen after three years of follow-up (Figure 5).

3. Discussion

The findings of direct immunofluorescence were sufficient for the diagnosis of MMP in the context of adequate clinical correlation [1]. Patients with MMP with oral involvement often exhibit bilateral lesions. We reported a unilateral presentation on the right buccal and hard palate mucosa, without additional involvement during a period of five years. A possible previous chronic inflammatory process of the mucosa associated with local trauma probably exposed hidden antigens of the BMZ and evoked a secondary autoimmune response, explaining this mosaic of disease [2]. Direct immunofluorescence findings and the complete response after IVIg also suggest an autoimmune etiology, here with unique presentation [3, 5]. Since management of MMP is often difficult, our case also shows a complete response to a therapeutic option not commonly used in the limited or less severe disease.

Conflict of Interests

The authors declare that there is no conflict of interests regarding the publication of this paper.

References

[1] L. S. Chan, A. Razzaque Ahmed, G. J. Anhalt et al., "The first international consensus on mucous membrane pemphigoid: definition, diagnostic criteria, pathogenic factors, medical treatment and prognostic indicators," *Archives of Dermatology*, vol. 138, no. 3, pp. 370–379, 2002.

[2] L. S. Chan, "Ocular and oral mucous membrane pemphigoid (cicatricial pemphigoid)," *Clinics in Dermatology*, vol. 30, no. 1, pp. 34–37, 2012.

[3] A. S. Kourosh and K. B. Yancey, "Pathogenesis of mucous membrane pemphigoid," *Dermatologic Clinics*, vol. 29, no. 3, pp. 479–484, 2011.

[4] K. A. Rashid, H. M. Gürcan, and A. R. Ahmed, "Antigen specificity in subsets of mucous membrane pemphigoid," *Journal of Investigative Dermatology*, vol. 126, no. 12, pp. 2631–2636, 2006.

[5] D. A. Culton and L. A. Diaz, "Treatment of subepidermal immunobullous diseases," *Clinics in Dermatology*, vol. 30, no. 1, pp. 95–102, 2012.

19

Majocchi's Granuloma after Topical Corticosteroids Therapy

Fu-qiu Li, Sha Lv, and Jian-xin Xia

The Second Hospital of Jilin University, Changchun, Jilin 130000, China

Correspondence should be addressed to Jian-xin Xia; 911469806@qq.com

Academic Editor: Alexander A. Navarini

Majocchi's granuloma (MG) is an unusual but not rare dermatophyte infection of dermal and subcutaneous tissues. Dermatophytes usually result in the infections of hair, epidermis, and nail, and are rarely involved in deep cutaneous and subcutaneous tissues. Now it is considered that MG includes two forms: one is a small perifollicular papular form and the other is a deep subcutaneous nodular form; the front one mainly occurs in healthy individuals and the latter one usually presents in immunocompromised hosts. The clinical manifestations of MG are many and varied, except the common presentations of erythema, papule and nodules, and Kaposi sarcoma-like and molluscum-like lesions have been reported in literatures (Kim et al. (2011), Bord et al. (2007), and Lillis et al. (2010)). This characteristic induces the difficulty of diagnosis, and thus it is so important and necessary to make direct microscopical and histological examinations. We describe a case of MG over the face in a patient who had been treated with topical corticosteroids over a long time.

1. Case Report

A 46-year-old male patient presented with one-year history of erythema, papule and nodules, and desquamation over his whole face, accompanied with pruritus. He had consulted doctors in some private clinics, was diagnosed with eczema and solar dermatitis and was treated with topical corticosteroids and systemic antibiotic or antiallergic drugs for several months intermittently. The patient had been treated with topical corticosteroids including fluocinolone, dexamethasone ointment, and mometasone furoate off and on for about three months. The lesions had been improved at one time and then grown worse. Skin examination reveals multiple variably sized red and firm nodules on his face accompanied with swelling; some were associated with surrounding erythema and desquamation on an erythematous base (Figure 1). The patient denied any history of trauma like shaving of the face or previous cutaneous fungal infections such as tinea pedis, onychomycosis, or fungal infections of other regions. There were no other systemic diseases. The HIV test was negative. KOH examination of the discharge materials reveals distinct hyphae. Histological examination of a punch biopsy specimen taken from the left face showed cell granulomas with lymphocytes, neutrophils, and monocytes around the follicle and vessels in the dermis, and yet no

hyphae and spores were detected. Only one spore was noted in the dermis which was stained with D-periodic acid-Schiff (D-PAS) (Figure 2). The fungal culture of biopsy specimen yielded the growth of spreading white colonies with a cottony surface and red reverse pigment. Based on clinical, KOH examination, and histopathological and culture findings, MG caused by *Trichophyton rubrum* was identified. Systemic treatment was with itraconazole 200 mg twice daily and topical sertaconazole olamine for 4 weeks; after that, the dose of itraconazole reduced to 100 mg twice daily for the following 4 weeks; then the lesions completely disappeared (Figure 3).

2. Discussion

MG was first described as a kind of deep granulomatous trichophytosis by Professor Majocchi in 1883 [1]. The initiating factors are usually divided into two types in literatures; one is thought to be physical trauma which is induced by shaving, pricking, and other external forced like that and the other is due to immunosuppression caused by immunosuppressive therapy or autoimmune diseases that had been reported in literatures [2–8]. These two factors lead to disruption of the follicle in the dermis and subcutaneous tissue when hosts are infected by dermatophytes which usually invade

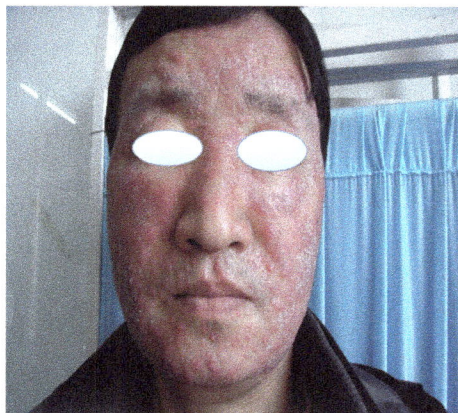

FIGURE 1: Erythema, papule and nodules, and desquamation over the whole face.

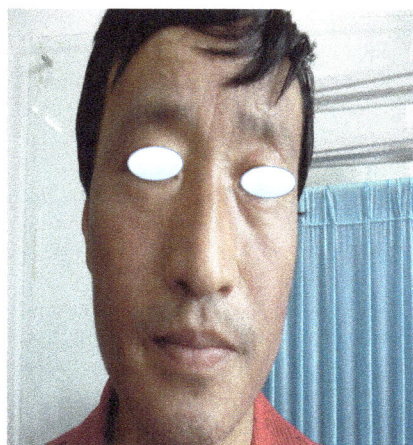

FIGURE 3: The lesions completely disappeared.

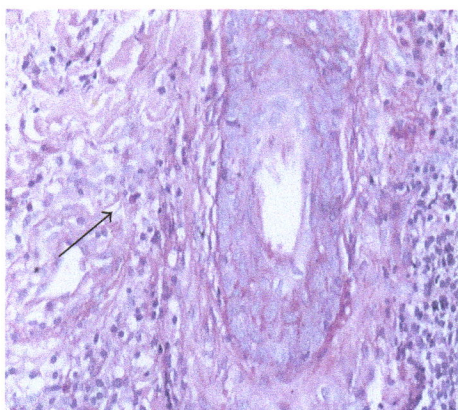

FIGURE 2: One spore was noted in the dermis which was stained with D-periodic acid-Schiff (D-PAS).

epidermis. The most common causative pathogen is *Trichophyton rubrum*, and *Microsporum canis* and *Aspergillus fumigatus* have also been reported in literatures [7, 9]. The pathogens generally exist in stratum corneum because keratinous material can potentially provide a substrate for the organism [10]. It is believed that keratin is carried by the severe inflammation into the dermis [3] and then provides a suitable living environment for the organism.

In our report, the patient had no history of trauma such as shaving of the face or previous cutaneous fungal infections and had no immunosuppression; in that way what is the initiating factor? Immunosuppressive drugs include corticosteroids, vincristine, cyclophosphamide, azathioprine, and tacrolimus, alone or in combination. Jacobs [11] thought that misapplication of topical corticosteroids over a long period can produce Majocchi granuloma. It was reported that MG was made by applying betamethasone ointment for 4 months by Meehan [12]. When it occurs to the patient, it might be eczema or allergic diseases at first, and he consulted doctors in private clinics and was given topical corticosteroids over a long time; then the host was occasionally infected by dermatophytes; the application of corticosteroids initially

suppressed the inflammatory component associated with dermatophytes while simultaneously accelerating dermatophyte growth [9].

Owing to the variety of MG's manifestations, it is necessary to make examinations including direct microscopical, histological examinations and the fungal culture. When the patient came to our clinic for diagnosis and treatment, these diagnoses including corticosteroid-dependent dermatitis, lupus miliaris disseminates, acne rosacea, fungal infective dermatoses, and skin tumour were considered by us. After a series of examinations, MG was diagnosed as being caused by *Trichophyton rubrum* which was identified by the features of fungal culture.

Reviewing the past literatures about MG's treatment, we can find that systemic antifungals such as itraconazole or terbinafine are a must because of the deep location of the infection. The duration of therapy does not have the same standard, from 3 weeks to 1 year in the literatures, and it takes more time for immunosuppressed individuals in general. For the treatment of Majocchi's granuloma, topical antifungals are usually ineffective [13]. Direct microscopical examinations of the discharge materials reveal obviously hyphae in our case that indicates the organism lives not only in deep cutaneous and subcutaneous tissues but also in epidermis, so it was assumed that topical antifungals are effective for this patient.

Conflict of Interests

The authors declare that there is no conflict of interests regarding the publication of this paper.

References

[1] D. Majocchi, "Spora una nuova trichofizia (granuloma tricofitico): studi clinici e micologici," *Bullettino Della Reale Accademia Medica di Roma*, vol. 9, pp. 220–223, 1883.

[2] J.-E. Kim, C.-H. Won, S. Chang, M.-W. Lee, J.-H. Choi, and K.-C. Moon, "Majocchi's granuloma mimicking Kaposi sarcoma in

a heart transplant patient," *Journal of Dermatology*, vol. 38, no. 9, pp. 927–929, 2011.

[3] C. Brod, F. Benedix, M. Röcken, and M. Schaller, "Trichophytic Majocchi granuloma mimicking Kaposi sarcoma," *Journal der Deutschen Dermatologischen Gesellschaft*, vol. 5, no. 7, pp. 591–593, 2007.

[4] J. V. Lillis, E. S. Dawson, R. Chang, and C. R. White Jr., "Disseminated dermal Trichophyton rubrum infection—an expression of dermatophyte dimorphism?" *Journal of Cutaneous Pathology*, vol. 37, no. 11, pp. 1168–1169, 2010.

[5] A. Gega, G. Ketsela, F. L. Glavin, C. Soldevilla-Pico, and D. Schain, "Majocchi's granuloma after antithymocyte globulin therapy in a liver transplant patient," *Transplant Infectious Disease*, vol. 12, no. 2, pp. 143–145, 2010.

[6] P. Saadat, S. Kappel, S. Young, M. Abrishami, and M. S. Vadmal, "*Aspergillus fumigatus* Majocchi's granuloma in a patient with acquired immunodeficiency syndrome," *Clinical and Experimental Dermatology*, vol. 33, no. 4, pp. 450–453, 2008.

[7] S. Gupta, B. Kumar, B. D. Radotra, and R. Rai, "Majocchi's granuloma trichophyticum in an immunocompromised patient," *International Journal of Dermatology*, vol. 39, no. 2, pp. 140–141, 2000.

[8] K. J. Smith, M. Welsh, and H. Skelton, "Trichophyton rubrum showing deep dermal invasion directly from the epidermis in immunosuppressed patients," *British Journal of Dermatology*, vol. 145, no. 2, pp. 344–348, 2001.

[9] B. G. Bae, H. J. Kim, D. J. Ryu, Y. S. Kwon, and K. H. Lee, "Majocchi granuloma caused by Microsporum canis as tinea incognito," *Mycoses*, vol. 54, no. 4, pp. 361–362, 2011.

[10] M. V. Dahl, "Dermatophytosis and the immune response," *Journal of the American Academy of Dermatology*, vol. 31, no. 3, pp. S34–S41, 1994.

[11] P. H. Jacobs, "Majocchi's granuloma (due to therapy with steroid and occlusion)," *Cutis*, vol. 38, no. 1, article 23, 1986.

[12] K. Meehan, "A growing, pruritic plaque on the thigh. Majocchi's granuloma with secondary tinea incognito," *Journal of the American Academy of Physician Assistants*, vol. 15, no. 3, pp. 16–65, 2002.

[13] H.-R. Cho, M.-H. Lee, and C.-R. Haw, "Majocchi's granuloma of the scrotum," *Mycoses*, vol. 50, no. 6, pp. 520–522, 2007.

20

Clinical Effects of Topical Tacrolimus on Fox-Fordyce Disease

Hilal Kaya Erdoğan,[1] Işıl Bulur,[1] and Zeliha Kaya[2]

[1]*Department of Dermatology, Eskisehir Osmangazi University, 26480 Eskisehir, Turkey*
[2]*Department of Pathology, Kırsehir Ahi Evran University, 40200 Kirsehir, Turkey*

Correspondence should be addressed to Hilal Kaya Erdoğan; hilalkayaerdogan@yahoo.com

Academic Editor: Akimichi Morita

Fox-Fordyce Disease (FFD) is a rare, chronic, pruritic, inflammatory disorder of apocrine glands. It is characterized by dome-shaped, firm, discrete, skin-colored, and monomorphic perifollicular papules. The most common sites of involvement are axillae and anogenital and periareolar regions which are rich in apocrine sweat glands. Treatment is difficult. Topical, intralesional steroids, topical tretinoin, adapalene, clindamycin, benzoyl peroxide, oral contraceptives, isotretinoin, phototherapy, electrocauterisation, excision-liposuction and curettage, and fractional carbon dioxide laser are among the treatment options. In the literature, there are articles reporting beneficial effects of pimecrolimus in FFD. Nevertheless, there have not been any reports about the use of tacrolimus in FFD. We report two patients diagnosed with FFD by clinical and histopathologic examination and discussed therapeutic effects of topical tacrolimus on FFD in the light of literature.

1. Introduction

Fox-Fordyce Disease (FFD) or "apocrine miliaria" is a chronic, pruritic, rare, inflammatory disorder of apocrine glands. It is observed primarily in women between the ages 15 and 35 and usually remits after menopause [1–3]. There are few reports of prepubescent patients in the literature [4].

Clinically it is characterized by dome-shaped, firm, discrete, skin-colored, and monomorphic perifollicular papules. Most common sites of involvement are axillae, anogenital, and periareolar regions which are rich in apocrine sweat glands. Less common locations include the medial thighs and periumbilical and sternal regions. The affected areas show reduction of sweating and hairs. The chief complaint generally is severe pruritus. Exercise, heat, and emotional stress can aggravate pruritus [1, 2].

Herein we report two patients diagnosed with FFD and discuss therapeutic effects of topical tacrolimus in the light of literature.

2. Report of Cases

2.1. Case 1. A 23-year-old woman presented with intensely pruritic lesions on her axillae for 3 years. She had been previously unsuccessfully treated with topical steroids, antifungals, and antibiotics. Her medical and family history was unremarkable. Dermatological examination revealed multiple, monomorphic, perifollicular, firm, skin-colored, and hyperpigmented papules confined to the bilateral axillary areas (Figure 1(a)). The remainder of her physical examination results was unremarkable. Histology from an axillary skin biopsy revealed hyperkeratosis and keratotic plug in follicular infundibulum, spongiosis, lymphocyte exocytosis, and perivascular and periadnexal lymphocytic infiltration. The diagnosis of FFD was made by clinical and histopathological findings. She was prescribed topical tacrolimus ointment (0,1%) twice daily for 3 months. After 3 months she had marked improvement of her lesions and pruritus (Figure 1(b)). There were no side effects of the treatment.

2.2. Case 2. A 32-year-old woman presented with papular lesions on her axillae for 10 years. Although the disease in this patient was subjectively asymptomatic, lesions were cosmetically disfiguring. She had been previously unsuccessfully treated with topical steroids. Dermatological examination revealed multiple, monomorphic, perifollicular, firm, skin-colored, and hyperpigmented perifollicular papules confined to the bilateral axillary areas. Also thinning of axillary hair

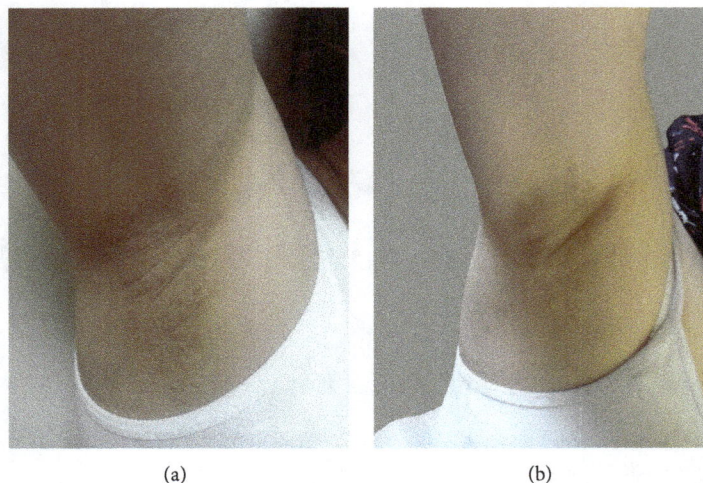

FIGURE 1: (a) Before treatment and (b) improvement of lesions after 3 months of topical tacrolimus.

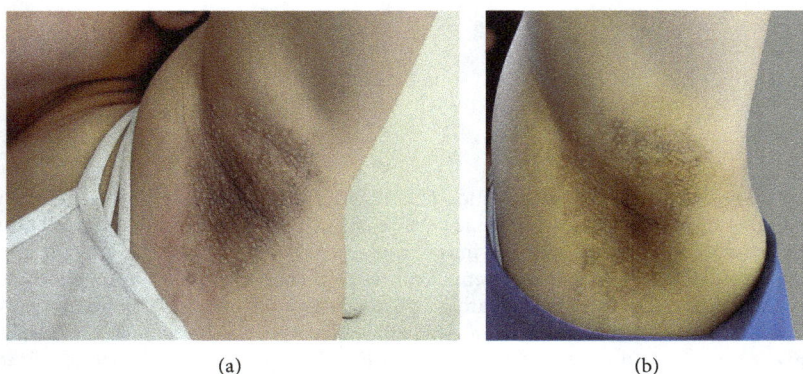

FIGURE 2: (a) Before treatment and (b) no change after 3 months of topical tacrolimus.

was noted (Figure 2(a)). The remainder of her physical examination results were unremarkable. Histologic examination of a 4 mm punch biopsy specimen taken from one of the papules revealed marked hyperkeratosis and keratotic plug in follicular infundibulum, spongiosis, lymphocyte exocytosis, and perivascular and periadnexal lymphocytic infiltration (Figure 3). The diagnosis of FFD was made by clinical and histopathological findings. She was prescribed topical tacrolimus ointment (0,1%) twice daily for 3 months. After 3 months, there was no change in lesions, and treatment was stopped (Figure 2(b)).

3. Discussion

FFD, first described by George Henry Fox and John Addison Fordyce in 1902, is a rare, pruritic, inflammatory disease of apocrine glands [2].

Etiology is not completely known. However, female predominance, start of symptoms with the onset of puberty, flare up in perimenstruel period, regress in pregnancy, postmenopausal period and by using oral contraceptives indicate hormonal factors. On the other hand, prepubertal FFD cases, lack of hormonal abnormalities, monozygotic twin, and familial case reports suggest that genetic and emotional factors may play role in etiology [2, 4, 5]. Besides, in literature, reported FFD cases after axillary hair removal suggest that physical factors also may play role [6].

Although the chronology of events is not proven in pathogenesis, the mechanism defined by Shelley and Levy is widely recognized. First event is obstruction of apocrine canal's distal part with keratin plug. It is considered that the keratin plug occurred by dysmaturation of keratinocytes. Canal is ruptured in epidermis because of apocrine sweat retention. This is followed by perifollicular and periadnexal infiltration [3, 6, 7].

Early histological finding is the keratin plug that blocks apocrine ductus in follicular infundibulum. Epidermal spongiosis and vesiculation occur. Perifollicular and periadnexal infiltration which consists of lymphocytes, few histiocytes, and eosinophils is accompanying finding. Mataix et al. noted that xanthomatosis due to phagocytosis of fat-rich apocrine material by macrophages was also an important histopathologic finding [3, 7].

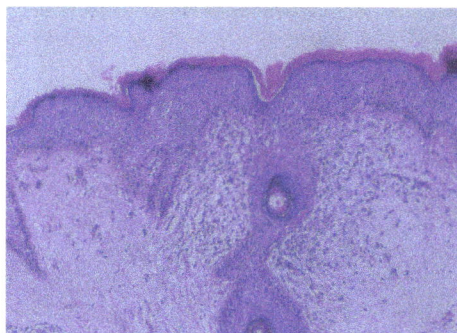

FIGURE 3: Hyperkeratosis, a keratotic plug in the follicular infundibulum, spongiosis, lymphocyte exocytosis, and perivascular and periadnexal lymphocytic infiltration.

Topical and intralesional steroids are first-line treatment in FFD, but their use is limited due to risk of cutaneous atrophy and striae. Topical tretinoin, adapalene, clindamycin, benzoyl peroxide, and pimecrolimus are used in the treatment. Oral contraceptives and oral isotretinoin treatment are also tried in the treatment. Phototherapy, electrocauterisation, excision-liposuction and curettage, and fractional carbon dioxide laser are also among the treatment options [8–11].

Tacrolimus is a calcineurin inhibitor and is apparently more effective than pimecrolimus in atopic dermatitis. Although there are articles reporting beneficial effects of pimecrolimus in FFD, there have not been any reports about the use of tacrolimus in FFD. We used tacrolimus pomade (0,1%) on our patients twice a day due to its strong anti-inflammatory effect and little side effect profile. While the first patient was successfully treated with tacrolimus, we did not observe any improvement in the second one. We think that the first patient responded well because she had more inflammatory disease with newer lesions and intense pruritus. On the other hand, the failure of the treatment in second patient can be explained by long duration of disease and marked keratinization. The difference in treatment response between two patients reminds us of the question that either keratin plug formation or inflammation is the primary pathogenetic event in pathogenesis [10, 11].

Consequently, topical calcineurin inhibitors should be noted as an option in the treatment of FFD patients with intense pruritus and short disease duration rather than patients with more chronic course and prominent keratinization.

Conflict of Interests

The authors declare that there is no conflict of interests regarding the publication of this paper.

References

[1] M. Schaller and G. Plewig, "Structure and function of eccrine, apocrine, apoeccrine and sebaceous glands," in *Dermatology*, chapter 35, pp. 489–494, Mosby-Elsevier, Barcelona, Spain, 2nd edition, 2008.

[2] J. Yost, M. Robinson, and S. A. Meehan, "Fox-Fordyce disease," *Dermatology Online Journal*, vol. 18, no. 12, p. 28, 2012.

[3] E. Arca, O. Köse, H. B. Taştan et al., "A case of Fox-Fordyce," *Turkiye Klinikleri Journal of Medical Sciences*, vol. 23, no. 1, pp. 49–52, 2003.

[4] G. T. Demirci, Ş. Yaşar, A. T. Mansur, I. E. Aydingöz, and S. Sever, "Prepubertal Fox-Fordyce disease: a case report," *Turkiye Klinikleri Journal of Medical Sciences*, vol. 26, no. 3, pp. 338–341, 2006.

[5] E. Erkek, M. Koçak, P. Atasoy et al., "Fox-Fordyce disease," *Turkderm*, vol. 36, no. 1, pp. 60–63, 2002.

[6] M. T. Tetzlaff, K. Evans, D. M. DeHoratius, R. Weiss, G. Cotsarelis, and R. Elenitsas, "Fox-Fordyce disease following axillary laser hair removal," *Archives of Dermatology*, vol. 147, no. 5, pp. 573–576, 2011.

[7] J. Mataix, J. F. Silvestre, M. Niveiro, A. Lucas, and M. Pérez-Crespo, "Perifollicular xanthomatosis as a key histological finding in Fox-Fordyce disease," *Actas Dermo-Sifiliográficas*, vol. 99, no. 2, pp. 145–148, 2008.

[8] L. E. D. B. P. Kassuga, M. M. Medrado, N. S. Chevrand, S. D. A. N. Salles, and E. G. Vilar, "Fox-Fordyce disease: response to adapalene 0.1%," *Anais Brasileiros de Dermatologia*, vol. 87, no. 2, pp. 329–331, 2012.

[9] K. M. Chae, M. A. Marschall, and S. F. Marschall, "Axillary Fox-Fordyce disease treated with liposuction-assisted curettage," *Archives of Dermatology*, vol. 138, no. 4, pp. 452–454, 2002.

[10] D. Milcic and M. Nikolic, "Clinical effects of topical pimecrolimus in a patient with Fox-Fordyce disease," *Australasian Journal of Dermatology*, vol. 53, no. 2, pp. 34–35, 2012.

[11] L. Pock, M. Švrčková, R. Macháčková, and J. Hercogová, "Pimecrolimus is effective in Fox-Fordyce disease," *International Journal of Dermatology*, vol. 45, no. 9, pp. 1134–1135, 2006.

Dyschromatosis Symmetrica Hereditaria of Late Onset?

Caroline Balvedi Gaiewski,[1] **Sergio Zuneda Serafini,**[1]
Betina Werner,[2] **and Janyana M. D. Deonizio**[1]

[1] _Dermatology Department, Federal University of Parana, 80530-905 Curitiba, PR, Brazil_
[2] _Pathology Department, Federal University of Parana, 80530-905 Curitiba, PR, Brazil_

Correspondence should be addressed to Janyana M. D. Deonizio; janyanadd@yahoo.com.br

Academic Editors: A. Morita and E. Schmidt

Dyschromatosis symmetrica hereditaria (DSH), also known as reticulated acropigmentation of Dohi, is an autosomal dominant disease with high penetrance, characterized by hypo- and hyperpigmented macules of varying sizes on the dorsal of the extremities with reticulated pattern. This paper presents a female patient with typical dermatological lesions, but only diagnosed in adulthood. It is necessary to perform differential diagnosis with other pigmentary disorders. This entity is not very common in South America, and the vast majority of cases were described in Japanese population. Since it is a benign disease, it is important to be aware of this diagnosis in order to establish the correct conduct for these patients.

1. Introduction

Dyschromatoses are characterized by the presence of hyper- and hypopigmented macules arranged in a reticular pattern. Dyschromatosis symmetric hereditaria (DSH) is a rare genodermatosis, autosomal dominant with high penetrance, with some sporadic reported cases. It is often reported in Japanese patients, but there have been also cases in India, Europe, and South America [1, 2]. After the literature review in PubMed database, this is the fourth case reported in Brazil [3, 4].

2. Case Report

A 40-year-old female patient presented with multiple small hyperchromic and hypochromic macules distributed symmetrically on the dorsum of the hands and feet (Figures 1 and 2). She noted these lesions when she was 26 years old, and they were asymptomatic. Moreover multiple freckle-like pigmented macules were also noted on her face (Figure 3). She denies other comorbidities. Investigation for autoimmune disease and other laboratory findings were negative. Family history was positive with a nephew with similar lesions.

Two different biopsies were performed from hypochromic and hyperchromic areas. From hypochromic lesion, histology demonstrated a compact stratum corneum and discrete acanthosis. Using Fontana Masson staining, hypochromic lesion demonstrated marked decrease, with almost absence, of melanin. On the other hand, the hyperchromic lesion demonstrated an intense pigmentation (Figures 4(a) and 4(b)). Those findings were compatible with the clinical hypothesis of DSH.

3. Discussion

DSH is a genodermatosis characterized by multiple small hypo- and hyperpigmented macules, with irregular size and shape, symmetrically distributed on the backs of the hands and feet. Some patients also show freckle-like macules on the face. Palms, plants, and mucous membranes are free from the disorder [5]. Lesions appear in childhood, usually before the age of six, remaining during life without any color or distribution changes after stabilization in adolescence. In general, the involvement is limited to skin, without systemic involvement or evidence of photosensitivity. However, there are isolated reports of association with neurofibromatosis type I, thalassemia, polydactyly, and torsion dystonia [6].

Since 2003, a genetic mutation has been identified on chromosome IqII-Iq2I as responsible for the production and

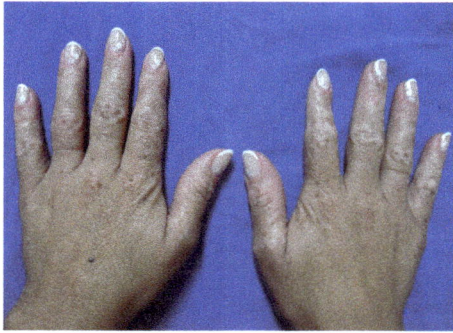

FIGURE 1: Hyper- and hypopigmented macules distributed symmetrically on the dorsum of the hands.

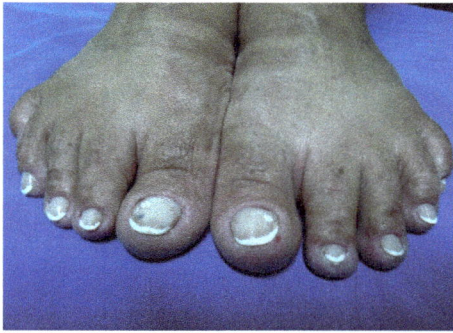

FIGURE 2: Hyper- and hypopigmented macules distributed symmetrically on the dorsum of the feet.

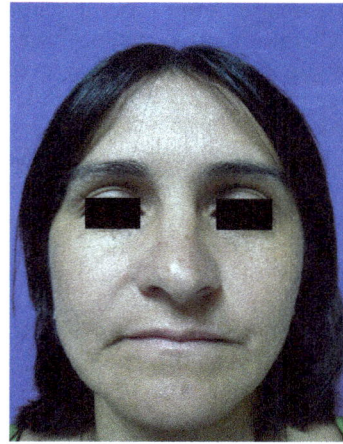

FIGURE 3: Multiple freckle-like pigmented macules on the face.

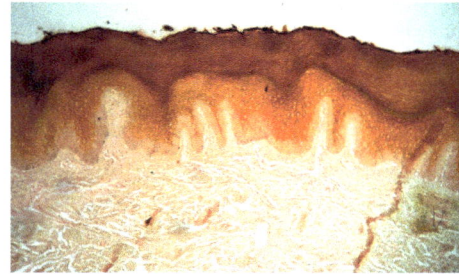

(a)

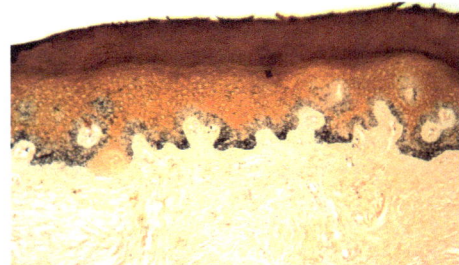

(b)

FIGURE 4: (a) Histology from hypochromic lesion showing decrease, with almost absence of melanin. (b) Histology from hyperchromic region showing intense amount of pigment (Fontana-Masson, 100X, 2X).

distribution changes of melanin. Miyamura et al. were the first to identify heterozygous mutations of the gene *DSRAD* or ADAR1, responsible for codifying the double-stranded adenosine deaminase specific RNA, as the cause of DSH [1, 6]. Despite more than 90 different mutations in the *DSRAD* gene having been described in the literature, it is still uncertain how these changes can cause the same phenotype [7].

Histologically, in hypopigmented areas, the deposit of melanin is scarce, in contrast to the areas of hyperpigmentation that contain melanocytes with an increased metabolic activity and high concentration of melanosomes [6]. The number of melanocytes in the areas of hypopigmentation is diminished compared to individuals without the disease [1].

This disease must be differentiated from other pigmentary disorders such as reticulate acropigmentation of Kitamura, which is marked by presence of atrophy and absence of hypopigmented lesions; Dowling-Degos disease by reticulate hyperpigmentation in the body's folds, accompanied by comedogenic lesions on back and neck, and depressed or pitted scars; initial cases of xeroderma pigmentosum distinguished by the development of more serious symptoms of xerosis, atrophy, telangiectasia, and tumors in photo-exposed areas; dyschromatosis universalis hereditaria with predominating lesions in trunk starting in childhood; vitiligo with repigmentation areas which can simulate hyperchromic macules of DSH but have perifollicular distribution [1, 2, 6, 8].

Interestingly the age of onset of DSH is 4.4 years old in average, which differs from our case (26 years old). Dowling-Degos disease and Galli-Galli disease are characterized by a later onset (24.5 and 45.6, resp.) and may be considered as a differential diagnosis [2]. Nevertheless, we favor the diagnosis of DSH once Dowling-Degos disease presents with reticulate hyperpigmented macules in the flexures and large body folds. Galli-Galli disease is characterized by reticulated pigmented and hyperkeratotic erythematous macules and papules, located in the same areas of Dowling-Degos disease, but has a very peculiar histology demonstrating moderate-to-severe acantholysis of the suprabasal epidermis, which was not observed in our case. Adult-onset dyschromatosis often is secondary to chemicals, drugs, physical agents, cutaneous lupus erythematous, or infection [9]. We excluded those causes by history and laboratory investigation. We believe that this is a true case of DSH since the patient has very typical clinical findings and positive family history of similar lesions. It is possible that lesions have been unnoticed until adulthood.

No treatment is effective for this genodermatosis [6]. The exact frequency of the DSH is unknown since the main changes are confined to the skin with no systemic involvement, and many cases remain unreported. Despite the several reports and genetic studies from East Asian countries, the DSH is a very rare diagnosis in Brazil. We report this case due to its rare occurrence in South America and in view of the need of proper diagnosis and guidance for these patients.

Conflict of Interests

The authors declare that there is no conflict of interests regarding the publication of this paper.

References

[1] M. Hayashi and T. Suzuki, "Dyschromatosis symmetrica hereditaria," *The Journal of Dermatology*, vol. 40, no. 5, pp. 336–343, 2013.

[2] C. S. Müller, L. Tremezaygues, C. Pföhler, and T. Vogt, "The spectrum of reticulate pigment disorders of the skin revisited," *European Journal of Dermatology*, vol. 22, no. 5, pp. 596–604, 2012.

[3] G. C. Froes, L. B. Pereira, and V. B. Rocha, "Case for diagnosis," *The Journal Brazilian Annals of Dermatology*, vol. 84, pp. 425–427, 2009.

[4] N. C. Fernandes and L. R. Andrade, "Case for diagnosis," *Anais Brasileiros de Dermatologia*, vol. 85, no. 1, pp. 109–110, 2010.

[5] V. Vachiramon, K. Thadanipon, and K. Chanprapaph, "Infancy- and childhood-onset dyschromatoses," *Clinical and Experimental Dermatology*, vol. 36, no. 8, pp. 833–839, 2011.

[6] J. Consigli, M. S. Gómez Zanni, L. Ragazzini, and C. Danielo, "Dyschromatosis symmetrica hereditaria: report of a sporadic case," *International Journal of Dermatology*, vol. 49, no. 8, pp. 918–920, 2010.

[7] Y. Liu, F. Liu, X. Wang et al., "Two novel frameshift mutations of the DSRAD gene in Chinese pedigrees with dyschromatosis symmetrica hereditaria," *International Journal of Dermatology*, vol. 51, pp. 920–922, 2012.

[8] D. Mohana, U. Verma, A. J. Amar, and R. K. P. Choudhary, "Reticulate acropigmentation of dohi: a case report with insight into genodermatoses with mottled pigmentation," *Indian Journal of Dermatology*, vol. 57, no. 1, pp. 42–44, 2012.

[9] V. Vachiramon, K. Thadanipon, and P. Rattanakaemakorn, "Adult-onset dyschromatoses," *Clinical and Experimental Dermatology*, vol. 37, no. 2, pp. 97–103, 2012.

22

A Case of Apparent Contact Dermatitis Caused by *Toxocara* Infection

Rosanna Qualizza,[1] **Eleni Makrì,**[2] **Laura Losappio,**[3] **and Cristoforo Incorvaia**[2]

[1]*Allergy Service, Istituti Clinici di Perfezionamento, 20100 Milan, Italy*
[2]*Allergy/Pulmonary Rehabilitation, Istituti Clinici di Perfezionamento, 20100 Milan, Italy*
[3]*General Medicine, University of Foggia, 71100 Foggia, Italy*

Correspondence should be addressed to Rosanna Qualizza; rosanna.qualizza@icp.mi.it

Academic Editor: Akimichi Morita

Infection from *Toxocara* species may give rise to a large array of clinical symptoms, including apparent manifestations of allergy such as asthma, urticaria/angioedema, and dermatitis. We report a case, thus far not described, of contact dermatitis attributed to nickel allergy but caused by *Toxocara* infection. The patient was a 53-year-old woman presenting from 10 years a dermatitis affecting head, neck, and thorax. Patch tests initially performed gave a positive result to nickel, but avoidance of contact with nickel did not result in recovery. The patient referred to our Allergy Service in 2010 because of dermatitis to feet. Patch testing confirmed the positive result for nickel, but expanding the investigation a positive result for IgG antibodies to *Toxocara* was detected by Western blotting and ELISA. Treatment with mebendazole achieved immediate efficacy on feet dermatitis. Then, two courses of treatment with albendazole resulted in complete regression of dermatitis accompanied by development of negative ELISA and Western blotting for *Toxocara* antibodies. This report adds another misleading presentation of *Toxocara* infection as apparent contact dermatitis caused by nickel and suggests bearing in mind, in cases of contact dermatitis not responding to avoidance of the responsible hapten and to medical treatment, the possible causative role of *Toxocara*.

1. Introduction

Toxocara species is an intestinal nematode mainly affecting dogs and cats, which causes human infection when embryonated eggs excreted in dog faeces are ingested but also by eating raw or undercooked meat (from chicken, cow, pigs, rabbits, and others), the latter being a frequent mode of infection in adults. In humans, the larvae do not develop into adult worms but may migrate to various tissues and organs where they can survive for years, giving rise to a number of clinical symptoms [1–3]. Among them, apparently allergic manifestations are reported, including asthma, urticaria/angioedema, and dermatitis [4–6]. We report a case, thus far not described, of contact dermatitis diagnosed as nickel allergy but caused by *Toxocara* infection.

2. Case Presentation

The patient was a 53-year-old woman presenting from 10 years a dermatitis affecting head, neck, and thorax. Patch tests initially performed gave a positive result only to nickel. The patient avoided any possible contact with nickel, but dermatitis recurred regularly at intervals of 6–8 months. In 2005 dermatitis also affected the sole of the right foot and was treated with topical steroids, but in the following years also edema of the foot with impaired walking occurred. The patient referred to our Allergy Service in 2010 because of the development of dermatitis also to the left foot (Figure 1(a)). Patch testing confirmed the positive result for nickel sulfate. The patients also complained about recurrent headache and asthenia especially in the morning. By routine blood tests, only peripheral eosinophilia and total IgE levels were

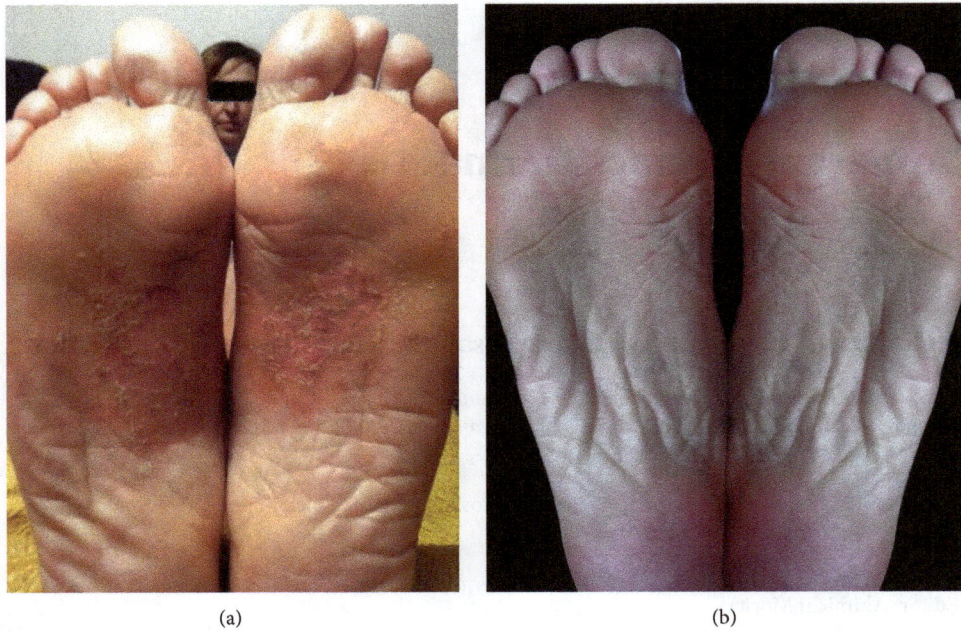

FIGURE 1: (a) Foot dermatitis before diagnosis of *Toxocara* infections. (b) Foot dermatitis after antiparasitic treatment.

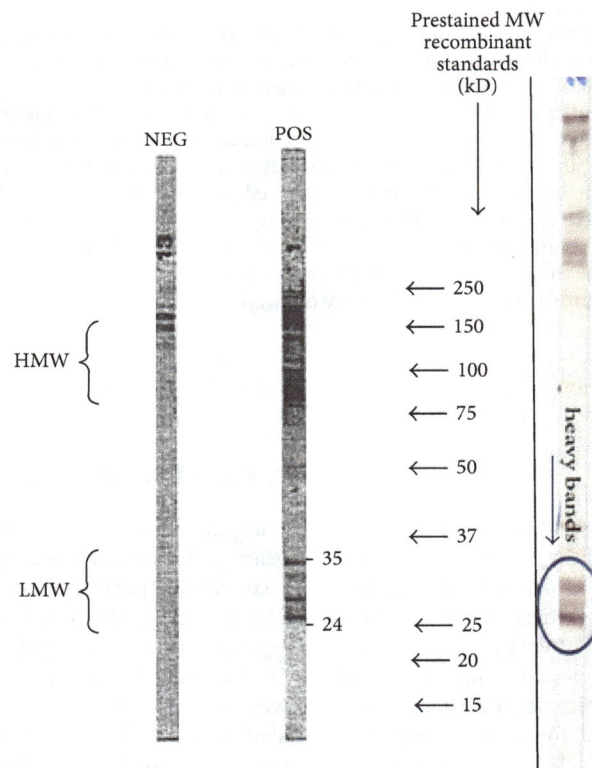

FIGURE 2: Result of Western blotting for anti-*Toxocara* IgG antibodies.

abnormal. We required other immunological tests including ANA, ENA, and anti-*Toxocara* IgG antibodies, yielding a positive result to the latter by Western blotting (Figure 2) and ELISA using material from LTBio Diagnostics (Lyon, France).

3. Results and Discussion

Following the diagnosis of *Toxocara* infection, treatment with mebendazole 100 mg b.i.d. for 3 days was started, achieving immediate efficacy on feet dermatitis and edema. Other 3 courses of mebendazole treatment were performed, with dermatitis showing a mild reoccurrence, while headache and asthenia disappeared. Also peripheral eosinophilia turned to normal value. Then, two courses of treatment with albendazole 400 mg b.i.d. for 5 days were performed that were followed by complete regression of dermatitis (Figure 1(b)), accompanied by development of negative ELISA and Western blotting for *Toxocara* antibodies. This observation differs from most reports in the literature that show persistence of ELISA and Western blotting positive results for a long period of time after treatment [7].

This report adds another misleading presentation of *Toxocara* infection as apparent contact dermatitis caused by nickel. Nickel allergy is quite common, its prevalence being estimated in around 12% in a recent study [8]. This makes understandable that in a patient with dermatitis and positive response to patch test with nickel an obvious diagnosis of nickel allergy is stated. The present case shows that also this kind of clinical presentation may be sustained by an unrecognized *Toxocara* infection. Only the correct diagnosis allowed curing the 10-year long dermatitis of the patient, the causative role of *Toxocara* being supported by the immunological laboratory results. This confirms that the role of *Toxocara* infection in causing clinical manifestations of apparent allergy is often overlooked [9] and suggests bearing in mind, at least in cases of apparent contact dermatitis not responding to avoidance of the responsible hapten and to medical treatment, that the possible agent may be *Toxocara*.

Conflict of Interests

The authors declare that there is no conflict of interests regarding the publication of this paper.

References

[1] P. A. Overgaauw, "Aspects of toxocara epidemiology: human toxocarosis," *Critical Reviews in Microbiology*, vol. 23, no. 3, pp. 215–231, 1997.

[2] D. Despommier, "Toxocariasis: clinical aspects, epidemiology, medical ecology, and molecular aspects," *Clinical Microbiology Reviews*, vol. 16, no. 2, pp. 265–272, 2003.

[3] G. Rubinsky-Elefant, C. E. Hirata, J. H. Yamamoto, and M. U. Ferreira, "Human toxocariasis: diagnosis, worldwide seroprevalences and clinical expression of the systemic and ocular forms," *Annals of Tropical Medicine and Parasitology*, vol. 104, no. 1, pp. 3–23, 2010.

[4] P. J. Cooper, "Toxocara *canis* infection: an important and neglected environmental risk factor for asthma?" *Clinical and Experimental Allergy*, vol. 38, no. 4, pp. 551–553, 2008.

[5] B. Gavignet, R. Piarroux, F. Aubin, L. Millon, and P. Humbert, "Cutaneous manifestations of human toxocariasis," *Journal of the American Academy of Dermatology*, vol. 59, no. 6, pp. 1031–1042, 2008.

[6] R. Qualizza, C. Incorvaia, R. Grande, E. Makrì, and L. Allegra, "Seroprevalence of IgG anti-Toxocara species antibodies in a population of patients with suspected allergy," *International Journal of General Medicine*, vol. 4, pp. 783–787, 2011.

[7] J. Fillaux and J.-F. Magnaval, "Laboratory diagnosis of human toxocariasis," *Veterinary Parasitology*, vol. 193, no. 4, pp. 327–336, 2013.

[8] C. G. Mortz, C. Bindslev-Jensen, and K. E. Andersen, "Nickel allergy from adolescence to adulthood in the TOACS cohort," *Contact Dermatitis*, vol. 68, no. 6, pp. 348–356, 2013.

[9] E. Pinelli and C. Aranzamendi, "Toxocara infection and its association with allergic manifestations," *Endocrine, Metabolic & Immune Disorders: Drug Targets*, vol. 12, no. 1, pp. 33–44, 2012.

23

Facial and Periorbital Cellulitis due to Skin Peeling with Jet Stream by an Unauthorized Person

Asli Feride Kaptanoglu,[1] Didem Mullaaziz,[1] and Kaya Suer[2]

[1] *Department of Dermatology, Near East University Hospital, Lefkosa, North Cyprus, Mersin 10, Turkey*
[2] *Department of Infectious Diseases and Clinical Microbiology, Near East University Hospital, Lefkosa, North Cyprus, Mersin 10, Turkey*

Correspondence should be addressed to Didem Mullaaziz; didem_mullaaziz@yahoo.com

Academic Editor: Gérald E. Piérard

Technologies and devices for cosmetic procedures are developing with each passing day. However, increased and unauthorized use of such emerging technologies may also lead to increases in unexpected results and complications as well. Here, we report a case of facial cellulitis after a "beauty parlor" session of skin cleaning with jet stream peeling device in 19-year old female patient for the first time. Complications due to improper and unauthorized use of jet stream peeling devices may also cause doubts about the safety and impair the reputation of the technology as well. In order to avoid irreversible complications, local authorities should follow the technology and update the regulations where the dermatologists should take an active role.

1. Introduction

Nowadays, cosmetic applications and medical devices that promise to improve the skin problems are popular and widely used and some of them are easily accessed due to the lack of government regulations in some countries. Peeling skin with a jet stream (shortly named as jet-peeling) is a new technology for cosmetic resurfacing and deep cleansing of the skin. It is reported as a safe and effective tool for the usual indications for facial peeling such as resurfacing, wrinkles, scars, and acne treatment [1]. Indications of jet-peeling are also developing, such as delivering antiseptic and anesthetic solutions to the deeper layers of skin [2]. However, increased and unauthorized use of such emerging technologies may also lead to increases in unexpected results and complications as well. Infectious complications after cosmetic procedures by unauthorized persons are commonly reported [3–5]. To the best of our literature search, facial cellulitis developing after a session of jet-peeling has not been reported previously. The aim of reporting this case is to draw attention to the possible complications which might be caused by the misuse of cosmetic devices.

2. Case Report

Nineteen-year-old previously healthy female patient was admitted with swelling, pain, and redness on the left side of her face and left eye region. Her admittance to our clinic was the first time of medical admittance. The patient declared the presence of only blackheads (comedones) until two days ago. However, she had a history of jet-peeling session in "*a beauty parlor*" for the facial skin cleansing and peeling 5 days ago. She had no other disease and was using neither a systemic nor a topical treatment for acne and did not use any medication for any other reason. She had no history of previous dentistry treatment. Two days prior to her admission, left side of her face got edematous and followed by increasing redness, swelling, and pain which spread to her eye and neck. Physical examination revealed unilateral diffuse edema including periorbital region, erythema, pustules, and cysts with a purulent discharge on the left side of the face (Figure 1). Palpation was painful and there were lymphadenopathies in the anterior cervical and submandibular chains. She had mild fever as 38.1 C. Laboratory tests showed elevated C Reactive Protein (CRP: 2.39 mg/dL) and white blood cells (12.900/uL). Her blood glucose, IgE levels, Blood Urea Nitrogen (BUN), creatinine, and liver tests were in normal ranges. A direct

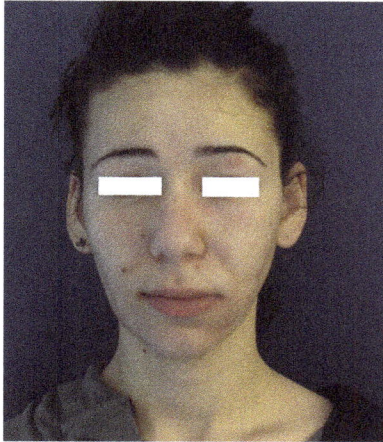

FIGURE 1: Erythema, edema, and pustules on the left side of the face.

smear and microbiological culture were performed from the purulent discharge. In the microscopic evaluation with gram stain polymorphonuclear leukocytes, gram (−) bacillus and gram (+) coccus were seen. Bacterial culture with blood agar revealed *Staphylococcus epidermidis* reproduction. In the antibiogram there was resistance to only clindamycin, penicillin, and erythromycin. She was diagnosed as facial-periorbital cellulitis and antibiotherapy was planned. She was initially given cefazolin and continued after the culture as the antibiogram revealed sensitivity to cefazolin. After 10 days of antibiotic regimen, her facial edema, erythema, and purulent lesions were recovered, with a residue of comedones and slightly erythematous papules of acne.

3. Discussion

Cellulitis is an infection of the deep dermis and subcutaneous tissue that manifest as areas of erythema, swelling, warmth, and tenderness. Bacteria typically gain access to the dermis via a break in the skin barrier in immunocompetent persons. Cellulitis in immunocompetent adults is mostly due to Streptococcus *spp.* and *Staph aureus* [6]. *Staphylococcus* is common colonizers of skin. Particularly, *Staphylococcus epidermidis* is a commensal bacterium of the human skin and regarded as an innocuous commensal microorganism. However, there are many reports regarding it as an "accidental pathogen" responsible for the nosocomial infections in immunocompromised or medical prosthesis inserted patients [7, 8]. In our patient, insertion of bacteria might not be with surgery, but with a strong jet stream pressure which even can enhance drug delivery from intact skin [2]. We were not the initial operator of the device. Hence, neither we nor the patient had information about the technique, depth of peel, number of passes, anestesia, or the type of the fluid. The patient reported that she had no knowledge if her skin has been well disinfected before the treatment.

Jet-peel seems to be a noninvasive, effective, and easy-to-apply facial peeling method and such "innocent" properties provide an attractive option for beauty salons. The success of

a treatment modality in facial resurfacing is based on patient selection as well as ability to manage the side effects even in most developed devices [9]. This unauthorized use and misuse of the device may lead to unexpected and worrisome complications as in our patient. All the techniques which break the epidermal barrier must be performed by a trained practitioner. Jet- peel may not be suitable if the patient has certain medical conditions, such as inflamed or infected skin, possibility of keloid scarring, or pressure urticaria. We strongly emphasize the importance of a good clinical exam before this procedure to avoid the risk of superficial but also deep infection. Also the physician should be aware of the risk of herpes outbreak. In our patient, there was unilateral facial cellulitis indicating an external inoculation of infection. Moreover, as jet-peel has effects on lymphatic drainage, inappropriate and improper use of the device might have caused the spread of the superficial skin infection into deeper skin tissues or the orbita.

4. Conclusion

Considering that the data in the literature is few, jet-peeling devices should be used with caution and under the supervision of a dermatologist or plastic surgeon. Whether severe or not, acne should only be treated by medical doctors. Beauticians' dare to treat acne is not only unlawful but also can result in permanent damage to the patients face. Bad complications due to improper use of the device may also cause doubts about the safety and impair the reputation of the technology as well.

Conflict of Interests

The authors declare that there is no conflict of interests regarding the publication of this paper.

References

[1] J. Golan and N. Hai, "JetPeel: a new technology for facial rejuvenation," *Annals of Plastic Surgery*, vol. 54, no. 4, pp. 369–374, 2005.

[2] T. Iannitti, S. Capone, and B. Palmieri, "Short review on face rejuvenation procedures: focus on preoperative antiseptic and anesthetic delivery by Jet Peel," *Minerva Chirurgica*, vol. 66, no. 3, supplement, pp. 1–8, 2011.

[3] J. Chwalek and D. J. Goldberg, "Ablative skin resurfacing," *Current Problems in Dermatology*, vol. 42, pp. 40–47, 2011.

[4] W. Ziebuhr, S. Hennig, M. Eckart, H. Kränzler, C. Batzilla, and S. Kozitskaya, "Nosocomial infections by *Staphylococcus epidermidis*: how a commensal bacterium turns into a pathogen," *International Journal of Antimicrobial Agents*, vol. 28, no. 1, pp. 14–20, 2006.

[5] M. Otto, "Staphylococcus *epidermidis*—the "accidental" pathogen," *Nature Reviews Microbiology*, vol. 7, no. 8, pp. 555–567, 2009.

[6] C. Quiñones, E. Ramalle-Gómara, M. Perucha et al., "An outbreak of *Mycobacterium fortuitum* cutaneous infection associated with mesotherapy," *Journal of the European Academy of Dermatology and Venereology*, vol. 24, no. 5, pp. 604–606, 2010.

[7] I. A. Rivera-Olivero, A. Guevara, A. Escalona et al., "Soft tissue infections due to non-tuberculous mycobacteria following mesotherapy. What is the price of beauty?" *Enfermedades Infecciosas y Microbiologia Clinica*, vol. 24, no. 5, pp. 302–306, 2006.

[8] P. Schütz, H. H. Ibrahim, S. S. Hussain, T. S. Ali, K. El-Bassuoni, and J. Thomas, "Infected facial tissue fillers: case series and review of the literature," *Journal of Oral and Maxillofacial Surgery*, vol. 70, no. 10, pp. 2403–2412, 2012.

[9] C. R. Millet, A. V. Halpern, and A. C. Reboli, "Bacterial disesase," in *Dermatology*, J. L. Bolognia, J. L. Jorizzo, J. W. Schaffer, and W. R. Heymann, Eds., p. 1198, Elsevier Saunders, 3rd edition, 2012.

24

Granulomatous Cheilitis: Successful Treatment of Two Recalcitrant Cases with Combination Drug Therapy

Ambika Gupta and Harneet Singh

Department of Oral Medicine and Radiology, Pandit B.D. Sharma UHS (PGIDS), Rohtak, Haryana, India

Correspondence should be addressed to Ambika Gupta; drambika79@rediffmail.com

Academic Editor: Bhushan Kumar

Granulomatous cheilitis is a rare, idiopathic, inflammatory disorder which usually affects young adults. It is characterized by persistent, diffuse, nontender, soft-to-firm swelling of one or both lips. Various treatment modalities have been suggested. In spite of the best treatment, recurrence of the disease is very common. We report two cases of granulomatous cheilitis treated with a combination of steroids, metronidazole, and minocycline with no signs of relapse at one-year follow-up.

1. Introduction

Orofacial granulomatosis comprises a group of diseases characterized by noncaseating granulomatous inflammation affecting the soft tissues of the oral and maxillofacial region [1]. The term, introduced by Wiesenfeld et al. in 1985, includes Melkersson-Rosenthal syndrome and cheilitis granulomatosa of Miescher [2]. Melkersson-Rosenthal syndrome manifest itself as a triad of recurrent or persistent lip or facial swelling, recurrent, partial, or complete facial paralysis, and fissured tongue [3, 4]. Cheilitis granulomatosa of Miescher is characterized by swelling restricted to the lips [5]. Granulomatous cheilitis is considered a monosymptomatic form of Melkersson-Rosenthal syndrome by some clinicians. The etiology of this disease is unclear, but the condition has been linked to an abnormal immune reaction. The available therapeutic options provide only limited and temporary remissions. Two cases of granulomatous cheilitis are being reported, who showed an excellent and sustained response to combination of intralesional steroids, metronidazole, and minocycline.

2. Case 1

A 17-year-old female reported in an outdoor department of Oral Medicine at Government Dental College, Rohtak, with a 2-year history of persistent asymptomatic swelling of the upper lip and occasional gingival swelling (Figure 1). Her medical history was noncontributory. There was no history suggestive of abdominal cramps, diarrhea, fatigue, weight loss, or any other gastrointestinal disorders. Systemic examination did not reveal any abnormalities. Examination revealed a nontender, diffuse, firm swelling of the upper lip. The surrounding facial skin showed diffuse erythematous swelling. The surface of the lip was smooth with no signs of scabs, bleeding, or exudation. No fissuring of the tongue, oral ulcers, or hypertrophy of the oral mucosa was noticed. There was no palsy of facial muscles. The patient had received intralesional triamcinolone injections in the past with temporary remissions and recurrences of the swelling. A chest radiograph, complete haemogram, erythrocyte sedimentation rate, serum folate, iron, and vitamin B12 levels, serum levels of angiotensin-converting enzyme, were ordered, which were in normal range. The tuberculin skin test for tuberculosis was negative. Ultrasonography of the upper lip revealed a mildly increased vascularity in the region. The diagnosis of cheilitis granulomatosa was confirmed on a histopathological examination, which revealed Langhans type giant cells, epithelioid cells, lymphocytes, and few neutrophils (Figure 2). We decided to treat her with a combination of intralesional weekly injections of triamcinolone acetonide 10 mg/mL in the upper lip for 4 weeks, along with oral metronidazole 400 mg three times a day

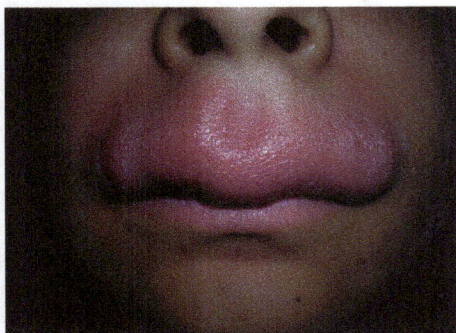

FIGURE 1: Pretreatment view of the swelling in the first patient showing diffuse, erythematous swelling of upper lip.

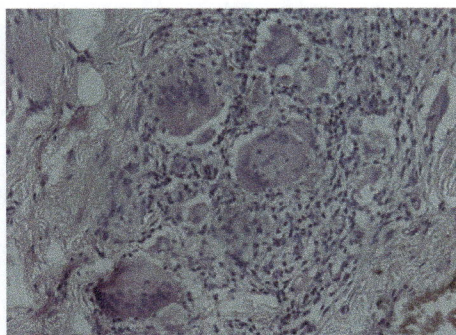

FIGURE 2: Histopathological pictures showing Langhans giant cells, epithelioid cells, lymphocytes, and neutrophils.

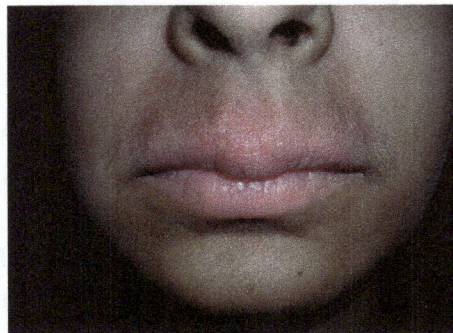

FIGURE 3: Posttreatment view of the first patient with marked improvement of swelling and erythema.

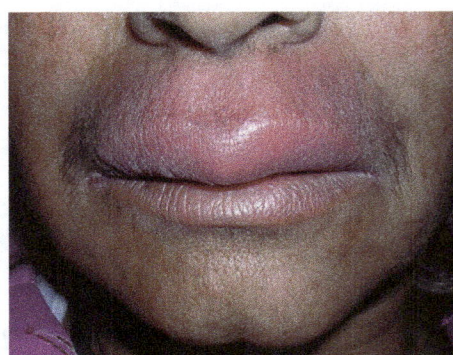

FIGURE 4: Pretreatment photograph of second patient showing diffuse swelling of upper lip.

and oral minocycline 100 mg daily. There was a significant improvement in the labial swelling and erythema after 15 days of treatment. The gingival swelling also subsided after 20 days. After one month, metronidazole was withdrawn and minocycline was continued on alternate days for an additional one month. A recurrence of swelling of the upper lip was noticed after 4 months, which subsided with an injection of intralesional triamcinolone acetonide solution 10 mg/mL. In a 1-year follow-up, there was no further recurrence (Figure 3).

3. Case 2

A 58-year-old female reported with a 6-month history of asymptomatic swelling of the upper lip. Her medical history was noncontributory. She reported no intestinal problems that would suggest Crohn's disease, nor did she complain of chronic fatigue. There was no history of tuberculosis. Examination revealed a nontender, diffuse, erythematous, and firm- to-soft swelling of the upper lip. The surface of the lip was dry and smooth (Figure 4). There were no appreciable changes in the tongue or any ulceration of the oral mucosa. All the investigations done to rule out other differential diagnoses were within normal ranges. These included chest radiography and assessment of serum levels of angiotensin-converting enzyme for sarcoidosis; complete blood count, erythrocyte sedimentation rate and serum levels

of folic acid, iron and vitamin B12 for Crohn's disease; and tuberculin skin test and chest radiography for tuberculosis. Histopathological findings revealed perivascular lymphocytic infiltration and noncaseating granulomas that were not well formed. Ziehl-Neelsen and periodic acid-Schiff (PAS) staining yielded negative results. We started the treatment with intralesional triamcinolone injections in the upper lip without any improvement. So, we decided to treat her with the same combination of intralesional triamcinolone acetonide 10 mg/mL, oral metronidazole 400 mg three times a day, and oral minocycline 100 mg daily, as in the previous case. We noticed a significant improvement in the labial swelling after 1 month of treatment. After one month, metronidazole was withdrawn and minocycline was continued on alternate days for an additional one month. At 1-year follow-up, there was no sign of recurrence (Figure 5).

4. Discussion

The exact etiology of orofacial granulomatosis is unknown [6]. Several theories have been postulated, including infection, genetic predisposition, and allergy [7–9]. A monoclonal lymphocytic expression, secondary to the chronic antigenic stimulation, cytokine production leading to granulomas formation, and a cell-mediated hypersensitivity reaction have also been suggested [10].

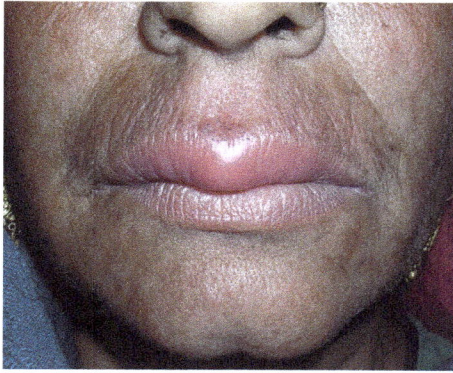

FIGURE 5: Posttreatment photograph of the second patient after 1 year.

The clinical features of orofacial granulomatosis are highly variable. The classical clinical presentation of cheilitis granulomatosa is recurrent labial swelling of one or both lips [11]. The swellings are soft-to-firm in its consistency and nontender and eventually become persistent. Sometimes, the swelling extends to the chin, cheeks, periorbital region, and eyelids [12]. Rarely, superficial amber colored vesicles, resembling lymphangiomas, may be seen [13]. Intraorally the disease may cause gingival hypertrophy, erythema, pain, and erosions. The predominant lesions are edema, ulcers, and papules. The tongue may develop fissures, edema, paresthesia, erosions, or taste alterations. Cobblestone appearance of buccal mucosa may be seen. The palate may have papules or hyperplastic tissue [13]. Both cases reported here had a persistent swelling of the upper lip with gingival enlargement in the first case.

Orofacial granulomatosis may occur as the oral manifestation of a systemic condition, such as Crohn's disease, Sarcoidosis, or more rarely Wegener's granulomatosis [14]. Other differential diagnoses include tuberculosis, leprosy, systemic fungal infections and foreign body reactions, amyloidosis, certain soft-tissue tumours, angioedema, minor salivary gland tumour, and Ascher's syndrome [11]. All these local and systemic conditions may be a diagnostic dilemma and must be excluded by appropriate clinical and laboratory investigations [6, 14]. In the present cases, as the history and initial investigations were not suggestive of any gastrointestinal involvement, an in-depth evaluation of the gastrointestinal system did not appear justified.

The management of granulomatous cheilitis becomes difficult in the absence of knowledge concerning its etiology. The treatment objectives are to improve the patient's clinical appearance and comfort. Although rare, spontaneous remission is possible [1]. The elimination of odontogenic infections may reduce the swelling in certain patients [15].

First-line treatment is local or systemic corticosteroids or both. Intralesional injections of triamcinolone 10–40 mg/mL are often helpful [16]. However, relapses are common, with the use of corticosteroids, and long-term treatment may be required. Other therapeutic measures have been reported in the literature, including hydroxychloroquine, methotrexate,

clofazimine, metronidazole, minocycline, thalidomide, dapsone, and danazol [17–19]. Cheiloplasty is reserved for resistant cases or those complicated by a major lip deformation.

Coskun et al. have reported successful results with a combination of intralesional steroids and metronidazole [20]. Similarly, Stein and Mancini treated two children successfully, with a combination of oral prednisolone and minocycline [21]. Dar et al. used a combination of intralesional triamcinolone, metronidazole, and minocycline to treat a patient and observed a marked improvement in the lip swelling after one month treatment [22]. We also decided to follow the same regimen as tried by Dar et al. in our two cases.

We injected the patient weekly with intralesional triamcinolone acetonide solution 10 mg/mL in the upper lip (0.25–0.50 mL at three points) for 4 weeks and prescribed oral metronidazole tablets 400 mg, three times a day, and oral minocycline 100 mg daily for one month. A significant decrease in swelling was noticed in both the patients after a period of 15 days. After one month, intralesional steroid and metronidazole were discontinued. Minocycline, however, was continued in a dose of 100 mg on alternate days for the next month. The dose of minocycline was tapered to look out for any relapse and to get sustained results. Both patients were followed up regularly for a period of one year without any relapses. The complete remission of the swelling may be attributable to the potent anti-inflammatory action of the drug combination used here. The treatment was well tolerated by both patients with no evidence of any side effects.

5. Conclusion

Based upon our experience with the two reported cases, we agree with the observations of Dar et al. We also recommend that a combination of intralesional triamcinolone injection, along with oral metronidazole and minocycline, seems to be an effective remedy for successful and sustained response in granulomatous cheilitis. Further, randomized case control trials are needed for establishing a universally accepted protocol for management of cheilitis granulomatosa.

Conflict of Interests

The authors declare that there is no conflict of interests regarding the publication of this paper.

References

[1] J. J. Sciubba and N. Said-Al-Naief, "Orofacial granulomatosis: presentation, pathology and management of 13 cases," *Journal of Oral Pathology and Medicine*, vol. 32, no. 10, pp. 576–585, 2003.

[2] D. Wiesenfeld, M. M. Ferguson, D. N. Mitchell et al., "Oro-facial granulomatosis—a clinical and pathological analysis," *Quarterly Journal of Medicine*, vol. 54, no. 213, pp. 101–113, 1985.

[3] R. M. Greene and R. S. Rogers III, "Melkersson-Rosenthal syndrome: a review of 36 patients," *Journal of the American Academy of Dermatology*, vol. 21, no. 6, pp. 1263–1270, 1989.

[4] A. C. Spielmann, F. Maury, and J. L. George, "Melkersson-Rosenthal syndrome: clinical, evolutive concepts," *Journal Francais d'Ophtalmologie*, vol. 23, no. 3, pp. 261–264, 2000.

[5] M. El-Hakim and P. Chauvin, "Orofacial granulomatosis presenting as persistent lip swelling: review of 6 new cases," *Journal of Oral and Maxillofacial Surgery*, vol. 62, no. 9, pp. 1114–1117, 2004.

[6] F. Alawi, "Granulomatous diseases of the oral tissues: differential diagnosis and update," *Dental Clinics of North America*, vol. 49, no. 1, pp. 203–221, 2005.

[7] D. W. Patton, M. M. Ferguson, A. Forsyth, and J. James, "ORO-facial granulomatosis: a possible allergic basis," *British Journal of Oral and Maxillofacial Surgery*, vol. 23, no. 4, pp. 235–242, 1985.

[8] R. D. Carr, "Is the Melkersson-Rosenthal syndrome hereditary?" *Archives of Dermatology*, vol. 93, no. 4, pp. 426–427, 1966.

[9] R. R. Muellegger, W. Weger, N. Zoechling et al., "Granulomatous cheilitis and *Borrelia burgdorferi*: polymerase chain reaction and serologic studies in a retrospective case series of 12 patients," *Archives of Dermatology*, vol. 136, no. 12, pp. 1502–1506, 2000.

[10] S. H. Lim, P. Stephens, Q.-X. Cao, S. Coleman, and D. W. Thomas, "Molecular analysis of T cell receptor β variability in a patient with orofacial granulomatosis," *Gut*, vol. 40, no. 5, pp. 683–686, 1997.

[11] C. M. Allen, C. Camisa, S. Hamzeh, and L. Stephens, "Cheilitis granulomatosa: report of six cases and review of the literature," *Journal of the American Academy of Dermatology*, vol. 23, no. 3, pp. 444–450, 1990.

[12] M. D. Mignogna, S. Fedele, L. Lo Russo, and L. Lo Muzlo, "The multiform and variable patterns of onset of orofacial granulomatosis," *Journal of Oral Pathology & Medicine*, vol. 32, no. 4, pp. 200–205, 2003.

[13] B. W. Neville, D. D. Damm, C. M. Allen, and J. E. Bouquot, Eds., *Oral and Maxillofacial Pathology*, W.B. Saunders Company, Toronto, Canada, 2nd edition, 2002.

[14] C. Girlich, T. Bogenrieder, K.-D. Palitzsch, J. Schölmerich, and G. Lock, "Orofacial granulomatosis as initial manifestation of Crohn's disease: a report of two cases," *European Journal of Gastroenterology and Hepatology*, vol. 14, no. 8, pp. 873–876, 2002.

[15] N. Worsaae, K. C. Christensen, M. Schiodt, and J. Reibel, "Melkersson-Rosenthal syndrome and cheilitis granulomatosa. A clinicopathologic study of thirty-three patients with special reference to their oral lesions," *Oral Surgery Oral Medicine and Oral Pathology*, vol. 54, no. 4, pp. 404–413, 1982.

[16] A. Sakuntabhai, R. I. MacLeod, and C. M. Lawrence, "Intralesional steroid injection after nerve block anesthesia in the treatment of orofacial granulomatosis," *Archives of Dermatology*, vol. 129, no. 4, pp. 477–480, 1993.

[17] R. I. F. van der Waal, E. A. J. M. Schulten, E. H. van der Meij, M. R. van de Scheur, T. M. Starink, and I. van der Waal, "Cheilitis granulomatosa: overview of 13 patients with long-term follow-up—results of management," *International Journal of Dermatology*, vol. 41, no. 4, pp. 225–229, 2002.

[18] M. Medeiros Jr., M. I. Araujo, N. S. Guimarães, L. A. Rodrigue, T. M. C. Silva, and E. M. Carvalho, "Therapeutic response to thalidomide in Melkersson-Rosenthal syndrome: a case report," *Annals of Allergy, Asthma and Immunology*, vol. 88, no. 4, pp. 421–424, 2002.

[19] A. Hegarty, T. Hodgson, and S. Porter, "Thalidomide for the treatment of recalcitrant oral Crohn's disease and orofacial granulomatosis," *Oral Surgery, Oral Medicine, Oral Pathology, Oral Radiology, and Endodontics*, vol. 95, no. 5, pp. 576–585, 2003.

[20] B. Coskun, Y. Saral, D. Cicek, and N. Akpolat, "Treatment and follow-up of persistent granulomatous cheilitis with intralesional steroid and metronidazole," *Journal of Dermatological Treatment*, vol. 15, no. 5, pp. 333–335, 2004.

[21] S. L. Stein and A. J. Mancini, "Melkersson-Rosenthal syndrome in childhood: successful management with combination steroid and minocycline therapy," *Journal of the American Academy of Dermatology*, vol. 41, no. 5, pp. 746–748, 1999.

[22] N. R. Dar, N. Raza, A. Nadeem, and A. Manzoor, "*Granulomatous cheilitis*: sustained response to combination of intralesional steroids, metronidazole and minocycline," *Journal of the College of Physicians and Surgeons—Pakistan*, vol. 17, pp. 566–567, 2007.

25

A Gigantic Anogenital Lesion: Buschke-Lowenstein Tumor

Rikinder Sandhu, Zaw Min, and Nitin Bhanot

Department of Medicine, Allegheny General Hospital, 420 East North Avenue, Allegheny Health Network, Pittsburgh, PA 15212, USA

Correspondence should be addressed to Nitin Bhanot; nitinbhanot@gmail.com

Academic Editor: Xing-Hua Gao

Buschke-Lowenstein tumor is a relatively rare sexually transmitted disease. It is a neoplasm of the anogenital region which has benign appearance on histopathology but is locally destructive. It carries a high recurrence rate and a significant potential for malignant transformation. Human papilloma virus has been implicated as an etiologic agent for this tumor. Since this disease is rare and no controlled studies exist, radical excision of this anogenital lesion is generally recommended as the first line therapy and close vigilance and followup are essential. We have discussed an overview of etiopathogenesis, clinical presentation, diagnosis, and management of this uncommonly encountered disease.

1. Case Presentation

A 65-year-old man presented to the hospital with 1-week history of bloody and foul smelling discharge from his groin. The patient had initially noticed a small lesion of approximate dimension of a pea in his right inguinal area about 20 years ago. Since the lesion did not bother him at that time, he did not seek medical care until when he started to notice blood oozing from it. The lesion had increased in size multifold over the years and had extended into the left groin and the perineal region. It was not painful, but caused some discomfort mainly during sitting. He reported no fevers, loss of weight, urinary symptoms, or difficulty in defecation and denied any other skin lesions elsewhere. All other reviews of systems were essentially unremarkable. He was in a monogamous relationship with his wife who had passed away 10 years prior to presentation. He denied previous promiscuous behavior.

On examination, patient was afebrile and hemodynamically stable. An extensive, foul-smelling cauliflower-shaped lesion was apparent in the inguinal regions bilaterally. It measured around 15 cm in width in each groin along the maximum dimension, and about 40 cm in length, extending from the waist line through the groin into the intergluteal cleft towards the rectum (Figure 1). It had also involved the lateral aspects and base of the scrotum. The lesion was not tender. Remainder of the physical examination was normal. Laboratory studies revealed leukocytosis (white blood cell

count 15,300 per mm^3), hemoglobin 14.3 gm/dL, and platelet count 284,000 per mm^3. Renal and liver function tests were normal.

Human immunodeficiency virus and rapid plasma reagin serological tests were nonreactive. Urine analysis and blood cultures were unremarkable. Contrast enhanced computed tomography of chest, abdomen, and pelvis was done that did not reveal any regional lymph node involvement or evidence of distant metastasis.

Based on the clinical presentation, a diagnosis of giant condyloma acuminatum of Buschke-Lowenstein was suspected. The lesion was radically excised and the entire specimen was sent for gross pathological examination (Figure 2) and histopathology (Figures 3 and 4). Grossly, the tumor appeared as fungating, exophytic, cauliflower-shaped like mass. It was hard in consistency and gave the look of a bulky tumor. On histopathology, there was evidence of epidermal hyperplasia, hyperkeratosis, and papillomatosis (Figure 3). Koilocytes (vacuolated cells with clear cytoplasm and perinuclear halo), a result of infection from HPV, were seen on higher magnification (Figure 4). There were no histopathologic features of malignant transformation.

A final diagnosis of condyloma acuminata of BLT (superficially invasive verrucous carcinoma with pathological staging T1) was made. The patient has not had a recurrence of the tumor for 3 years from the time of radical excision.

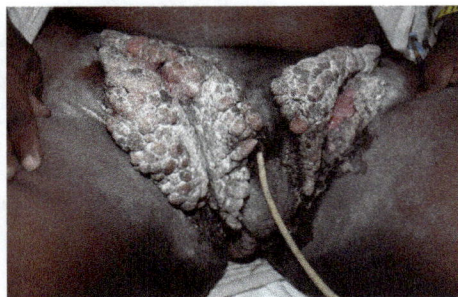

FIGURE 1

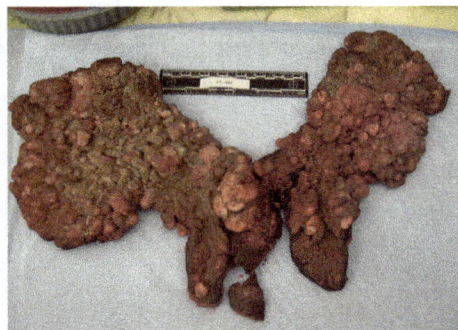

FIGURE 2

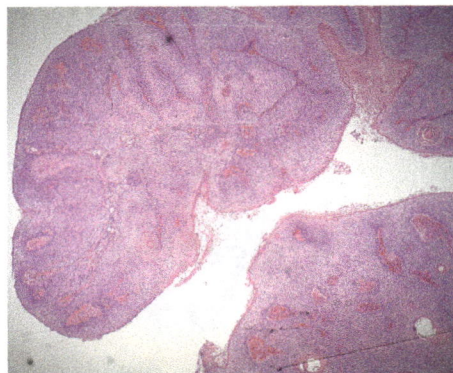

FIGURE 3

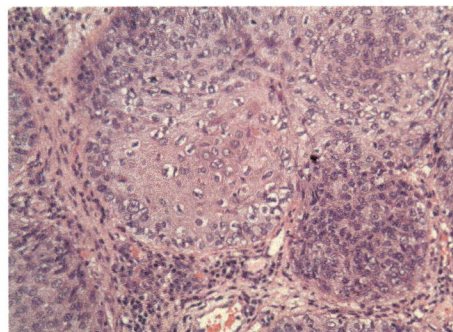

FIGURE 4

2. Discussion

Giant condyloma acuminata was first described by Buschke and Loewenstein in 1925 in the penis and they named it "condyloma acuminate carcinoma-like" [1]. Since then, it has also been reported in the anorectal and perineal regions [2]. The vulva is the predominant location in females [3]. While the characteristic feature of Buschke-Lowenstein tumor (BLT) is benign appearance on histopathology, the lesion has locally destructive behaviour and may undergo malignant transformation [2, 4]. Therefore, some authors support the hypothesis that BLT is an intermediary lesion between condyloma acuminata and squamous cell carcinoma [4]. However, others and probably a majority of them, equate it to verrucous carcinoma (a well-differentiated variety of squamous cell carcinoma) of the anogenital region [3].

It is a sexually transmitted disease with an estimated incidence of about 0.1% in the general population [3]. Human papilloma virus (HPV) has been linked to the etiopathogenesis of BLT [3]. HPV DNA types 6 and 11 have been most commonly recovered from pathological specimens of BLT, suggesting a pathogenic role [2].

To confirm histopathologically, deeper tissue must be biopsied to ensure that no malignant cytological characteristics are missed in superficially biopsied specimens [3]. Radical excision of the entire lesion is suggested because it serves the dual purpose of making the diagnosis and helping therapeutically with the highest chances of cure [3].

While a variety of treatment modalities (surgery, chemotherapy (systemic and intralesional), carbon dioxide laser therapy, and photodynamic therapy) have been used for the treatment of BLT, wide surgical excision by Mohs technique is recommended as the most important therapeutic intervention [2]. Since this is a rare disease and no robust controlled studies have been conducted, no standardized management strategies exist. Chemoradiation has been recommended in cases when malignant transformation may occur [3]. Intra-arterial chemotherapy with agents such as methotrexate has also been successfully utilized in verrucous carcinoma of different parts of the body, including the anogenital region [5, 6]. This modality may be used as neoadjuvant therapy before surgical intervention and in certain cases may obviate the need for surgery [5, 6]. Radiation therapy alone has generally been discouraged because of potential risk of transformation into anaplastic carcinoma [7].

Since radical excision was achieved with peripheral and deep margins free of tumor and no regional lymphadenopathy was noted, the oncologist did not recommend additional modalities such as chemotherapy in our patient. Vigilant and prolonged surveillance was suggested. This is important because this tumor has been reported to have a significant rate of recurrence (66%) and malignant transformation (56%) with an overall mortality of 20% [8]. The tumor may also form abscesses and fistulae in the perianal region [9].

Since all lesions of BLT initially start as condyloma acuminata and progress over many years, this entity is likely preventable to an extent by vaccination against certain strains of HPV and seeking timely medical attention. Our case adds to this relatively rare disease and highlights the importance of timely detection, aggressive management, and close surveillance to improve patient outcomes.

Conflict of Interests

The authors declare that there is no conflict of interests regarding the publication of this paper.

Authors' Contribution

All authors had access to the paper and a role in writing and editing it.

References

[1] A. Buschke and L. Loewenstein, "Über carcinomahnliche condylomata acuminata des penis," *Klinische Wochenschrift*, vol. 4, no. 36, pp. 1726–1728, 1925.

[2] M. Ahsaini, Y. Tahiri, M. F. Tazi et al., "Verrucous carcinoma arising in an extended giant condyloma acuminatum (Buschke-Löwenstein tumor): a case report and review of the literature," *Journal of Medical Case Reports*, vol. 7, article 273, 2013.

[3] A. Lévy and C. Lebbe, "Buschke-Löwenstein tumour: diagnosis and treatment," *Annales d'Urologie*, vol. 40, no. 3, pp. 175–178, 2006.

[4] C. Creasman, P. A. Haas, T. A. Fox Jr., and M. Balazs, "Malignant transformation of anorectal giant condyloma acuminatum (Buschke-Loewenstein tumor)," *Diseases of the Colon & Rectum*, vol. 32, no. 6, pp. 481–487, 1989.

[5] P. H. Chiang, C. H. Chen, and Y. C. Shen, "Intraarterial chemotherapy as the first-line therapy in penile cancer," *The British Journal of Cancer*, vol. 111, no. 6, pp. 1089–1094, 2014.

[6] C.-F. Wu, C.-M. Chen, Y.-S. Shen et al., "Effective eradication of oral verrucous carcinoma with continuous intraarterial infusion chemotherapy," *Head and Neck*, vol. 30, no. 5, pp. 611–617, 2008.

[7] M. Fukunaga, K. Yokoi, Y. Miyazawa, T. Harada, and S. Ushigome, "Penile verrucous carcinoma with anaplastic transformation following radiotherapy: a case report with human papillomavirus typing and flow cytometric DNA studies," *The American Journal of Surgical Pathology*, vol. 18, no. 5, pp. 501–505, 1994.

[8] Q. D. Chu, M. P. Vezeridis, N. P. Libbey, and H. J. Wanebo, "Giant condyloma acuminatum (Buschke-Lowenstein tumor) of the anorectal and perianal regions: analysis of 42 cases," *Diseases of the Colon and Rectum*, vol. 37, no. 9, pp. 950–957, 1994.

[9] M. Bjorck, L. Athlin, and B. A. Lundskog, "Giant consyloma acuminatum (Buschke Lowenstein tumor of the anrectum with malignant transformation)," *European Journal of Surgery*, vol. 161, pp. 691–694, 1995.

26

Keloidal Scleroderma: Case Report and Review

Sama Kassira, Tarannum Jaleel, Peter Pavlidakey, and Naveed Sami

Department of Dermatology, University of Alabama at Birmingham, EFH 414, 1530 3rd Avenue S, Birmingham, AL 35294, USA

Correspondence should be addressed to Naveed Sami; nsami@uab.edu

Academic Editor: Jacek Cezary Szepietowski

Objective. We report a rare case of keloidal scleroderma and provide an analysis of similar cases. *Results.* A 41 year-old woman presented with dark brown, indurated, exophytic nodules over the chest along with smaller hyperpigmented plaques scattered over the abdomen, with concomitant sclerodactyly. The clinical, laboratory, and pathological findings were consistent with a diagnosis of keloidal scleroderma. The patient was treated with methotrexate, resulting in reduced firmness of her plaques and no new lesions. A literature review of previously reported cases was performed using keywords including keloidal morphea, keloidal scleroderma, nodular morphea, and nodular scleroderma. In our review, the majority of patients were African American and female. 91% of cases had nodular lesions with distribution on the trunk. The majority of patients exhibited sclerodactyly and pulmonary involvement was reported in 28%1. The majority of patients were ANA positive (63%) and only 10% demonstrated anti-SCL-70 positivity. *Conclusion.* Keloidal scleroderma is a rare presentation, which can often be clinically confused with keloid and scar formation. Due to this being a rare variant, our knowledge of treatment options and efficacy is limited. Methotrexate could be considered as an initial treatment option for patients with progressive keloidal scleroderma.

1. Introduction

Keloidal scleroderma is a very rare diagnosis, which has been also reported with alternate nomenclature including keloidal morphea, nodular morphea, and nodular sclero-derma. Keloidal scleroderma presents as multiple keloid-like lesions that occur in the absence of preceding trauma or injury and can be associated with localized or systemic symptoms of scleroderma. This is in contrast to the flat and/or depressed plaques with associated tightening of the skin that is seen in classical cutaneous scleroderma. Histopathological findings in keloidal scleroderma can be variable. We report a 41-year-old woman with keloidal scleroderma and provide a review of 43 reported cases of this variant of scleroderma.

2. Case

A 41-year-old African American woman presented with initial symptoms of burning and stinging of the upper body for over 4 weeks, progressing to dark firm painful areas on her chest, neck, and abdomen with concomitant sclerodactyly. She denied tightening around her mouth, dry eyes or mouth, arthritis, dysphagia, or signs of Raynaud's phenomenon.

Physical examination revealed dark brown indurated nodules with a slightly violaceous border over the chest and breasts along with smaller hyperpigmented plaques scattered over the abdomen (Figure 1). There was also extensive hyperpigmentation and skin tightening over the anterior neck, chest, axillae, and abdomen. A hypertrophic, exophytic papule overlying a hyperpigmented plaque was present over the center of the chest. Examination of the hands showed a contracture of the left hand 4th and 5th digits with slight tapering of the fingertips. There was sparing of the face and telangiectasias were absent.

Complete blood count, metabolic panel, and hepatitis serologies did not reveal any abnormalities. Serum ANA (antinuclear antibody) titer was elevated (1:1280). Anti-SSA and anti-SSB serum antibodies were both elevated, while SCL70 and anti-Smith autoantibody titers were within normal limits.

Histologic sections show an acanthotic epidermis with overlying basilar hyperpigmentation. Within the dermis there is a proliferation of myofibroblasts and thickened collagen bundles. There is a lack of vertically oriented blood vessels and a lack of atrophy of the overlying epidermis speaking against that of a keloid or scar. At low power biopsy

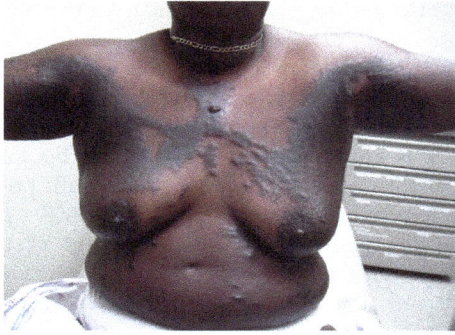

FIGURE 1: Keloidal scleroderma. Multiple, scattered, and hyperpigmented nodules overlying plaques along the trunk and upper extremities.

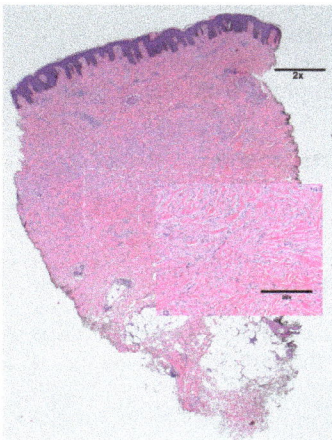

FIGURE 2: Keloidal scleroderma. Histologic sections show an acanthotic epidermis with overlying basilar hyperpigmentation. Within the dermis there is a proliferation of myofibroblasts and thickened collagen bundles. There is a lack of vertically oriented blood vessels and a lack of atrophy of the overlying epidermis speaking against that of a keloid or scar. At low power (2x) biopsy has a barrel-shaped appearance. The dermal component is expansile and extends beyond that of the epidermal component.

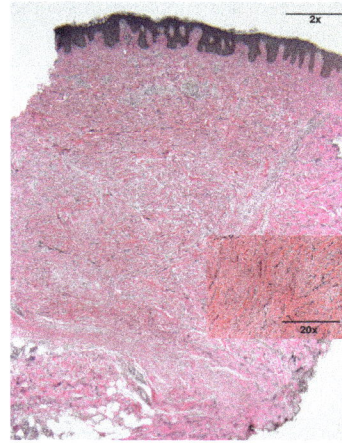

FIGURE 3: A tissue elastic stain shows preserved elastic fibers within areas of scleroderma. In areas of keloid these elastic fibers are typically absent, thus supporting the diagnosis of keloidal scleroderma and not that of a keloid.

has a barrel-shaped appearance. The dermal component is expansile and extends beyond that of the epidermal component (Figure 2). A tissue elastic stain shows preserved elastic fibers within areas of scleroderma (Figure 3). In areas of keloid these elastic fibers are typically absent, thus supporting the diagnosis of keloidal scleroderma and not that of a keloid.

The clinical and pathological findings were consistent with a diagnosis of keloidal scleroderma. The patient was treated with methotrexate (17.5 mg/week) for six weeks resulting in reduced firmness of her plaques and no new lesions.

3. Discussion

Keloidal scleroderma is a rare presentation, which can often be clinically confused with keloid and scar formation. Although there have been some reports suggesting that keloidal scleroderma may represent two distinct processes with keloid formation causally unrelated to sclerosis, others suggest that there is a combined mechanism with a dermal inflammatory process of sclerosis forming keloidal lesions [1]. High levels of tenascin have been histologically observed in keloidal scleroderma lesions as well as increased levels of TFG-beta cytokines [1, 2]. Tenascin has been shown to have distinct mid-dermal distribution in sclerodermal lesions, reflecting active fibrosis [1]. A strikingly different tenascin distribution in the nodular lesions of a single case as compared to sclerotic tissue has been shown, suggesting a differing pathological course between the nodular and sclerotic lesions [1]. However, keloidal scleroderma lesions have shown increased levels of TGF-beta and connective tissue growth factor (CTF), which is similarly seen in fibroblasts of classic sclerodermal lesions suggesting analogous pathogenesis of collagen synthesis [1, 2].

We performed a literature review for previously reported cases using keywords, which have been used to describe similar clinical presentations, including keloidal morphea, keloidal scleroderma, nodular morphea, and nodular scleroderma. All cases where the clinical presentation was confirmed by a histopathological diagnosis were included. Clinical data of 43 patients from 29 different publications is presented in Table 1.

In our review, the majority of patients were African American and female. Ages ranged from 3 to 70 years (median 41). 91% of cases had nodular lesions with distribution on the trunk, while one case had lesions in the intertriginous areas. The majority of patients presented with sclerodactyly as well as extracutaneous manifestations of systemic scleroderma (Table 1). Pulmonary involvement was reported in 28% and renal involvement in 5% [1]. Ten percent of cases noted an external trigger prior to the onset of keloidal plaques, including infection, D-penicillamine, tetanus vaccine, and environmental exposures. One patient, who already had a diagnosis of keloidal scleroderma, did not have any involvement at a recent surgical site [1].

TABLE 1: Patient characteristics, clinical manifestations, and laboratory findings in keloidal scleroderma.

Patient characteristics	% of total patients
Gender	
Female	70
Male	30
Race	
African American	59
Caucasian	30
Hispanic	7
Middle Eastern	4
Clinical manifestation	58
Sclerodactyly	58
Raynaud's	47
Arthritis	30
Pulmonary involvement	28
Esophageal dysmotility	23
Renal involvement	5
Distribution	
Trunk	91
Acral	60
Head/neck	35
Intertriginous	2
External trigger	10
Laboratory results	
ANA	63
Elevated ESR	15
Anti-Scl-70	10

Laboratory values demonstrated the majority of patients were ANA positive (63%) and only 10% demonstrated anti-SCL-70 positivity. A single case noted positive anti-*Borrelia* antibodies and two cases were seropositive for anti-SSB [1].

Current treatments for cutaneous and systemic sclerosis include topical or intralesional corticosteroids, a topical vitamin D analog, topical tacrolimus or imiquimod, UV light therapy, methotrexate, and systemic steroids [3–5].

Thirteen out of 22 cases were treated with local and/or systemic steroids. The majority reported no response to treatment. Only three cases showed partial response with local and/or systemic steroid therapy and one case showed complete response to systemic steroids. D-penicillamine was used in 6 patients and only one patient had full resolution with 5 years of oral D-penicillamine in combination with topical steroids. However, one patient showed progression while on therapy [1, 6–9]. Both patients who showed complete response to D-penicillamine and systemic steroids had systemic scleroderma with pulmonary involvement [1]. Azathioprine (100 mg daily) was also used in a case for an unknown duration with no resolution. Surgical removal of several large nodules showed complete resolution in one patient [1, 10]. Multiple studies using PUVA showed partial response. However, one case using PUVA in combination with methotrexate and systemic steroids reported no response [2]. Our patient reported a partial response with six weeks of methotrexate

with a decrease in firmness of the keloidal plaques and no new active lesions.

In conclusion, diagnosis of scleroderma should be considered in a patient with extensive keloids. Due to this being a rare variant, our knowledge of treatment options and efficacy is limited. Methotrexate could be considered as an initial treatment option for patients with progressive keloidal scleroderma. Further research is still needed to understand the pathogenesis and treatment of this rare variant of scleroderma.

Abbreviations

ANA: Antinuclear antibody
SSA: Anti-Ro antibody
SSB: Anti-La antibody
TGF: Transforming growth factor
CTF: Connective tissue factor
UV: Ultraviolet
PUVA: Psoralen plus Ultraviolet-A treatment.

Conflict of Interests

The authors have no conflict of interests to declare.

Acknowledgments

All authors have contributed equally to this work and are in agreement with the content of this paper.

References

[1] J. Labandeira, A. León-Mateos, J. M. Suárez-Peñaranda, M. T. Garea, and J. Toribio, "What is nodular-keloidal scleroderma?" *Dermatology*, vol. 207, no. 2, pp. 130–132, 2003.

[2] B. Stadler, M. T. Fontana, A. P. B. Somacal, T. L. Skare, and E. Weingraber, "Systemic sclerosis with keloidal nodules," *Anais Brasileiros de Dermatologia*, vol. 88, supplement 1, no. 6, pp. 75–77, 2013.

[3] B. A. Zwischenberger and H. T. Jacobe, "A systematic review of morphea treatments and therapeutic algorithm," *Journal of the American Academy of Dermatology*, vol. 65, no. 5, pp. 925–941, 2011.

[4] F. H. J. van den Hoogen, A. M. T. Boerbooms, A. J. G. Swaak, J. J. Rasker, H. J. J. van Lier, and L. B. A. van de Putte, "Comparison of methotrexate with placebo in the treatment of systemic sclerosis: a 24 week randomized double-blind trial, followed by a 24 week observational trial," *British Journal of Rheumatology*, vol. 35, no. 4, pp. 364–372, 1996.

[5] J. E. Pope, N. Bellamy, J. R. Seibold et al., "A randomized, controlled trial of methotrexate versus placebo in early diffuse scleroderma," *Arthritis and Rheumatism*, vol. 44, no. 6, pp. 1351–1358, 2001.

[6] L. Melani, M. Caproni, C. Cardinali et al., "A case of nodular scleroderma," *The Journal of Dermatology*, vol. 32, no. 12, pp. 1028–1031, 2005.

[7] H. Mizutani, H. Taniguchi, T. Sakakura, and M. Shimizu, "Nodular scleroderma: focally increased tenascin expression differing from that in the surrounding scleroderma skin," *Journal of Dermatology*, vol. 22, no. 4, pp. 267–271, 1995.

[8] M. Santiago, D. O. de Castro Jr., C. A. Costa, E. S. Passos, and A. Paixão, "Keloidal scleroderma," *Clinical Rheumatology*, vol. 23, no. 1, pp. 50–51, 2004.

[9] T. Sasaki, K. Denpo, H. Ono, and H. Nakajima, "Nodular scleroderma in systemic sclerosis under D-penicillamine therapy," *The Journal of Dermatology*, vol. 19, no. 12, pp. 968–971, 1992.

[10] E. N. Le, J. M. Junkins-Hopkins, N. S. Sherber, and F. M. Wigley, "Nodular/keloidal scleroderma: acquired collagenous nodules in systemic sclerosis," *The Journal of Rheumatology*, vol. 39, no. 3, pp. 660–661, 2012.

27

Perianal Median Raphe Cyst: A Rare Lesion with Unusual Histology and Localization

Betül Ünal, Cumhur İbrahim Başsorgun,
Meryem İlkay Eren Karanis, and Gülsüm Özlem Elpek

School of Medicine, Department of Pathology, Akdeniz University, 07070 Antalya, Turkey

Correspondence should be addressed to Betül Ünal; betulunalmd@gmail.com

Academic Editor: Akimichi Morita

Median raphe cysts present anywhere between the external urethral meatus and the anus. The cysts can occur at parameatus, glans penis, penile shaft, scrotum, or perineum. Perianal region is an extremely rare location for these lesions. Here we present a 50-year-old male patient who presented with a cystic, fluctuant lesion, located at 12 o'clock in perianal region. Microscopic examination revealed a cystic lesion with keratinized and nonkeratinized stratified squamous epithelium, pseudostratified ciliated epithelium, and scattered goblet cells. The final diagnosis of the lesion was median raphe cyst. Ciliated cells and perianal localization in median raphe cysts are extremely rare characteristics.

1. Introduction

Median raphe cysts are common benign lesions that present anywhere between the external urethral meatus and the anus, along midline [1]. It appears commonly in childhood or adolescents [2]. In most patients it is usually asymptomatic or unrecognized during childhood. The cysts become symptomatic with advancing age due to infection or trauma, which make diagnosis difficult. The cysts can occur at any site including parameatus, glans penis, penile shaft, scrotum, or perineum. Presentation of median raphe cyst in the perianal region is exceptional [2]. The epithelial lining of median raphe cysts includes urethral type, epidermoid type, glandular type, and mixed type epithelium [3]. Ciliated epithelium in median raphe cysts is an extremely rare finding [4–6].

According to our knowledge, in English literature our case represents the sixth case of median raphe cyst with ciliated epithelium. In addition, also this is the third case of ciliated median raphe cyst in the perianal region.

2. Case Presentation

A 50-year-old male patient presented with a cystic, fluctuant lesion, located at 12 o'clock in perianal region. Any other pathology was not detected in perineal, scrotal, and perineal area. Surgical procedure was performed and cystic lesion was excised. Microscopic examination revealed a cystic lesion with a diameter of 37 mm and 3 mm wall thickness which was located in the dermis (Figure 1(a)). The epithelial lining of cyst consisted of keratinized and nonkeratinized stratified squamous epithelium (Figure 1(b)), pseudostratified ciliated epithelium (Figure 2), and scattered goblet cells (Figure 3(a)). Under the cyst epithelium, in some areas, hemosiderin laden macrophages, pigment of melanin, were seen. Immunohistochemical Melan-A and histochemical Prussian blue were performed for these areas (Figures 4(a) and 4(b)). Mucin secretion in goblet cells was shown by histochemical mucicarmine staining (Figure 3(b)). At 4 years of followup there was no evidence of recurrence.

3. Discussion

Median raphe cysts are rare congenital lesions along the male external genitalia. Until today, these cases were reported with different terms including mucoid cyst of the penile skin, genitoperineal cyst of the median raphe, parameatal cyst, hydrocystoma, and apocrine cystadenoma. It presents

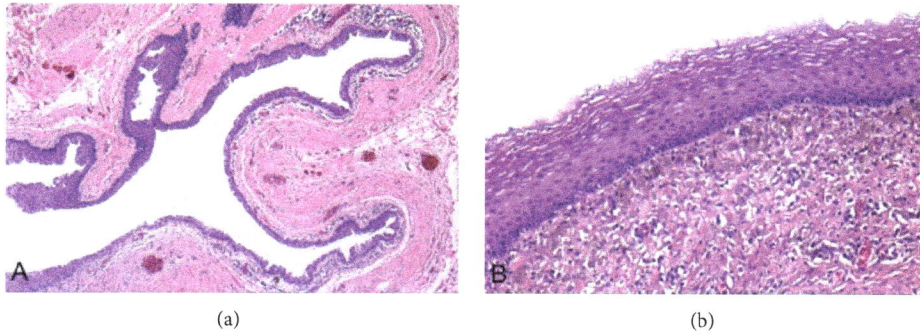

FIGURE 1: (a) Invaginated intradermal cyst. (b) Paved areas with stratified squamous epithelium (hematoxylin and eosin, magnifications (a) ×50, (b) ×200).

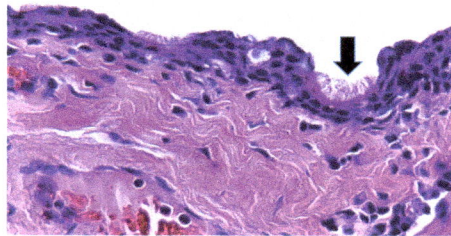

FIGURE 2: Cyst lining ciliated epithelium (arrow) (hematoxylin and eosin, magnification ×200).

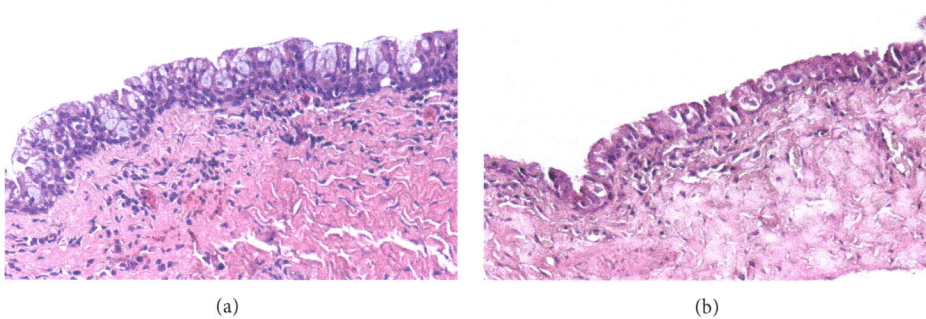

FIGURE 3: (a) Columnar epithelium with scattered goblet cells. (b) Bright pink mucin secretion in goblet cells ((a) hematoxylin and eosin and (b) mucicarmine, magnifications (a) and (b) ×200).

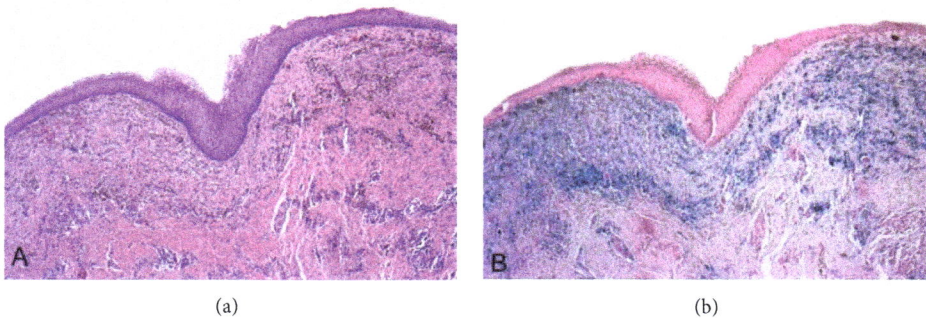

FIGURE 4: (a) Pigmented macrophages under stratified squamous epithelium. (b) This pigmented area consisted of blue colored hemosiderin and brown colored melanin ((a) hematoxylin and eosin and (b) Prussian blue, magnifications (a) and (b) ×100).

TABLE 1: Summary of median raphe cysts with ciliated epithelium.

Literature	Age	Localization
Koga et al., 2007 [11]	27	Penis
Sagar et al., 2006 [5]	65	Perineum (perianal)
Fernández Aceñero and García-González, 2003 [6]	24	Penis
Scelwyn, 1996 [2]	62	Perineum (perianal)
Romani et al., 1995 [4]	N/A	Penis

N/A: not available.

most commonly in the penile shaft [3, 5]. These types of cysts have been reported since 1910 [7] and such cases have been described in case reports. Shao et al. studied this issue in 55 patients with 56 median raphe cysts. According to their study, most (72.7%) of the patients were asymptomatic whereas 9 patients (16.4%) had infectious cysts. They stated that difficulty voiding in patients with cysts located on parameatus and distal prepuce. Respectively, cysts were found on the penile shaft, parameatus, prepuce, glans penis, and scrotum. In addition histopathological types of epithelium were urethral (55.4%), mixed (35.7%), epidermoid (5.4%), and glandular (3.4%) [3]. These findings support that our case is worthy of publication because of perianal location and presence of ciliated epithelium.

Ciliated cells in median raphe cysts are extremely rare and there were only 5 cases reported in the English literature (Table 1). Ciliated cells in median raphe cysts are probably a metaplastic change secondary to local irritation [3].

Median raphe cysts should be differentiated from other conditions such as epidermal cysts, pilonidal cysts, dermoid cysts, and urethral diverticula and especially for perianal location condyloma, viral wart, hemorrhoid, hypertrophied papilla, and neoplastic lesions [2, 8].

The pathogenesis of these cysts was not fully understood. Three different mechanisms have been described including fusion defect of urethral folds, development of the ectopic periurethral glands of Littre, and development from urethral columnar epithelium followed by separation [3].

Immunohistochemistry may be helpful for differential diagnosis in problematic cases.

The treatment of median raphe cysts is simple surgical excision and primary closure [9]. Median raphe cysts may regress spontaneously. Medical intervention may be required due to secondary infection and pain. Also small and asymptomatic cysts in infants can be observed without excision [10].

Conflict of Interests

The authors declare that there is no conflict of interests regarding the publication of this paper.

References

[1] J. G. LeVasseur and V. E. Perry, "Perineal median raphe cyst," *Pediatric Dermatology*, vol. 14, no. 5, pp. 391–392, 1997.

[2] M. Scelwyn, "Median raphe cyst of the perineum presenting as a perianal polyp," *Pathology*, vol. 28, no. 2, pp. 201–202, 1996.

[3] I. H. Shao, T. D. Chen, H. T. Shao, and H. W. Chen, "Male median raphe cysts: serial retrospective analysis and histopathological classification," *Diagnostic Pathology*, vol. 7, article 121, 2012.

[4] J. Romani, M. A. Barnadas, J. Miralles, R. Curell, and J. M. De Moragas, "Median raphe cyst of the penis with ciliated cells," *Journal of Cutaneous Pathology*, vol. 22, no. 4, pp. 378–381, 1995.

[5] J. Sagar, B. Sagar, A. F. Patel, and D. K. Shak, "Ciliated median raphe cyst of perineum presenting as perianal polyp: a case report with immunohistochemical study, review of literature, and pathogenesis," *TheScientificWorldJournal*, vol. 6, pp. 2339–2344, 2006.

[6] M. J. Fernández Aceñero and J. García-González, "Median raphe cyst with ciliated cells: report of a case," *The American Journal of Dermatopathology*, vol. 25, no. 2, pp. 175–176, 2003.

[7] T. Otsuka, Y. Ueda, M. Terauchi, and Y. Kinoshita, "Median raphe (parameatal) cysts of the penis," *The Journal of Urology*, vol. 159, no. 6, pp. 1918–1920, 1998.

[8] E. Nagore, J. M. Sánchez-Motilla, M. I. Febrer, and A. Aliaga, "Median raphe cysts of the penis: a report of five cases," *Pediatric Dermatology*, vol. 15, no. 3, pp. 191–193, 1998.

[9] T. Soyer, A. A. Karabulut, Ö. Boybeyi, and Y. D. Günal, "Scrotal pearl is not always a sign of anorectal malformation: median raphe cyst," *Turkish Journal of Pediatrics*, vol. 55, no. 6, pp. 665–666, 2013.

[10] C. O. Park, E. Y. Chun, and J. H. Lee, "Median raphe cyst on the scrotum and perineum," *Journal of the American Academy of Dermatology*, vol. 55, no. 5, pp. S114–S115, 2006.

[11] K. Koga, Y. Yoshida, M. Koga, M. Takeshita, and J. Nakayama, "Median raphe cyst with ciliated cells of the penis," *Acta Dermato-Venereologica*, vol. 87, no. 6, pp. 542–543, 2007.

28

Methylprednisolone Therapy in Acute Hemorrhagic Edema of Infancy

Jeyanthini Risikesan,[1] **Uffe Koppelhus,**[2] **Torben Steiniche,**[3]
Mette Deleuran,[2] **and Troels Herlin**[1]

[1] *Department of Pediatrics, Aarhus University Hospital, 8200 Aarhus N, Denmark*
[2] *Department of Dermatology, Aarhus University Hospital, Aarhus C, 8000 Aarhus, Denmark*
[3] *Department of Pathology, Aarhus University Hospital, Aarhus C, 8000 Aarhus, Denmark*

Correspondence should be addressed to Troels Herlin; troeherl@rm.dk

Academic Editors: A. Firooz, J. A. Tschen, and T.-W. Wong

We present a case of an 18-month-old boy who showed severe clinical signs indicative of acute hemorrhagic edema of infancy (AHEI) with painful purpuric skin affection primarily of the face and marked edema of the ears. The histological findings were diagnostic for leukocytoclastic vasculitis and thus met the histological criteria for AHEI. Indicative of infection as causative agent for the condition were symptoms of gastroenteritis. High-dose intravenous corticosteroids led to a fast resolution of symptoms and normalization of laboratory parameters. AHEI is usually not described as being very responsive to corticosteroids. The case presented here indicates that severe cases of AHEI can be treated with high-dose intravenous corticosteroids resulting in significant relief and shortening of the symptoms. Clinical followup showed no underlying malignancy or other severe chronic systemic diseases thus confirming earlier reports that AHEI is not associated with such conditions. The differential diagnoses with AHEI are discussed.

1. Introduction

Acute hemorrhagic edema of infancy (AHEI) is an uncommon benign form of cutaneous small-vessel leukocytoclastic vasculitis, which typically affects children from 4 to 24 months of age [1]. AHEI was first described by Snow in 1913 [2]. A case series and systematic review by Fiore et al. [3] has reported approximately 300 patients with AHEI, with a male predominance. The pathogenesis is not fully understood, but a prodromal phase with various infections has been documented in children with AHEI. These include upper respiratory infections, pharyngitis, conjunctivitis, otitis media, bronchitis, urinary tract infections, and pneumonia [4].

AHEI is characterized by the clinical triad of fever; edema of the face, auricles, and extremities; and rosette-shaped purpura. Unlike Henoch-Schönlein purpura (HSP) visceral involvement is infrequent [1]. A correct diagnosis of the disorder is important to distinguish it from other vasculitides. The clinical features of AHEI may be confused with the symptoms seen in (HSP), erythema multiforme (EM), meningococcemia, and septicemia. The diagnostic criteria for AHEI are (1) age younger than 2 years; (2) purpuric or ecchymotic "bruise-like" skin lesions with edema of the face, auricles, and extremities with or without mucosal involvement; (3) lack of systemic disease or visceral involvement and spontaneous recovery within a few days or weeks [5].

AHEI is self-limiting (lasting from one to three weeks) and is not usually considered responsive to corticosteroids [1]. We present a severe case of AHEI in an 18-months-old boy who responded rapidly to high-dose systemic corticosteroids.

2. Case Report

An 18-month-old boy was admitted to the pediatric department with fever and rash. Prior to admission he had a four-day history of gastroenteritis, fever, and incipient skin eruption on the ear and purpuric elements on the extremities.

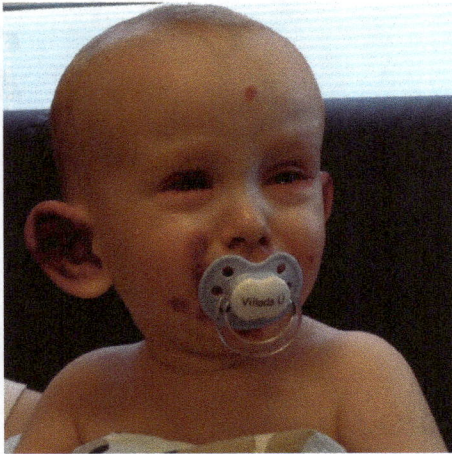

FIGURE 1: Purpura lesions distributed over the face and both ears in an 18-month-old boy. The ears were edematous and had a bright-red, nearly purple color.

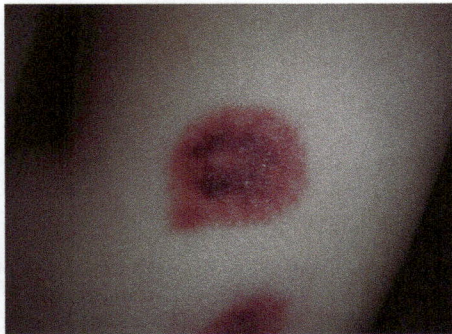

FIGURE 2: Tender, bright-red, infiltrated papules and nodules were found on the extremities and trunk.

On suspicion of meningococcal disease lumbar puncture was performed which revealed normal spinal fluid. Treatment with ceftriaxone was started. The skin lesions progressed, especially in the perioral area, in numbers and size and became bright-red and circular. Moreover, they became increasingly painful for the patient. Also, periorbital blushing was observed. The ears were edematous and had a bright-red, nearly purple color (Figure 1). Furthermore, tender, bright-red, slightly infiltrated papules and nodules were found on the extremities and trunk (Figure 2). The skin was otherwise intact. Temperature was 38.2°C. C-reactive protein (CRP) increased to max. of 135.9 mg/L and erythrocyte sedimentation rate (ESR) to 38 mm/hr. Leukocyte and platelet counts were within normal range. Skin biopsy was performed and high-dose corticosteroid treatment with intravenous (i.v.) methylprednisolone 20 mg/kg/day for 4 days was given. Histology of skin lesion was described as a well-established leukocytoclastic vasculitis with marked fibrinoid necrosis and granulocyte infiltration in the vessel wall (Figure 3). The treatment resulted in immediate declining of the edema and bleaching of the skin lesions and normalization of laboratory parameters. Over the next days a general improvement of

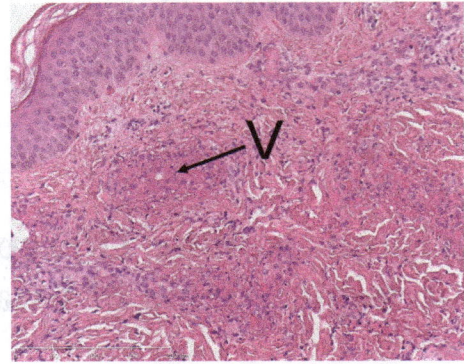

FIGURE 3: Biopsy from cutaneous lesion showed a neutrophilic infiltrate and exudation of fibrin (fibrinoid necrosis) in the walls of small vessels (V) and in their vicinity concordant with leukocytoclastic vasculitis.

the skin symptoms was seen even though a few new skin lesions appeared. Following pulse-steroid treatment with oral prednisolone, 2 mg/kg/day, was continued. Ten days after treatment was started he was readmitted with relapse of fever and relapse of an ecchymosis and several palpable purpura on both lower legs. Pulse-steroid treatment was repeated for 3 days, and all symptoms improved within two days. Prednisolone was then continued and tapered over 12 days. Clinical followup during the next 30 months did not show any episodes of relapse, and the patient appears completely well without any signs of sequelae.

3. Discussion

We present a case of an 18-month-old boy with severe vasculitis-like affection primarily of the face and marked edema of the ears. He had a prodromal period with gastroenteritis and the histological findings were diagnostic for leukocytoclastic vasculitis. The clinical findings met the criteria for the diagnosis of AHEI. Prompt recognition of this rare disease is important to differentiate it from other manifestations that require specific therapy. The main differential diagnosis of AHEI of young children includes HSP [6, 7]. In Table 1 the main characteristics and differences between the two diseases are outlined.

As seen from Table 1, there is no internal organ involvement in AHEI. The cutaneous findings are dramatic, both in appearance and rapidity of onset, and may therefore cause significant anxiety for parents as well as clinicians. Both AHEI and HSP are leukocytoclastic vasculitides, but the immunohistology in AHEI is different from the pattern of HSP. In AHEI there is more extensive vasculitis with fibrin deposits; IgA deposits are seen in a minority of cases. The target lesions of erythema multiforme (EM) often first appear over the dorsum of the hands progressing centripetally to involve the proximal extremities and the trunk. The severe form of erythema multiforme, Stevens-Johnson syndrome, may have hemorrhagic and papular lesions resembling AHEI, but it includes ulcerating lesions of the mucous membranes. Other differential diagnoses of AHEI include meningococcal

TABLE 1: Clinical differences between acute hemorrhagic edema of infancy (AHEI) and Henoch-Schönleins purpura (HSP).

Clinical findings	AHEI	HSP
Peak incidence	4 to 24 months	4 to 7 years
Skin distribution	Faces, auricles, and extremities	Extensor surfaces of the legs and buttocks
Edema	Consistent, nonpitting	Inconsistent
Gastrointestinal involvement	Rare	Common
Articular involvement	Rare	Common
Renal involvement	Extremely rare	Common
Skin histology	Leukocytoclastic vasculitis, frequently with fibrinoid necrosis	Leukocytoclastic vasculitis
Perivascular deposits	C1q	IgA
Duration	2-3 weeks	1 month or more
Relapses	Rare	Frequent

sepsis, purpura fulminans, eruptions of viral infections, drug-induced vasculitis, and Sweet's syndrome [8]. All these disorders can be differentiated from AHEI by results of history, physical examination, and appropriate laboratory studies, including histological examination of a skin biopsy. There is no specific treatment for patients with AHEI. In a recent review, corticosteroids and antihistamines were not reported to alter the course of the disease [8]. However, few publications have reported beneficial effect of steroids in AHEI [9], and nonsteroidal anti-inflammatory drugs are recommended for tender skin lesions or in cases with musculoskeletal pain [8, 9]. Furthermore, antibiotics are indicated when bacterial infection is suspected [10].

In the case reported here a clear improvement of the disease was seen immediately after high-dose therapy with i.v. methylprednisolone was started. However, after lowering the corticosteroid dose a relapse was observed but rapid improvement was obtained after repeating the high-dose i.v. methylprednisolone. Our results suggest that in severe cases of AHEI high-dose corticosteroids should be considered.

Conflict of Interests

There are no conflicts of interest.

References

[1] F. Savino, M. M. Lupica, V. Tarasco et al., "Acute hemorrhagic edema of infancy: a troubling cutaneous presentation with a self-limiting course," *Pediatric Dermatology*, vol. 30, no. 6, pp. e149–e152, 2013.

[2] Z. Javidi, M. Maleki, V. Mashayekhi, N. Tayebi-Maybodi, and Y. Nahidi, "Acute hemorrhagic edema of infancy," *Archives of Iranian Medicine*, vol. 11, no. 1, pp. 103–106, 2008.

[3] E. Fiore, M. Rizzi, M. Ragazzi et al., "Acute hemorrhagic edema of young children (cockade purpura and edema): a case series and systematic review," *Journal of the American Academy of Dermatology*, vol. 59, no. 4, pp. 684–695, 2008.

[4] R. R. Morrison and F. T. Saulsbury, "Acute hemorrhagic edema of infancy associated with pneumococcal bacteremia," *Pediatric Infectious Disease Journal*, vol. 18, no. 9, pp. 832–833, 1999.

[5] I. Krause, A. Lazarov, A. Rachmel et al., "Acute haemorrhagic oedema of infancy, a benign variant of leucocytoclastic vasculitis," *Acta Paediatrica*, vol. 85, no. 1, pp. 114–117, 1996.

[6] S. M. Salman and A.-G. Kibbi, "Vascular reactions in children," *Clinics in Dermatology*, vol. 20, no. 1, pp. 11–15, 2002.

[7] R. M. Villiger, R. O. von Vigier, G. P. Ramelli, R. I. Hassink, and M. G. Bianchetti, "Precipitants in 42 cases of erythema multiforme," *European Journal of Pediatrics*, vol. 158, no. 11, pp. 929–932, 1999.

[8] E. Fiore, M. Rizzi, G. D. Simonetti, L. Garzoni, M. G. Bianchetti, and A. Bettinelli, "Acute hemorrhagic edema of young children: a concise narrative review," *European Journal of Pediatrics*, vol. 170, no. 12, pp. 1507–1511, 2011.

[9] A. P. D. da Silva Manzoni, J. B. Viecili, C. B. de Andrade, R. L. Kruse, L. Bakos, and T. F. Cestari, "Acute hemorrhagic edema of infancy: a case report," *International Journal of Dermatology*, vol. 43, no. 1, pp. 48–51, 2004.

[10] H. M. Poyrazoğlu, H. Per, Z. Gündüz et al., "Acute hemorrhagic edema of infancy," *Pediatrics International*, vol. 45, no. 6, pp. 697–700, 2003.

29

A Rare Colocalization of Lichen Planus and Vitiligo

David Veitch,[1] Georgios Kravvas,[1] Sian Hughes,[2] and Christopher Bunker[1]

[1]*Department of Dermatology, University College London Hospitals, London NW1 2BU, UK*
[2]*Department of Histopathology, University College London Hospitals, London NW1 2BU, UK*

Correspondence should be addressed to Christopher Bunker; chris.bunker@uclh.nhs.uk

Academic Editor: Jacek Cezary Szepietowski

We report an unusual manifestation of vitiligo colocalizing with lichen planus (LP). A 76-year-old Greek male presented with a history of a red, scaly, itchy, asymmetrical patch located at the umbilicus within a well-demarcated depigmented macule of vitiligo. Histology showed features of a lichenoid interface dermatitis, favouring a diagnosis of LP. Colocalization of LP and vitiligo has rarely been reported in the literature. After reviewing the literature, we believe that at present there is insufficient evidence to resolve the uncertainties in the aetiology of this colocalization. It seems to us that the association between LP and vitiligo is more than coincidental, but none of the theories discussed in this paper can sufficiently account for it. Rather, the association is likely to be multifactorial in its pathogenesis.

1. Introduction

Colocalization of lichen planus (LP) and vitiligo has rarely been reported in the literature. A number of different patterns of association have been recognised.

The fact that both LP and vitiligo are common, each said to affect 1-2% of the general population, may mean that their association is merely a coincidence and may not represent any mutual interrelationship [1, 2]. On the other hand, a number of publications suggest that a causal link must be present since similar immunological mechanisms are shared by both conditions [3–6]. The aetiology of neither LP nor vitiligo is known. We discuss the theories below.

2. Case Report

A 76-year-old Greek male (retired plumber) presented with a 5-6-year history of a red, scaly, itchy, asymmetrical patch (more prominent after sun exposure, he averred) located at the umbilicus within a well-demarcated depigmented macule of vitiligo: he gave a 30-year history of generalized vitiligo affecting the genitals, umbilicus, axillae, and hands (Figure 1). The vitiligo was inactive, stable, and nonprogressive. He also had a solitary red, itchy papule of the glans penis present for over 3 years (Figure 2). Hair, scalp, nails, and mucosae were otherwise completely normal.

His medical background included ischaemic heart disease, paroxysmal atrial fibrillation (with multiple failed ablations), moderate aortic stenosis, obstructive sleep apnoea, bleeding duodenal ulcer (emergency laparotomy), benign prostatic hypertrophy, and thalassaemia trait. There was no history of autoimmune disease in the patient or his family. His medication consisted of atorvastatin, spironolactone, losartan, lansoprazole, finasteride, and warfarin. He was not on topical or systemic therapy for vitiligo due to the longstanding, stable nature of the disease and relative lack of psychosocial morbidity. He was given sun protection advice.

Bowen's disease was suspected and a 4 mm punch biopsy of the lesion on the umbilicus was performed. Histology showed hyperkeratosis and cytoid bodies: Civatte (epidermal) and colloid (dermal). There was some epidermal flattening suggestive of resolving lichen planus. There was a band-like inflammatory cell infiltrate composed of lymphocytes, histiocytes, and occasional eosinophils (Figure 3). The features were those of a lichenoid interface dermatitis, favouring a diagnosis of lichen planus.

He was prescribed clobetasol propionate ointment which he applied once daily for 4 weeks to both the umbilicus and glans. Both lesions completely resolved leaving only mild telangiectatic change over the umbilicus.

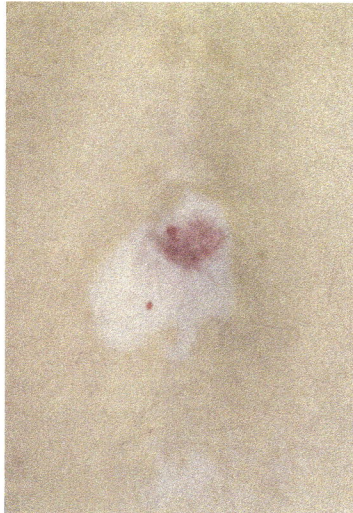

FIGURE 1: Umbilicus demonstrating vitiligo with overlying lichen planus.

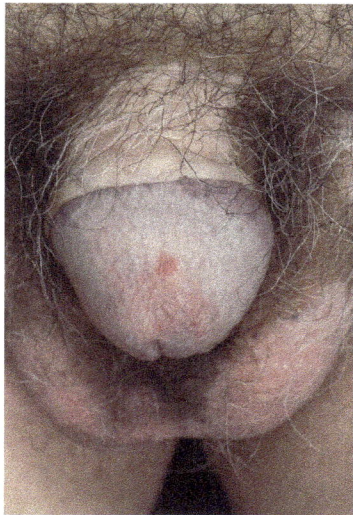

FIGURE 2: Scrotal and penile vitiligo with a region of lichen planus lesion on the glans.

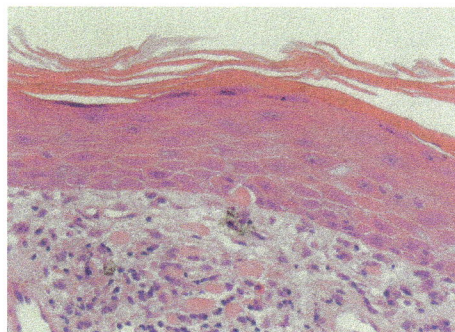

FIGURE 3: Umbilical 4 mm punch biopsy magnification ×200, Hematoxylin and Eosin stain. Features described in text.

3. Discussion

A number of associations between LP and vitiligo have been reported.

LP lesions have been described as confined to vitiliginous areas alone or even affecting both normal and vitiliginous skin [3, 4]. They have been said to be more severe on sun-exposed vitiliginous areas, less so on sun-exposed normally pigmented skin, and the least severe on covered areas [7]. In most cases vitiligo is described as the precursor disease but concomitant onset and progression of both conditions has also been noted [1].

Various theories for the aetiology of vitiligo have been advanced and the autoimmune hypothesis is the prevailing view. This is because of the association of vitiligo with other autoimmune disorders, the higher frequency of organ specific antibodies found in patients with vitiligo compared with the general public, and the detection of melanocyte-specific antibodies detected in patients with vitiligo [8].

LP also occurs in patients with autoimmune diseases other than vitiligo. Within lesions CD4 and CD8 cells accumulate in the dermis where they cause lysis of keratinocytes. LP is thought to be an immunologically mediated disorder driven by a T cell response to an unknown antigen or antigens [4, 9].

Baghestani et al. have suggested that sun-exposed depigmented areas play an important part in the initiation of LP that then extends to involve normal skin. A popular hypothesis holds that photodamage within areas of vitiligo causes the release of inflammatory mediators, thus promoting the accumulation of effector T cells as are seen in LP. According to this theory, in vitiligo-affected patients, LP is more likely to be encountered in abnormally pigmented skin and in sun-exposed areas [4, 7]. To support this further, it has been well documented that psoralen and UVA- (PUVA-) induced lichenoid changes can occur in vitiliginous skin [2, 4].

In contrast to the actinic damage theory, there have been descriptions of cases in which LP is confined solely on nonexposed areas of the skin, such as the scrotum, inguinal folds, and thighs [4].

Another theory is based on the evident manifestation of the Koebner phenomenon in LP; koebnerisation describes the eruption of an inflammatory skin disease following mechanical injury of the skin [10]. It has been proposed that cellular injury in vitiligo-affected skin, augmented by the effects of solar damage, modifies the mechanisms responsible for the Koebner phenomenon, resulting in LP on sun-exposed skin [1]. However, the presentation in our patient may represent Wolf's isotopic response, a subtype of the Koebner phenomenon, in which one skin disease may trigger a second, pathogenically unrelated skin lesion [10].

Yet another conjecture is that long-standing vitiligo alters the expression of antigens identified by effector T cells in LP or inactivates suppressor T cells, thus leading to the pathophenotype of LP [4].

Göktay et al. have suggested that tumor necrosis factor (TNF) may be the crucial mediator in the colocalization of LP and vitiligo. The rationale is that TNF-α immunoreactivity has often been detected in oral and cutaneous LP and that enhanced levels of TNF-α production from melanocytes have also been detected in patients with vitiligo [4].

But the literature also contains cases of associated LP and vitiligo that are not readily accommodated by these theories. Baran et al. described lesions of LP, in the shape of a rim with sharp borders, affecting only the pigmented skin around several vitiliginous patches [6]. Wayte and Wilkinson reported a case in which widespread LP spared all areas of long-standing vitiligo, with sharp borders separating the two types of lesions. Indeed, Wayte and Wilkinson proposed that changes in vitiliginous skin actually protected against lichenoid transformation [5].

After reviewing the literature, we believe that at present there is insufficient evidence to resolve the uncertainties. It seems to us that the association between LP and vitiligo is more than coincidental, but none of the above theories can sufficiently account for it. Rather, the association is likely to be multifactorial in its pathogenesis.

Conflict of Interests

The authors declare that there is no conflict of interests regarding the publication of this paper.

References

[1] M. T. Hefazi, H. Mosiehi, E. Amir, and N. Ostradahimi, "Colocalization of Lichen Planus and vitiligo: challenging the universality of current theories," *Iranian Journal of Dermatology*, vol. 12, supplement 3, pp. S16–S18, 2009.

[2] S. R. Porter, C. Scully, and J. W. Eveson, "Coexistence of lichen planus and vitiligo is coincidental," *Clinical and Experimental Dermatology*, vol. 19, no. 4, p. 366, 1994.

[3] H. Ujiie, D. Sawamura, and H. Shimizu, "Development of lichen planus and psoriasis on lesions of vitiligo vulgaris," *Clinical and Experimental Dermatology*, vol. 57, no. 4, pp. 690–699, 2006.

[4] F. Göktay, A. T. Mansur, and I. E. Aydingöz, "Colocalization of vitiligo and lichen planus on scrotal skin: a finding contrary to the actinic damage theory," *Dermatology*, vol. 212, no. 4, pp. 390–392, 2006.

[5] J. Wayte and J. D. Wilkinson, "Unilateral lichen planus, sparing vitiliginous skin," *British Journal of Dermatology*, vol. 133, no. 5, pp. 817–818, 1995.

[6] R. Baran, J. P. Ortonne, and C. Perrin, "Vitiligo associated with a lichen planus border," *Dermatology*, vol. 194, no. 2, article 199, 1997.

[7] S. Baghestani, A. Moosavi, and T. Eftekhari, "Familial colocalization of lichen planus and vitiligo on sun exposed areas," *Annals of Dermatology*, vol. 25, no. 2, pp. 223–225, 2013.

[8] A. V. Anstey, "Disorders of skin colour," in *Rook's Textbook of Dermatology*, T. Bruns, S. Breathnach, and C. Griffiths, Eds., pp. 58.1–58.59, Wiley-Blackwell, West Sussex, UK, 8th edition, 2010.

[9] S. M. Breathnach, "Lichen planus and lichenoid disorders," in *Rook's Textbook of Dermatology*, T. Bruns, S. Breathnach, and C. Griffiths, Eds., pp. 41.1–41.28, Wiley-Blackwell, West Sussex, UK, 8th edition, 2010.

[10] J. Kroth, J. Tischer, W. Samtleben, C. Weiss, T. Ruzicka, and A. Wollenberg, "Isotopic response, Köbner phenomenon and Renbök phenomenon following herpes zoster," *Journal of Dermatology*, vol. 38, no. 11, pp. 1058–1061, 2011.

30

Paraneoplastic Dermatomyositis with Carcinoma Cervix: A Rare Clinical Association

Sumir Kumar,[1] **B. B. Mahajan,**[1] **Sandeep Kaur,**[1,2] **and Amarbir Singh**[1]

[1]*GGS Medical College & Hospital, Sadiq Road, Faridkot, Punjab 151203, India*
[2]*Skin OPD, GGS Medical College & Hospital, OPD Block, 1st Floor, Sadiq Road, Faridkot, Punjab 151203, India*

Correspondence should be addressed to Sandeep Kaur; docsandeep_2005@yahoo.com

Academic Editor: Mario Vaccaro

Dermatomyositis is an uncommon inflammatory myopathy associated with cutaneous manifestations. It may also occur as paraneoplastic syndrome associated with various malignancies, most common of which being lung, breast, stomach, rectum, kidney, or testicular cancer. A postmenopausal woman presented to us with generalized itching along with skin rash and proximal muscle weakness of 2 years' duration. Examination revealed heliotrope rash and mechanic hands and muscle power 2/5 in proximal muscle groups of both upper and lower limbs. A clinical diagnosis of dermatomyositis was made which was supported by raised lactate dehydrogenase levels and skin biopsy findings. Past history was significant for vaginal discharge and bleeding per vagina. Further work-up revealed carcinoma cervix and she was referred to oncology department for further management. Temporal relationship and improvement of muscle weakness with treatment of underlying neoplasm supported its paraneoplastic nature. So, final diagnosis of keratinizing squamous cell carcinoma of cervix with paraneoplastic dermatomyositis was made. A nationwide cohort study of 1,012 patients with dermatomyositis in Taiwan revealed only 3 patients with cervical cancer. So this case is being reported for its rare association with carcinoma cervix and to highlight the need of detailed evaluation for underlying malignancies in patients with dermatomyositis.

1. Introduction

Dermatomyositis (DM) is a multisystem disorder characterized clinically by muscle weakness and cutaneous rash. It has a well-recognized relationship with various types of cancers, most common of which being lung, breast, female genital tract, stomach, rectum, kidney, or testis cancer. Dermatomyositis precedes the neoplasm in 40%; both conditions may occur together (26%) or the neoplasm may occur first (34%). The incidence of carcinoma in association with DM varies from 15 to 34% [1].

A nationwide cohort study of 1,012 patients with DM revealed only 3 patients with cervical cancer [2]. We here present a case of cervical carcinoma with paraneoplastic DM for its rarity.

2. Case Report

A 65-year-old nonhypertensive, nondiabetic woman presented with generalized itching since 2 years. She developed rash on body with photo aggravation. She complained of muscle weakness for the last 2 years for which she had been taking treatment from a local doctor without being investigated. She had difficulty in standing from sitting position and climbing up the stairs as well as combing her hair. There was no history of dysphagia, oral ulcers, or joint pains. She had vaginal discharge for the last 6 months and vaginal bleeding of few days duration. She was nonalcoholic and nonsmoker. She achieved menopause 15 years back.

Examination revealed presence of heliotrope rash around eyelids characterized by periorbital, confluent, and violaceous erythema (Figure 1(a)). Poikilodermatous changes were evident on V-area of neck and dorsolateral aspects of bilateral forearms and shins (Figure 1(b)). Trunk was relatively spared. On examination of hands, hyperkeratotic lesions were seen predominantly involving the centre of palms (mechanics hands) along with presence of Gottron's papules on proximal interphalangeal joints. Muscle power was 2/5 in both upper and lower limb proximal muscle groups. Per vaginal

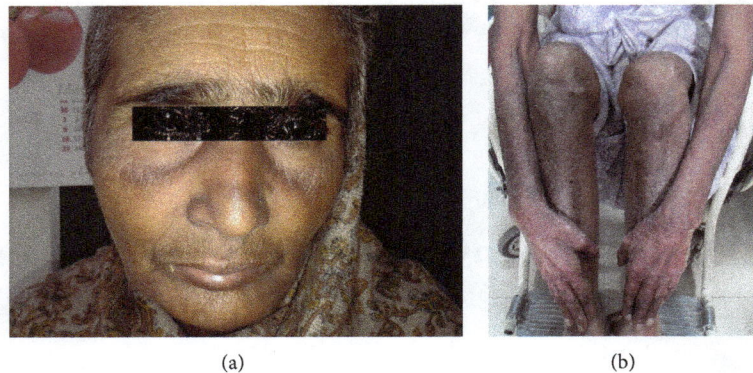

(a)

(b)

FIGURE 1: (a) Heliotrope rash in periorbital region. (b) Poikilodermatous changes evident on dorsolateral aspects of bilateral forearms.

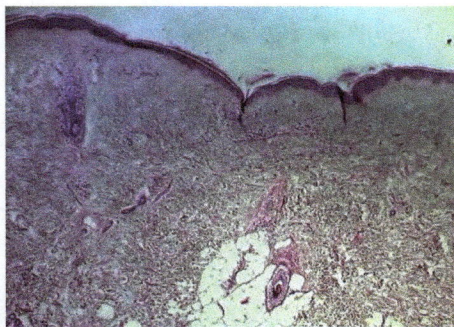

FIGURE 2: Histopathology of skin: focal thinning of epidermis along with hydropic degeneration of the basal keratinocytes. Deposition of eosinophilic material was seen particularly at dermoepidermal junction. There was sparse perivascular lymphomononuclear cell infiltrate in the dermis.

examination revealed an exfoliative growth extending into upper half of vagina. On per speculum examination, growth was seen in vagina protruding out of external cervical os. About 5 × 6 cm mass at the level of cervix with involvement of bilateral parametrium just short of pelvic wall was felt on per rectum palpation. Clinical findings strongly suggested the possibility of underlying genital tract malignancy, so oncology consultation was sought.

Results of investigations showed Hb = 7.8 g/dL, total leukocyte count = $5.25 \times 10^3/\mu L$, LDH = 960 IU/L, s. creatine kinase = 18 IU/L, and negative ANA and anti-dsDNA.

Skin biopsy was consistent with DM (Figure 2). Cervical biopsy showed keratinizing squamous cell carcinoma (SCC). CT scan of pelvis showed heterogeneous enhancing mass (69 × 89 mm) in the region of cervix and proximal part of vagina and distal part of body of uterus. Few soft tissue density lesions at both iliac fossa regions were seen. Chest X-ray and bone scintigraphy were normal. Thus, a diagnosis of keratinizing SCC uterine cervix stage III A with paraneoplastic DM was made for which she was started on PTF (Paclitaxel, Cisplatin, 5-Fluorouracil) chemotherapy followed by external beam radiation therapy. She was started on oral steroids (prednisolone 1 mg/kg), topical steroids, antihistamines, emollients, sunscreens, and physiotherapy for the treatment of dermatomyositis. After 6 weeks of treatment, she reported improvement in her muscle power without much improvement in dermatological manifestations. She also developed anagen effluvium secondary to chemotherapy and prominent follicular pluggings on scalp and forehead. After that, the patient was lost to follow-up.

3. Discussion

Dermatomyositis is a rare idiopathic inflammatory myopathy (IIM). It occurs at least twice as frequently in females as in males. In adults, onset is predominantly between the ages of 40 and 60 years. The mean age of onset is later in men than in women [3]. Paraneoplastic DM generally occurs in middle to elderly age group.

As malignancy in our case was diagnosed at such an advanced stage, onset of the malignancy must be few years back, and onset of DM was about 2 years back; these two events can be correlated temporally and DM occurring as paraneoplastic syndrome can, thus, be justified.

A model of crossover immunity for cancer-associated myositis has been suggested recently [4–6]. Common antigenic myositis-specific autoantigens expressed in both tumor cells and undifferentiated myoblasts lead to the generation of both specific T cells and B cells against those antigens and then to successful antitumor immunity. In a subset of patients, subsequent muscle damage from a variety of causes (such as viral infection and trauma) may lead to muscle damage and regeneration and may reactivate immune responses previously generated in the antitumor response. The crossover immunity between tumor cells and myofibroblasts may explain the parallel clinical course of both diseases [7].

A variety of investigations are available for the work-up of DM.

Serum creatine kinase (CK) level is usually the first step. About 80% to 90% of adult myositis patients show an increase in CK, but our patient had normal CK. Although muscle enzymes are frequently elevated in DM, they can be normal even in active disease with myositis [8]. Normal CK is relatively more common in DM than in PM [9]. Hence, measurement of other serum muscle enzymes, including aldolase, aspartate transaminase, alanine transaminase, and lactate dehydrogenase (LDH), significantly improves the chance of diagnosing active myositis, like in our patient with elevated LDH. This patient had normal liver function tests which help to rule out liver as source of these elevated enzymes.

Histopathologic findings of skin in DM are hyperkeratosis, vacuolization of the basal keratinocytes, melanin incontinence, perivascular lymphocytic infiltrate, and epidermal atrophy. However, histopathologic features are shared among DM and SLE. So, histopathology should be used to support the clinical diagnosis rather than being utilized as a diagnostic test.

Muscle biopsy remains the "gold standard" for the diagnosis of inflammatory myopathies such as DM. The features specific to DM include loss of capillaries, altered morphology of capillaries, capillary necrosis, complement deposition in the vessel walls and, rarely, muscle infarcts, and perifascicular atrophy. Bohan-Peter diagnostic criteria do not require muscle biopsy as a must to do investigation. Also, it is given the same weight as the other clinical criteria. So, in our patient diagnosis of DM can be justified on the basis of other findings as we were not able to do a muscle biopsy.

Electromyogram (EMG) changes are usually nonspecific but can serve as useful indicator of myopathic changes, to monitor disease activity and practical guide for biopsy sampling.

Identification of specific autoantibody strengthens the diagnosis. ANA has a low specificity for DM and has a sensitivity of 40–60%. Our patient had negative ANA. Autoantibodies in DM are now categorized into two groups: (1) myositis-specific autoantibodies which include Jo-1, PL-7, PL-12, OJ, Mi-2, and signal-recognition particle; (2) myositis-associated autoantibodies such as PM/Scl, Ro/SSA, and U1RNP.

The course is variable. Patients without muscle involvement have a better prognosis [10]. The overall mortality is approximately one-quarter [11]. Death usually occurs from respiratory infection, cardiac failure, and malnutrition due to difficulty in swallowing, malignancy, or from the side effects of therapy. The worst prognosis is seen in cancer-associated DM. The underlying malignancy, not the DM, accounts for the poor outcome. Removal of an underlying carcinoma in adults can lead to regression of the dermatomyositis [12]. Relapse of underlying neoplasm may be associated with exacerbation of DM.

4. Conclusion

This case report highlights the occurrence of DM as a paraneoplastic manifestation of cervical carcinoma with which it is rarely associated. Marked poikilodermatous changes on both upper and lower limbs, failure of full therapeutic response to conventional treatment of DM, and absence of elevation of usual muscle enzymes like creatine kinase were the unusual features in our case.

Abbreviations

DM: Dermatomyositis
SLE: Systemic lupus erythematosus
SCC: Squamous cell carcinoma
CK: Creatine kinase
PM: Polymyositis
IIM: Idiopathic inflammatory myositis
ANA: Antinuclear antibodies.

Conflict of Interests

The authors declare no conflict of interests.

References

[1] T. Burns, S. Breathnach, N. Cox, and C. Griffiths, *Rook's Textbook of Dermatology*, chapter 51: the connective tissue diseases, John Wiley & Sons, 8th edition, 2004.

[2] Y. J. Chen, C. Y. Wu, Y. L. Huang, C. B. Wang, J. L. Shen, and Y. T. Chang, "Cancer risks of dermatomyositis and polymyositis: a nationwide cohort study in Taiwan," *Arthritis Research & Therapy*, vol. 12, no. 2, p. R70, 2010.

[3] R. Degos, J. Civatte, S. Belaich, and A. Delarue, "The prognosis of adult dermatomyositis," *Transactions of the St. John's Hospital Dermatological Society*, vol. 57, no. 1, pp. 98–104, 1971.

[4] L. Casciola-Rosen, K. Nagaraju, P. Plotz et al., "Enhanced autoantigen expression in regenerating muscle cells in idiopathic inflammatory myopathy," *The Journal of Experimental Medicine*, vol. 201, no. 4, pp. 591–601, 2005.

[5] K. Danko, A. Ponyi, A. P. Molnar, C. Andras, and T. Constantin, "Paraneoplastic myopathy," *Current Opinion in Rheumatology*, vol. 21, no. 6, pp. 594–598, 2009.

[6] S. M. Levine, "Cancer and myositis: new insights into an old association," *Current Opinion in Rheumatology*, vol. 18, pp. 620–624, 2006.

[7] I. N. Targoff, "Idiopathic inflammatory myopathy: autoantibody update," *Current Rheumatology Reports*, vol. 4, no. 5, pp. 434–441, 2002.

[8] T. Takken, E. Elst, N. Spermon, P. J. M. Helders, A. B. J. Prakken, and J. van der Net, "The physiological and physical determinants of functional ability measures in children with juvenile dermatomyositis," *Rheumatology*, vol. 42, no. 4, pp. 591–595, 2003.

[9] G. S. Firestein, R. C. Budd, and E. D. Harris, *Kelly's Textbook of Rheumatology*, W.B.Saunders, Philadelphia, Pa, USA, 8th edition, 2008.

[10] E. Genth, "Inflammatory muscle diseases: dermatomyositis, polymyositis, and inclusion body myositis," *Internist*, vol. 46, no. 11, pp. 1218–1232, 2005.

[11] A. Airio, H. Kautiainen, and M. Hakala, "Prognosis and mortality of polymyositis and dermatomyositis patients," *Clinical Rheumatology*, vol. 25, no. 2, pp. 234–239, 2006.

[12] M. J. Brunner and R. V. Lobraico Jr., "Dermatomyositis as an index of malignant neoplasm: report of a case and review of the literature," *Annals of Internal Medicine*, vol. 34, no. 5, pp. 1269–1273, 1951.

31

Cutaneous Plasmacytosis with Perineural Involvement

Elizabeth A. Brezinski, Maxwell A. Fung, and Nasim Fazel

Department of Dermatology, Davis Health System, University of California, 3301 C Street, Suite 1400, Sacramento, CA 95816, USA

Correspondence should be addressed to Nasim Fazel; nasim.fazel@ucdmc.ucdavis.edu

Academic Editors: I. D. Bassukas, I. Kurokawa, J.-H. Lee, and J. Y. Lee

Importance. Cutaneous and systemic plasmacytosis are rare conditions of unknown etiology with characteristic red-brown skin lesions and a mature polyclonal plasma cell infiltrate within the dermis. Perineural plasma cell infiltrates may be a histologic clue to the diagnosis of cutaneous plasmacytosis. *Observations.* Our patient had a five-year history of persistent reddish-brown plaques on the neck and trunk without systemic symptoms. Histologic examination showed dermal perivascular and perineural plasma cells with excess lambda light chain expression. Due to decreased quality of life caused by his skin lesions, he was placed on a chemotherapeutic regimen with bortezomib. *Conclusions and Relevance.* The patient was diagnosed with cutaneous plasmacytosis based on classic histopathology results with a recently characterized pattern of perineural involvement. Bortezomib therapy was initiated to manage his skin eruption, which has not been previously described as a treatment for this chronic condition.

1. Introduction

Cutaneous and systemic plasmacytosis are rare, lympho-plasmacytic disorders characterized by red-brown poorly circumscribed plaques and nodules occurring mainly on the trunk primarily in patients of Japanese descent [1, 2]. The disease can be accompanied by fever, lymphadenopathy, anemia, and a polyclonal hypergammaglobulinemia [2, 3]. The characteristic histopathology is dermal perivascular infiltrates of mature polyclonal plasma cells [2, 4]. Herein we present a Hispanic patient with chronic red-brown macules and plaques on the trunk where these distinctive biopsy findings supported the diagnosis of cutaneous plasmacytosis. We discuss the classical histopathologic features of cutaneous plasmacytosis and evidence for cutaneous-only involvement of this condition.

2. Case

A 39-year-old Hispanic man presented with a five-year history of persistent red plaques on his neck and a two-year history of similar lesions that had spread to his trunk, sparing the upper and lower extremities. His past medical history included untreated latent tuberculosis infection and allergic rhinitis. Clinical examination revealed brownish-red macules and mildly indurated plaques on his trunk (Figure 1) and pink-to-violaceous plaques with fine scale on his neck. He was afebrile and had no lymphadenopathy. Laboratory examination showed normal complete blood count, serum protein, and erythrocyte sedimentation rate, no monoclonal protein on immunofixation, and hyperimmunoglobulin (Ig) E (199 KU/L—normal: <25 KU/L). The serum level of interleukin-(IL-) 6 was normal and antinuclear antibodies were negative. Free kappa and lambda chains and the kappa: lambda ratio were normal. Urinalysis was without blood or protein with no measurable Bence Jones protein in the urine. Human immunodeficiency virus, rapid plasma reagin, and Borrelia burgdorferi IgM were negative. Positron emission tomography/computed tomography (PET/CT) showed no evidence of fluorodeoxyglucose (FDG) avid cutaneous lesions or other areas of active disease.

3. Histology, Molecular Studies, and Therapeutic Trials

Skin biopsies from the abdomen, neck/shoulder, flank, and cervical region were obtained. The distinctive feature was a

(a)

(b)

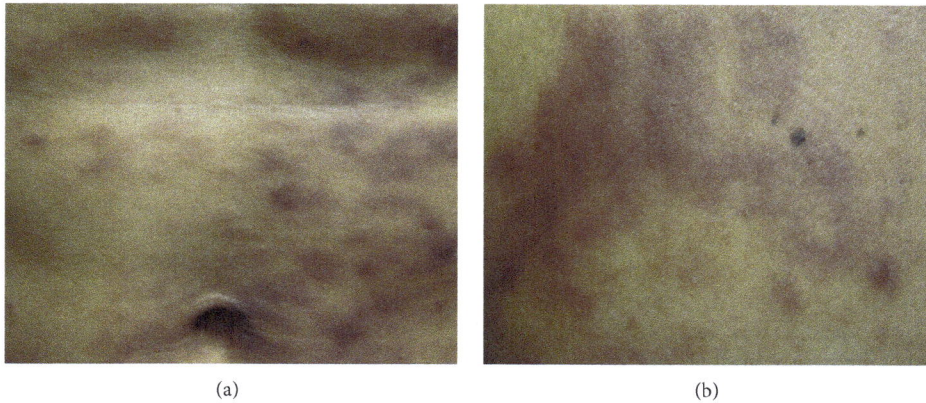

FIGURE 1: (a) The patient presented with brownish-red macules and mildly indurated plaques on his abdomen. (b) Similar lesions were present on his chest.

superficial and deep perivascular and perineural dermatitis with prominent plasma cells (Figures 2 and 3). The plasma cells were highlighted by IgG but negative for IgG4. There were evidence of B-cell clonality by PCR gene rearrangement analysis (two of two specimens) and evidence of slight lambda excess by immunohistochemistry and *in situ* hybridization. Other small B cells were highlighted by CD20 but negative for Bcl-6. Small CD3-positive T cells were intermixed with the plasma cells. CD117 marked background levels of mast cells. Immunohistochemical staining for *T. pallidum* was negative. PAS, Fite, and Warthin-Starry stains were negative. Tissue cultures for bacteria, mycobacteria, viruses, and fungi were negative. These skin biopsies were reviewed by our institution's dermatopathologists and hematopathologists and subsequently in consultation at the National Institutes of Health. Bone marrow aspirate demonstrated normocellular marrow with mildly increased numbers of plasma cells seen by CD138 and a minute kappa dominant plasma cell population detected by flow cytometry. Occasional small groups of plasma cells were seen which were predominantly associated with vessels. This distribution with only 5-6% plasma cells in the absence of atypia favored a reactive etiology. Chromosome analysis showed a normal male chromosome complement.

After evaluation by hematology and oncology, the patient was prescribed a one-month course of doxycycline to eliminate a possible nidus of infection with subsequent worsening of his cutaneous plaques on this therapy. He was later treated with a three-week course of clobetasol ointment with continued worsening. Since this patient did not tolerate a trial of clobetasol ointment and there is not currently an FDA-approved pharmacologic therapy for cutaneous plasmacytosis, an alternative therapy was investigated. After extrapolating from cutaneous T- and B-cell malignancy data as well as other plasma cell disorder therapies, the decision was made to start bortezomib. He subsequently was put on subcutaneous bortezomib 1.3 mg/m^2. His chemotherapy regimen included twice weekly injections over two weeks for

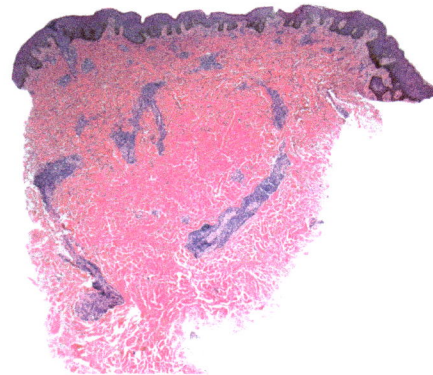

FIGURE 2: Abdominal biopsy highlighting dermal plasmacytes, which were evident in biopsies of the patient's abdomen, flank, and neck (hematoxylin & eosin stain; original magnification: ×40).

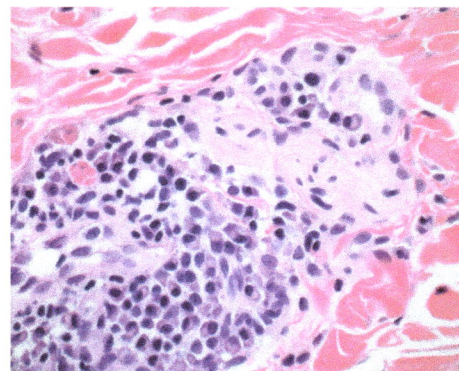

FIGURE 3: Abdominal biopsy was notable for perineural plasmacytes (hematoxylin & eosin stain; original magnification: ×600).

a total of four treatments per cycle, which he tolerated with mild nausea and myalgias. The skin lesions did not progress and he did not develop any new eruptions after two cycles of therapy; however, his rash showed partial regression after a total of eight treatments.

4. Discussion

Cutaneous plasmacytosis is a disorder of unknown etiology, which was first described by Yashiro as a "kind of plasmacytosis" and later redefined by Kitamura et al. as "cutaneous plasmacytosis" [1, 5]. Whether pure cutaneous plasmacytosis is a condition distinct from systemic involvement has been debated. It has been proposed that asymptomatic patients with manifestations of cutaneous plasmacytosis may have systemic involvement [6, 7]. Thus, these patients may warrant additional work-up, such as a superficial lymph node biopsy, to exclude the disorder of cutaneous and systemic plasmacytosis. Similar to prior case reports of cutaneous plasmacytosis, our patient had no palpable lymphadenopathy to suggest systemic involvement and PET/CT with FDG did not highlight any extracutaneous activity. Further evaluation by bone marrow biopsy revealed slightly increased plasma cells, which was thought to be reactive. It was determined that lymph node biopsy for histopathologic examination to rule out this largely benign, chronic, and indolent condition was not clinically warranted in this patient given the imaging and bone marrow biopsy results and selection of aggressive treatment.

Histopathology characteristically demonstrates a moderately dense, superficial, and deep perivascular and periadnexal infiltrate of plasma cells without atypia [3, 4]. The plasma cells are typically polyclonal and mature. In a minority of cases, accompanying small reactive germinal centers are found [2, 8]. Recently, focal infiltrates of perineural plasma cells were described in six patients with cutaneous plasmacytosis [8]. Intraneural plasma cells were also observed in a subset of these patients. In biopsies from our patient, marked perivascular and perineural plasmacytosis in the dermis was present. After no infectious etiologies were identified, this patient with normal IL-6 and gammaglobulin levels was diagnosed with cutaneous plasmacytosis by clinical correlation between the skin lesions and confirmatory histopathology. This case adds to the spectrum of histopathologic presentations that cutaneous plasmacytosis may take on in the absence of systemic signs and characteristic laboratory findings.

Although this condition is primarily described in middle-aged patients of Japanese descent, there have been case reports of cutaneous plasmacytosis occurring in patients of other Asian ethnicities and Caucasian descent [7]. Our patient is the first Hispanic individual reported to have cutaneous plasmacytosis.

Cutaneous plasmacytosis typically follows a benign clinical course, which does not require treatment; however, decreased quality of life due to the appearance of the lesions was a significant concern for this patient. Various treatment approaches have been tried to induce clinical remission. Topical and systemic corticosteroids, topical tacrolimus, antibiotics, and systemic chemotherapy have produced variable long-term clinical results [3, 9]. Treatment with intralesional

steroids, combination prednisone and cyclophosphamide, photodynamic therapy with long-pulse ruby laser, psoralen-UVA, and topical pimecrolimus have reportedly improved skin lesions of cutaneous plasmacytosis [10–14].

Bortezomib is FDA-approved for the treatment of multiple myeloma and mantle cell lymphoma in patients who have received at least one prior therapy [15]. This chemotherapeutic agent acts by inhibiting the 26S proteasome, which prevents selective proteolysis and can lead to cell death. The pathophysiology of cutaneous plasmacytosis has not yet been elucidated and it is uncertain whether therapy that targets other plasma cell malignancies will be effective for plasmacytosis. This patient was placed on a regimen of twice weekly subcutaneous bortezomib followed by a 10-day rest period. After two cycles, the patient developed no new lesions and the persistent plaques had evidence of regression. Additional cycles of chemotherapy are planned and longer-term follow-up is needed. The patient experienced a mild adverse reaction during the course of therapy.

5. Conclusion

Cutaneous and systemic plasmacytosis are largely benign conditions with unknown pathophysiology that occur mainly in Japanese patients and can have a wide range of clinical and histopathologic presentations. We report a case of cutaneous plasmacytosis with distinctive perineural involvement, a histopathologic feature that may aid in the diagnosis of this disorder when used with clinical correlation. This is also the first case of a Hispanic patient presenting with cutaneous plasmacytosis. Further, this patient was treated with bortezomib with partial improvement after two cycles of therapy. Additional long-term studies are needed to determine the potential efficacy of targeted chemotherapeutic medications for the management of cutaneous plasmacytosis.

Abbreviations

Ig: Immunoglobulin
IL: Interleukin
PET/CT: Positron emission tomography/computed
          tomography
FDG: Fluorodeoxyglucose.

Conflict of Interests

The authors declare that there is no conflict of interests regarding the publication of this paper.

Acknowledgments

The authors are indebted to Dr. Elaine Jaffe and Dr. Xiangrong Zhao at the National Institutes of Health for reviewing the skin biopsies of the patient.

References

[1] K. Kitamura, N. Tamura, and H. Hatano, "A case of plasmacytosis with multiple peculiar eruptions," *Journal of Dermatology*, vol. 7, no. 5, pp. 341–349, 1980.

[2] S. Watanabe, K. Ohara, A. Kukita, and S. Mori, "Systemic plasmacytosis: a syndrome of peculiar multiple skin eruptions, generalized lymphadenopathy, and polyclonal hypergammaglobulinemia," *Archives of Dermatology*, vol. 122, no. 11, pp. 1314–1320, 1986.

[3] H. Uhara, T. Saida, S. Ikegawa et al., "Primary cutaneous plasmacytosis: report of three cases and review of the literature," *Dermatology*, vol. 189, no. 3, pp. 251–255, 1994.

[4] S. Shimizu, M. Tanaka, H. Shimizu, and H. Han-Yaku, "Is cutaneous plasmacytosis a distinct clinical entity?" *Journal of the American Academy of Dermatology*, vol. 36, no. 5, part 2, pp. 876–880, 1997.

[5] A. Yashiro, "A kind of plasmacytosis: primary cutaneous plasmacytoma?" *Japanese Journal of Dermatology*, vol. 86, p. 910, 1976.

[6] Y. Tada, M. Komine, S. Suzuki et al., "Plasmacytosis: systemic or cutaneous, are they distinct?" *Acta Dermato-Venereologica*, vol. 80, no. 3, pp. 233–235, 2000.

[7] A. L. Leonard, S. A. Meehan, D. Ramsey, L. Brown, and F. Sen, "Cutaneous and systemic plasmacytosis," *Journal of the American Academy of Dermatology*, vol. 56, supplement 2, pp. S38–S40, 2007.

[8] R. Honda, L. Cerroni, A. Tanikawa, T. Ebihara, M. Amagai, and A. Ishiko, "Cutaneous plamacytosis: report of 6 cases with or without systemic involvement," *Journal of the American Academy of Dermatology*, vol. 68, no. 6, pp. 978–985, 2013.

[9] H. Miura, S. Itami, and K. Yoshikawa, "Treatment of facial lesion of cutaneous plasmacytosis with tacrolimus ointment," *Journal of the American Academy of Dermatology*, vol. 49, no. 6, pp. 1195–1196, 2003.

[10] T. Yamamoto, K. Soejima, I. Katayama, and K. Nishioka, "Intralesional steroid-therapy-induced reduction of plasma interleukin-6 and improvement of cutaneous plasmacytosis," *Dermatology*, vol. 190, no. 3, pp. 242–244, 1995.

[11] W. P. Carey, M. J. Rico, M. Nierodzik, and G. Sidhu, "Systemic plasmacytosis with cutaneous manifestations in a white man: successful therapy with cyclophosphamide/prednisone," *Journal of the American Academy of Dermatology*, vol. 38, no. 4, pp. 629–631, 1998.

[12] T. Tzung, K. Wu, J. Wu, and H. Tseng, "Primary cutaneous plasmacytosis successfully treated with topical photodynamic therapy," *Acta Dermato-Venereologica*, vol. 85, no. 6, pp. 542–543, 2005.

[13] M. Kaneda, K. Kuroda, M. Fujita, and H. Shinkai, "Successful treatment with topical PUVA of nodular cutaneous plasmacytosis associated with alopecia of the scalp," *Clinical and Experimental Dermatology*, vol. 21, no. 5, pp. 360–364, 1996.

[14] C. Hafner, U. Hohenleutner, P. Babilas, M. Landthaler, and T. Vogt, "Targeting T cells to hit B cells: successful treatment of cutaneous plasmacytosis with topical pimecrolimus," *Dermatology*, vol. 213, no. 2, pp. 163–165, 2006.

[15] Millennium Pharmaceuticals, *Velcade (Bortezomib) Package Insert*, Millennium Pharmaceuticals, Cambridge, Mass, USA, 2003.

32

Successful Treatment of Disseminated Subcutaneous Panniculitis-Like T-Cell Lymphoma with Single Agent Oral Cyclosporine as a First Line Therapy

Nida Iqbal and Vinod Raina

Department of Medical Oncology, Dr. B. R. A. Institute Rotary Cancer Hospital, All India Institute of Medical Sciences, New Delhi 110029, India

Correspondence should be addressed to Nida Iqbal; nida.iqbal55@yahoo.com

Academic Editor: Alireza Firooz

Subcutaneous panniculitis-like T-cell lymphoma (SPTL) is a rare cutaneous neoplasm of mature cytotoxic T-cells. Currently there are no standardized therapies for SPTL; however good responses have been seen with chemotherapy regimens generally employed for B-cell lymphomas. Cyclosporine, an immunosuppressant, has shown good responses in relapsed/refractory SPTL; however its use in first line setting is not well established. We, herein, describe a 22-year-old girl with disseminated SPTL who attained complete clinical remission with single agent oral cyclosporine used as a first line therapy.

1. Introduction

Subcutaneous panniculitis-like T-cell lymphoma (SPTL) is a type of T-cell lymphoma with clinicopathologic features simulating panniculitis and associated with an aggressive clinical course [1]. There are two subtypes, TCR alpha/beta and TCR gamma/delta [2]. While TCR alpha/beta generally have a CD4−, CD8+, CD56− phenotype and a favorable prognosis, TCR gamma/delta typically have a CD4−, CD8− T-cell phenotype with frequent coexpression of CD56 and a poor prognosis [3]. SPTL most commonly affects patients in 4th decade of life with a female predominance [4]. Patients present with subcutaneous nodules or plaques most commonly on extremities and trunk that, on pathologic evaluation, demonstrate cellular infiltrates in the subcutaneous fat, generally with sparing of the overlying epidermis. Metastatic disease is very rare. Clinical and systemic symptoms are nonspecific. There is no standardized treatment for SPTL [4]. CHOP-like chemotherapy is generally used as an initial therapy. Cyclosporine, an immunosuppressant, has shown activity in relapsed/refractory SPTL [5, 6]. However, it is still not clear whether cyclosporine as a single agent is able to induce remissions in patients with disseminated SPTL

and the question of its use as first line therapy remains unanswered.

In this report, we describe complete clinical remission of disseminated SPTL (TCR alpha/beta) in a 22-year-old girl with single agent oral cyclosporine used as a first line therapy.

2. Case Report

A 22-year-old girl presented with the complaints of intermittent fever, decreased appetite, and progressively increasing nodular swellings over both cheeks, lower back, both gluteal areas, and lower limbs. On physical examination, the patient was febrile with ECOG performance status of 2. There was mild hepatosplenomegaly with no peripheral lymphadenopathy. Skin examination revealed nodular swelling 3-4 cm over both cheeks and 2-3 cm swellings over lower back, both gluteal areas, and right thigh. There was an ulcerative lesion approximately 3 cm over left calf with surrounding hyperpigmented area (Figure 1(a)). The laboratory investigations revealed haemoglobin level of 8.7 g/dL, white blood cell count of 4.1×10^9/L, platelet count of 275×10^9/L, serum LDH of 228 U/L, and normal renal and liver function tests.

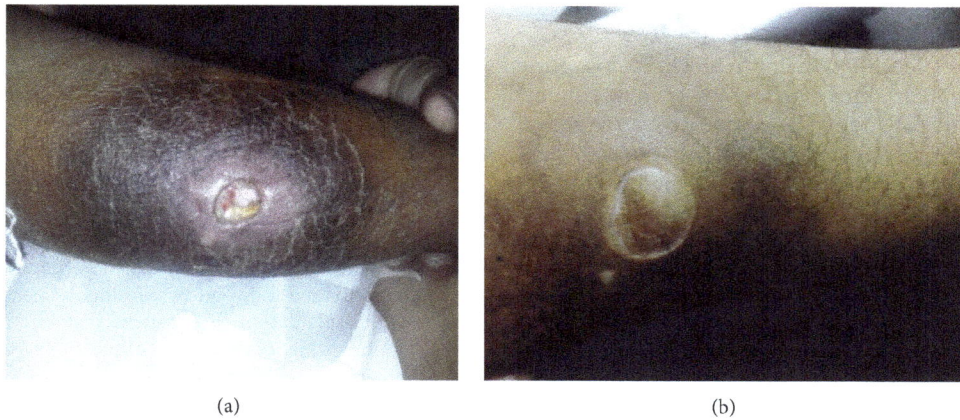

(a)   (b)

FIGURE 1: (a) Ulcerative lesion with surrounding hyperpigmented area over left calf before treatment. (b) Healed lesion 18 months after completion of therapy.

The serologic tests for human immunodeficiency virus and hepatitis B and C were negative. Contrast enhanced CT chest and abdomen did not reveal any abnormality. PET scan revealed diffuse uptake in subcutaneous fat, left breast, liver, and spleen. Bone marrow examination was normal. There was no evidence of hemophagocytic syndrome. An excisional biopsy from the skin nodule showed septal and interstitial panniculitis with fat necrosis and atypical lymphoid cell infiltrate focally lining the adipocytes, mainly limited to subcutaneous tissue and lower dermis. Foamy histiocytes with beanbag cells were also identified in the interstitium. Immunohistochemistry analysis showed that tumor cells expressed CD3 and CD8 but were negative for CD20, CD4, and CD 56. Ki-67 was not measured. These findings were consistent with the diagnosis of subcutaneous panniculitis-like T-cell lymphoma (alpha/beta subtype).

She was started on oral cyclosporine 4 mg/kg/d as a single agent. Patient responded well with resolution of all systemic manifestations of disease within two weeks of initiation of therapy. All skin nodules resolved completely within two months. She was continued on same dose of cyclosporine for next 5 months and finally the drug was tapered over 1 month. She tolerated the therapy well except for mild hirsutism. PET scan done at 6 months of treatment showed complete resolution of all subcutaneous nodules with mild uptake in left calf. Currently, the patient is in clinical remission 18 months after completion of therapy (Figure 1(b)).

3. Discussion

Subcutaneous panniculitis-like T-cell lymphoma (SPTL) was first described by Gonzalez et al. in 1991 [1] and defined as a distinct entity by the World Health Organization (WHO) classification in 2001 [7, 8]. SPTL is a cutaneous condition and metastatic disease or visceral involvement is uncommon. CD56 is an important marker in T-cell lymphomas as CD56 positive tumors have worse outcome in view of disseminated disease and hemophagocytosis [9]. Only cases with TCR

gamma/delta phenotype (mostly CD56 positive) tend to have metastasis to various organs, including lungs, liver, kidneys, and the central nervous system. Hemophagocytic syndrome (HPS) characterized by fever, pancytopenia, hepatosplenomegaly, and coagulopathy is most commonly seen in TCR gamma/delta phenotype and associated with aggressive outcome [10]. TCR alpha/beta phenotype is generally CD56 negative and associated with favourable outcome. The overall five-year survival rate for TCR alpha/beta exceeds 80%; however, in the presence of HPS, it reduces to less than 50%. In cases of TCR gamma/delta, the five-year survival rate is less than 20% in either group [4].

Due to rarity of disease, no standardized therapy for SPTL currently exists. For indolent local disease, local radiotherapy can be used as an effective treatment modality. For indolent disease with a more generalized distribution, systemic biologic agents may be used, such as bexarotene and interferon, as well as low-dose chemotherapy with agents such as methotrexate. For aggressive presentations, doxorubicin-based therapies are most commonly used, with overall complete or partial remission rates of 50%. Fludarabine-based chemotherapies have shown an overall remission rates of more than 70% in a few case reports [11, 12]. A case of SPTL with HPS resistant to CHOP regimen achieved complete remission after combination chemotherapy using BFM-90 protocol [11]. High-dose chemotherapy followed by stem cell transplantation have been reported to produce the highest response rates [13, 14].

Immunosuppressive therapy with steroids and cyclosporine have shown good results in the treatment of relapsed/refractory SPTL in a few case reports [5, 6]. Cyclosporine, a calcineurin inhibitor, is a potent immunosuppressant. The mechanism of action of cyclosporine in SPTL is downregulation of cytokines. Despite its magical effects in a few cases of relapsed/refractory SPTL, we could not find any report of its use in upfront setting. Our case is the first of its kind in which upfront use of cyclosporine was able to maintain durable remission in patient with disseminated SPTL.

4. Conclusion

Because of lack of standard treatment to SPTL, cyclosporine may be a good option as a first line therapy even in patients with disseminated disease due to lack of side effects and ease of administration. However, its benefit in patients with TCR gamma/delta phenotype needs to be confirmed by further studies.

Conflict of Interests

The authors declare that there is no conflict of interests regarding the publication of this paper.

References

[1] C. L. Gonzalez, L. J. Medeiros, R. M. Braziel, and E. S. Jaffe, "T-cell lymphoma involving subcutaneous tissue: a clinico-pathologic entity commonly associated with hemophagocytic syndrome," *The American Journal of Surgical Pathology*, vol. 15, no. 1, pp. 17–27, 1991.

[2] K. E. Salhany, W. R. Macon, J. K. Choi et al., "Subcuta-neous panniculitis-like T-cell lymphoma: clinicopathologic, immunophenotypic, and genotypic analysis of alpha/beta and gamma/delta subtypes," *The American Journal of Surgical Pathology*, vol. 22, no. 7, pp. 881–893, 1998.

[3] C. Massone, A. Chott, D. Metze et al., "Subcutaneous, blastic natural killer (NK), NK/T-cell, and other cytotoxic lymphomas of the skin: a morphologic, immunophenotypic, and molecular study of 50 patients," *The American Journal of Surgical Pathology*, vol. 28, no. 6, pp. 719–735, 2004.

[4] R. Willemze, P. M. Jansen, L. Cerroni et al., "Subcutaneous panniculitis-like T-cell lymphoma: definition, classification, and prognostic factors: an EORTC Cutaneous Lymphoma Group Study of 83 cases," *Blood*, vol. 111, no. 2, pp. 838–845, 2008.

[5] P. Rojnuckarin, T. N. Nakorn, T. Assanasen, P. Wannakrairot, and T. Intragumtornchai, "Cyclosporin in subcutaneous panniculitis-like T-cell lymphoma," *Leukemia & Lymphoma*, vol. 48, no. 3, pp. 560–563, 2007.

[6] S. I. Go, W. S. Lee, M. H. Kang, D. C. Kim, J. H. Lee, and I. S. Kim, "Cyclosporine a treatment for relapsed subcuta-neous panniculitis-like T-cell lymphoma: a case with long-term follow-up," *Korean Journal of Hematology*, vol. 47, no. 2, pp. 146–149, 2012.

[7] E. S. Jaffe, N. L. Harris, H. Stein, and J. W. Vardiman, Eds., *Pathology and Genetics of Tumours of Haematopoietic and Lymphoid Tissues*, World Health Organization Classification of Tumours, IARC Press, Lyon, France, 2001.

[8] R. Willemze, E. S. Jaffe, G. Burg et al., "WHO-EORTC classi-fication for cutaneous lymphomas," *Blood*, vol. 105, no. 10, pp. 3768–3785, 2005.

[9] M. Takeshita, S. Okamura, Y. Oshiro et al., "Clinicopathologic differences between 22 cases of CD56-negative and CD56-positive subcutaneous panniculitis -like lymphoma in Japan," *Human Pathology*, vol. 35, no. 2, pp. 231–239, 2004.

[10] R. S. Go and S. M. Wester, "Immunophenotypic and molec-ular features, clinical outcomes, treatments, and prognostic factors associated with subcutaneous panniculitis-like T-cell lymphoma: a systematic analysis of 156 patients reported in the literature," *Cancer*, vol. 101, no. 6, pp. 1404–1413, 2004.

[11] C.-S. Chim, F. Loong, W.-K. Ng, and Y.-L. Kwong, "Use of fludarabine-containing chemotherapeutic regimen results in durable complete remission of subcutaneous panniculitis-like T-cell lymphoma," *American Journal of Clinical Dermatology*, vol. 9, no. 6, pp. 396–398, 2008.

[12] K. Medhi, R. Kumar, A. Rishi, L. Kumar, and S. Bakhshi, "Sub-cutaneous panniculitislike T-cell lymphoma with hemophago-cytosis: complete remission with BFM-90 protocol," *Journal of Pediatric Hematology/Oncology*, vol. 30, no. 7, pp. 558–561, 2008.

[13] K. Koizumi, K. Sawada, M. Nishio et al., "Effective high-dose chemotherapy followed by autologous peripheral blood stem cell transplantation in a patient with the aggressive form of cytophagic histiocytic panniculitis," *Bone Marrow Transplanta-tion*, vol. 20, no. 2, pp. 171–173, 1997.

[14] P. Reimer, T. Rüdiger, J. Müller, C. Rose, M. Wilhelm, and F. Weissinger, "Subcutaneous panniculitis-like T-cell lymphoma during pregnancy with successful autologous stem cell trans-plantation," *Annals of Hematology*, vol. 82, no. 5, pp. 305–309, 2003.

33

Methotrexate Treatment in Children with Febrile Ulceronecrotic Mucha-Habermann Disease: Case Report and Literature Review

Isil Bulur,[1] Hilal Kaya Erdoğan,[1] Zeynep Nurhan Saracoglu,[1] and Deniz Arık[2]

[1]*Department of Dermatology and Venereology, Faculty of Medicine, Osmangazi University, Eskişehir, Turkey*
[2]*Department of Pathology, Faculty of Medicine, Osmangazi University, Eskişehir, Turkey*

Correspondence should be addressed to Isil Bulur; isilbulur@yahoo.com

Academic Editor: Thomas Berger

Febrile Ulceronecrotic Mucha-Habermann disease is a rare and potentially fatal variant of pityriasis lichenoides et varioliformis acuta and is characterized by high fever, constitutional symptoms, and acute oncet of ulceronecrotic lesions. We present an 11-year-old male with Febrile Ulceronecrotic Mucha-Habermann disease who was cured with methotrexate and review the use of methotrexate for this disorder in the pediatric age group with the relevant literature.

1. Introduction

Pityriasis lichenoides et varioliformis acuta (PLEVA) is a rare idiopathic dermatosis. Febrile Ulceronecrotic Mucha-Habermann disease (FUMHD), first defined by Degos et al. in 1966, is a severe variant of PLEVA that is characterized by destructive ulceronecrotic lesions and frequently accompanied by systemic findings [1].

Systemic steroids, oral antibiotics (erythromycin, tetracycline), phototherapy, and immunosuppressive agents are used for treatment but the results are mostly in the form of case reports. Methotrexate treatment has been reported as an effective option in a few cases in the literature. We report here an 11-year-old boy with FUMHD who was treated with methotrexate.

2. Case Report

An 11-year-old male presented at our clinic with a 15-day history of body rash. There was no history of medication use and drug or food allergies. He had a history of Guillain-Barre syndrome at the age of 9 years. Dermatological examination revealed a widespread polymorphic rash with erythematous macules, papules with a central punctum, and pustules on the trunk and extremities (Figure 1(a)). There was not any involvement in oral mucosa and conjunctiva. Laboratory tests revealed normal complete blood count, erythrocyte sedimentation rate, C reactive protein, and biochemistry values. Serologies for *hepatitis B virus, hepatitis C virus, HIV, cytomegalovirus (CMV), rubeola, toxoplasma, parvovirus,* and *herpes simplex virus* were negative. *Rubella, varicella,* and *Epstein–Barr virus* were negative for IgM but positive for IgG, suggesting a past infection. Serum IgA and IgM were within the normal range and IgG was slightly decreased (610 mg/dL, normal: 700–1600 mg/dL). Analysis of peripheral lymphocyte subsets revealed slightly decreased numbers of CD3+CD4 cells (21.2%, normal: 30–60%). The percentage of B cells (CD19+) was slightly elevated (35.8%; normal 1–35%).

The skin biopsy taken from the body lesion revealed parakeratosis in the epidermis with neutrophil groups within, mixed inflammatory cell infiltration around the vessels and the interstitial area in the upper dermis, and vacuolar degeneration in the basal layer (Figure 1(b)). We diagnosed our patient with PLEVA in the presence of these clinicopathological findings and started oral methylprednisolone 32 mg/day and oral erythromycin 500 mg 2 times a day in addition to topical supportive treatment. However, we noticed an exacerbation of the patient's lesions on the 10th day of treatment. The erythematous papular lesions covered almost all the body including the face and extremities,

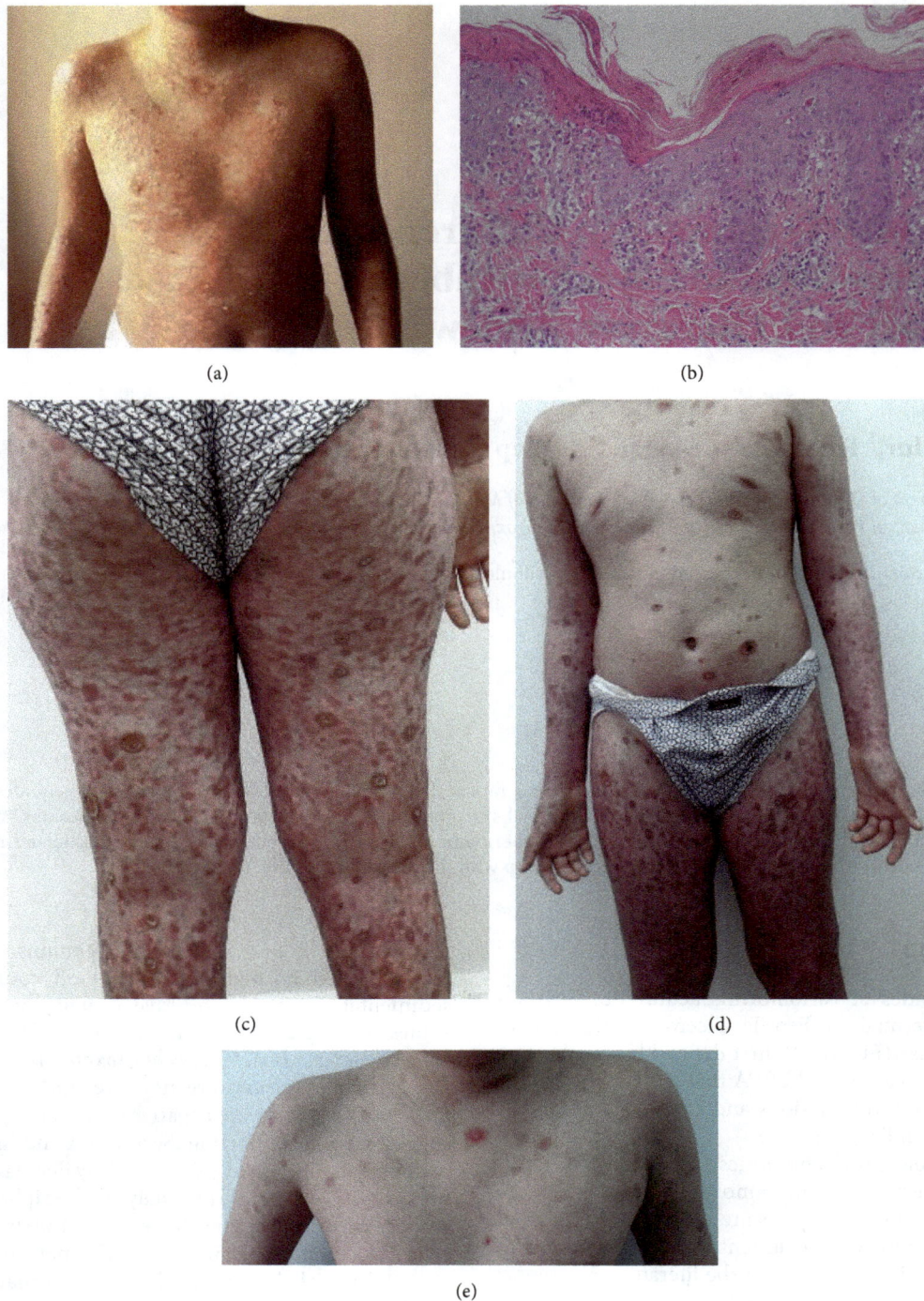

(a)

(b)

(c)

(d)

(e)

FIGURE 1: (a) Erythematous macules, papules, and pustules on the trunk. (b) Histopathology of the skin lesion showing parakeratosis, extension of infiltrate into epidermis, vacuolization of basal layer with necrotic keratinocytes, and mixed inflammatory cell infiltration around the vessels and in the upper dermis (HE ×200). (c) Necrotic ulcers, erythematous papules, and plaques on the limbs. (d) Clinical appearance after six doses of methotrexate. (e) Clinical appearance five months after the patient's initial visit.

together with an AST value of 73 U/L (normal: 0–37) and ALT value of 262 U/L (normal: 0–41). We discontinued the erythromycin treatment and continued with methylpred-nisolone 48 mg/day and topical supportive treatment. The liver function test results recovered to normal limits 10 days after discontinuation of erythromycin, but the patient continued to develop new ulceronecrotic lesions (Figure 1(c)). The second biopsy taken from the new developing lesion was also consistent with PLEVA, and methotrexate 15 mg/week was added to the systemic steroid treatment. The systemic

TABLE 1: Literature review.

Reference (first author)	Age	Sex	Systemic involvement	Therapy	Outcome
Lopez-Estebaranz, 1993 [4]	18 y	M	Liver dysfunction	SS, ATB, MTX, and PUVA	Cure
Fink-Puches, 1994 [5]	16 y	M	(—)	SS, ATB, and MTX	Cure
Romaní, 1998 [6]	12 y	F	(—)	ATB, MTX, and PUVA	Cure
Ito, 2003 [7]	12 y	M	Anemia, abdominal pain, and lymphadenopathy	SS, MTX	Cure
Tsianakas, 2005 [8]	9 y	M	(—)	SS, ATB, and MTX	Cure
Herron, 2005 [9]	8 y	F	Sepsis, DIG, ARDS, and gastrointestinal hemorrhage	SS, MTX, ATB, and cyclosporine	Cure
Pyrpasopoulou, 2007 [10]	17 y	F	Sepsis, anemia, and diarrhea	SS, ATB, IVIG, acyclovir, and MTX	Cure
Helbling, 2009 [11]	17 y	M	Lymphadenopathy	ATB, MTX	
Zhang, 2010 [12]	12 y	M	Pulmonary involvement	SS, ATB, and MTX	Cure
Kaufman, 2012 [13]	21 m	F	Laryngeal edema	SS, MTX	Cure
Kaufman, 2012 [13]	22 m	F	(—)	SS, ATB, acyclovir, and MTX	
Perrin, 2012 [14]	34 m	M	(—)	SS, ATB, acyclovir, dapsone, IVIG, and MTX	Cure
Lin, 2012 [15]	11 y	M	Fever, arthritis, fatigue	SS, MTX	Cure
Rosman, 2013 [16]	11 y	M	Central nervous system vasculitis	SS, ATB, MTX, and cyclophosphamide	Cure
Our patient	11 y	M	Liver dysfunction	SS, ATB, and MTX	Cure

F: female, M: male, y: year, m: month, SS: systemic steroid, ATB: antibiotic, MTX: methotrexate, IVIG: intravenous immunoglobulin, and PUVA: psoralen UVA.

steroid treatment was gradually tapered and stopped. There was marked improvement in the lesions at the 6th week of methotrexate treatment (Figure 1(d)). Methotrexate was stopped after 5 months. We did not observe any secondary side effect due to the methotrexate treatment. The lesions healed with a postinflammatory hyperpigmentation and hypertrophic scar (Figure 1(e)).

3. Discussion

PLEVA is characterized by acute onset of scaly erythematous papules that might become vesicles and pustules with hemorrhagic necrosis and ulceration [2]. FUMHD is a rare and potential fatal form of PLEVA with a severe course and ulceronecrotic involvement [3]. PUBMED data reveal that only a limited number of pediatric FUMHD cases have been reported, and there is no clear treatment algorithm in this disorder.

Topical corticosteroids, immunomodulators, and oral antibiotics (erythromycin, tetracycline) have been used as a first-step treatment and PUVA and UVB as a second-step treatment for PLEVA, while systemic steroid, methotrexate, cyclosporine, dapsone, and acitretin are third-step treatment [2]. However, third-step treatment for PLEVA should be started as soon as possible in FUMHD cases [3].

When we reviewed the literature data, we observed that methotrexate treatment has been used in 15 pediatric FUMHD cases and the results of methotrexate treatment have been successful together with systemic steroids in 13 patients [4–16] (Table 1). Cyclosporine and cyclophosphamide were used in addition to the methotrexate treatment in two patients with severe systemic involvement. Herron et al. have

reported clinical recovery with the addition of cyclosporine 3 mg/kg/day to methotrexate 15 mg/week in an FUMHD case accompanied by sepsis and ARDS [9]. Rosman et al. reported control of FUMDH with central nervous system vasculitis using systemic steroids and 15 mg/week methotrexate treatment supported by 1000 mg/m² cyclophosphamide treatment. They also emphasized that systemic steroids and methotrexate were added again to control the cutaneous findings that flared at the 5-year follow-up [16]. We observed that methotrexate was given in a dose of 7,5–20 mg/week for FUMDH cases. Neither our case nor any of patients reported in the literature developed liver dysfunction or blood level abnormalities secondary to the methotrexate treatment.

The primary mechanism of action of methotrexate is inhibiting DNA, RNA, thymidylate, and protein synthesis through dihydrofolate reductase inhibition. In addition, it is also effective in lymphoproliferative disorders through its anti-inflammatory features as a result of its effects on T cell activation [17]. FUMDH is considered to be within the lymphoproliferative disorder spectrum and therefore the effect of methotrexate on T cells may be responsible for these results in FUMHD cases.

In conclusion, we think that methotrexate treatment is more effective and reliable treatment option than steroid therapy for pediatric FUMHD cases. Therefore, methotrexate should be considered as first-line treatment in FUMHD.

Disclosure

Hilal Kaya Erdoğan, Zeynep Nurhan Saracoglu, and Deniz Arık are coauthors.

Conflict of Interests

The authors declare no conflict of interests.

Authors' Contribution

All authors have made substantial contributions to all of the following: the concept and design of the case report, drafting the paper or revising it critically for important intellectual content, and final approval of the version to be submitted.

References

[1] R. Degos, B. Duperrat, and F. Daniel, "Hyperthermic ulceronecrotic parapsoriasis. Subacute form of parapsoriasis guttata," *Annales de Dermatologie et de Syphiligraphie (Paris)*, vol. 93, no. 5, pp. 481–496, 1966.

[2] N. F. Fernandes, P. J. Rozdeba, R. A. Schwartz, G. Kihiczak, and W. C. Lambert, "Pityriasis lichenoides et varioliformis acuta: a disease spectrum," *International Journal of Dermatology*, vol. 49, no. 3, pp. 257–261, 2010.

[3] L. Meziane, A. Caudron, F. Dhaille et al., "Febrile ulceronecrotic mucha-habermann disease: treatment with infliximab and intravenous immunoglobulins and review of the literature," *Dermatology*, vol. 225, no. 4, pp. 344–348, 2013.

[4] J. L. Lopez-Estebaranz, F. Vanaclocha, R. Gil, B. Garcia, and L. Iglesias, "Febrile ulceronecrotic Mucha-Habermann disease," *Journal of the American Academy of Dermatology*, vol. 29, no. 5, pp. 903–906, 1993.

[5] R. Fink-Puches, H. P. Soyer, and H. Kerl, "Febrile ulceronecrotic pityriasis lichenoides et varioliformis acuta," *Journal of the American Academy of Dermatology*, vol. 30, no. 2, pp. 261–263, 1994.

[6] J. Romaní, L. Puig, M. T. Fernández-Figueras, and J. M. De Moragas, "Pityriasis lichenoides in children: clinicopathologic review of 22 patients," *Pediatric Dermatology*, vol. 15, no. 1, pp. 1–6, 1998.

[7] N. Ito, A. Ohshima, H. Hashizume, M. Takigawa, and Y. Tokura, "Febrile ulceronecrotic Mucha-Habermann's disease managed with methylprednisolone semipulse and subsequent methotrexate therapies," *Journal of the American Academy of Dermatology*, vol. 49, no. 6, pp. 1142–1148, 2003.

[8] A. Tsianakas and P. H. Hoeger, "Transition of pityriasis lichenoides et varioliformis acuta to febrile ulceronecrotic Mucha-Habermann disease is associated with elevated serum tumour necrosis factor-α," *British Journal of Dermatology*, vol. 152, no. 4, pp. 794–799, 2005.

[9] M. D. Herron, J. F. Bohnsack, and S. L. Vanderhooft, "Septic, CD-30 positive febrile ulceronecrotic pityriasis lichenoides et varioliformis acuta," *Pediatric Dermatology*, vol. 22, no. 4, pp. 360–365, 2005.

[10] A. Pyrpasopoulou, V. G. Athyros, A. Karagiannis, F. Chrysomallis, and C. Zamboulis, "Intravenous immunoglobulins: a valuable asset in the treatment of a case of septic febrile ulceronecrotic Mucha-Habermann disease," *Dermatology*, vol. 215, no. 2, pp. 164–165, 2007.

[11] I. Helbling, R. J. G. Chalmers, and V. M. Yates, "Febrile ulceronecrotic Mucha-Habermann disease: a rare dermatological emergency," *Clinical and Experimental Dermatology*, vol. 34, no. 8, pp. e1006–e1007, 2009.

[12] L.-X. Zhang, Y. Liang, Y. Liu, and L. Ma, "Febrile ulceronecrotic mucha-habermann's disease with pulmonary involvement," *Pediatric Dermatology*, vol. 27, no. 3, pp. 290–293, 2010.

[13] W. S. Kaufman, E. K. McNamara, A. R. Curtis, P. Kosari, J. L. Jorizzo, and D. P. Krowchuk, "Febrile ulceronecrotic Mucha-Habermann disease (*pityriasis lichenoides et varioliformis acuta fulminans*) presenting as Stevens-Johnson syndrome," *Pediatric Dermatology*, vol. 29, no. 2, pp. 135–140, 2012.

[14] B. S. Perrin, A. C. Yan, and J. R. Treat, "Febrile ulceronecrotic mucha-habermann disease in a 34-month-old boy: a case report and review of the literature," *Pediatric Dermatology*, vol. 29, no. 1, pp. 53–58, 2012.

[15] C.-Y. Lin, J. Cook, and D. Purvis, "Febrile ulceronecrotic Mucha-Habermann disease: a case with systemic symptoms managed with subcutaneous methotrexate," *Australasian Journal of Dermatology*, vol. 53, no. 4, pp. e83–e86, 2012.

[16] I. S. Rosman, L.-C. Liang, S. Patil, S. J. Bayliss, and A. J. White, "Febrile ulceronecrotic mucha-habermann disease with central nervous system vasculitis," *Pediatric Dermatology*, vol. 30, no. 1, pp. 90–93, 2013.

[17] A. Johnston, J. E. Gudjonsson, H. Sigmundsdottir, B. Runar Ludviksson, and H. Valdimarsson, "The anti-inflammatory action of methotrexate is not mediated by lymphocyte apoptosis, but by the suppression of activation and adhesion molecules," *Clinical Immunology*, vol. 114, no. 2, pp. 154–163, 2005.

34

An Uncommon Side Effect of Bupropion:
A Case of Acute Generalized Exanthematous Pustulosis

Hasan Tak,[1] Cengiz Koçak,[2] Gülben Sarıcı,[1] Nazlı Dizen Namdar,[1] and Mehtap Kıdır[1]

[1]*Department of Dermatology, Faculty of Medicine, Dumlupinar University, 43100 Kutahya, Turkey*
[2]*Department of Pathology, Faculty of Medicine, Dumlupinar University, 43100 Kutahya, Turkey*

Correspondence should be addressed to Hasan Tak; htak70@yahoo.com

Academic Editor: Akimichi Morita

Acute generalized exanthematous pustulosis (AGEP) is a rare inflammatory dermatosis characterized by multiple nonfollicular pustules that occur on erythematous skin. Despite its similarity to pustular psoriasis and association with fever and leukocytosis, AGEP typically heals quickly. Etiologically, drugs and viruses have been suspected in most cases. Here, we present a case of AGEP, in a woman, that developed 1 day after starting bupropion for smoking cessation, as a rare side effect of the treatment.

1. Introduction

Acute generalized exanthematous pustulosis (AGEP) is a rare inflammatory eruption characterized by the sudden development of multiple small sterile pustules on erythematous skin. It is accompanied by fever and leukocytosis. The disease has typical histopathological findings and recovers spontaneously within 15 days [1]. Mucosal membrane involvement occurs in about 20% of the cases and the majority of patients have mild oral lesions [2].

Etiologically, antibiotics, mostly aminopenicillins and macrolides, play a role in more than 90% of the cases [2].

The differential diagnosis of AGEP includes generalized pustular psoriasis, subcorneal pustular dermatosis, pemphigus foliaceus, toxic epidermal necrolysis, drug reaction with eosinophilia, systemic symptoms syndrome, and other follicular eruptions such as acneiform and bacterial folliculitis [1, 2].

Bupropion is a dopamine reuptake inhibitor that is used as an antidepressant and for smoking cessation. There are 28 reports of dermatological side effects from bupropion, including angioedema, erythema multiforme, Stevens-Johnson syndrome, exfoliative dermatitis, urticaria, and serum disease [3].

Here, we report a case of AGEP that developed as a rare side effect of bupropion.

2. Case Report

A 30-year-old woman visited our outpatient clinic with acute eruptions that appeared 4 days earlier on her face and trunk and then spread to her extremities. She took a bupropion tablet for smoking cessation 1 day before beginning of the eruptions and had a fever for the past 4 days. There was no history of psoriasis, previous drug allergy, or use of another drug with bupropion. She denied the use of any over-the-counter medications, supplements, or herbal remedies. She had not used a new soap, shampoo, or laundry soap before the skin reaction appeared.

Dermatological examination revealed numerous pustules on her face, trunk, and legs. The erythematous areas tended to fuse and were not characterized by follicular localization (Figure 1). There were no lesions on the oral mucosa and the examination of other systems was unremarkable. Her axillary temperature was 38.2°C.

The laboratory results showed leukocytosis (12.90 × 109/L, 88.8% neutrophils) and an increased C-reactive protein level. There was no eosinophilia. Her liver enzymes, serum protein, albumin, and electrolytes were normal.

To confirm the diagnosis of AGEP and to rule out generalized pustular psoriasis, a 4 mm punch biopsy was taken from the skin. The histopathology showed neutrophilic pustular lesions (red arrow) together with epidermal spongiosis,

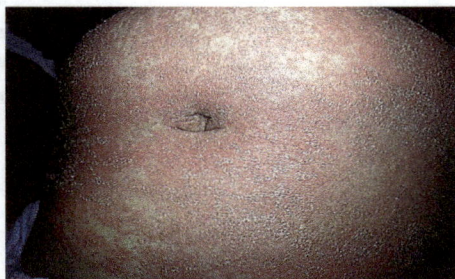

FIGURE 1: Revealed pustules on erythematous areas that tended to unite and did not display a follicular localization on the abdomen.

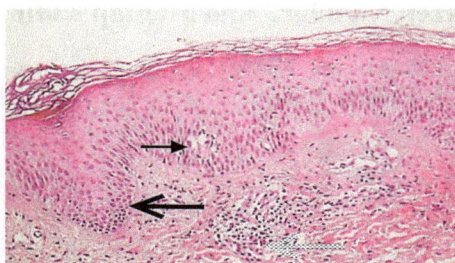

FIGURE 2: A photomicrograph of the biopsy showing neutrophilic pustular lesion together with epidermal spongiosis (thin arrow), minimal irregular acanthosis in epidermis (thick arrow), and neutrophilic and eosinophilic infiltration around dermal vessels (dashed arrow) (H&E ×200).

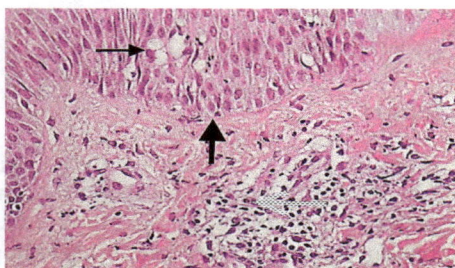

FIGURE 3: A photomicrograph of the biopsy showing neutrophilic pustular lesion together with epidermal spongiosis (thin arrow), minimal irregular acanthosis in epidermis (thick arrow), and neutrophilic and eosinophilic infiltration around dermal vessels (dashed arrow) (H&E ×400).

minimal irregular acanthosis (black arrow) in the epidermis, and neutrophilic and eosinophilic infiltration (blue arrow) around dermal vessels (Figures 2 and 3).

The diagnosis of AGEP was made histopathologically, combined with the clinical findings (a fever for 4 days and an eruption that spreads from the face and trunk to the extremities) and a history of the absence of psoriasis or other drug use. The patient discontinued the bupropion treatment after the fever and eruption appeared. Intravenous methylprednisolone (40 mg/day) was administered for 4 days. In addition, topical corticosteroid and oral analgesic and antihistaminic were used. Within 4 days of the treatment,

there were no new pustules and the healing was complete within 10 days with exfoliation.

3. Discussion

In 1980, Beylot et al. first described AGEP as a different entity from a drug eruption, characterized by sterile pustules on erythematous skin and usually confused with generalized pustular psoriasis [4]. Then, in 1991, Roujeau et al. outlined the characteristic features of AGEP in 63 cases [5]. These characteristic features were nonfollicular sterile pustules (5 mm) that were intraepidermal or subcorneal on histopathology (together with one or more additional findings like dermal edema, vasculitis, perivascular eosinophilia, or focal keratinocyte necrosis), disappearance of the eruptions within 15 days after drug cessation, presence of fever over 38°C, and neutrophilia over 7×109/L.

There are several theories on the pathogenesis of AGEP. Britschgi et al. suggested a T-cell mediated mechanism, as evidenced by positive findings on patch tests and lymphocyte transformation tests [6]. Moreau et al. proposed that AGEP is a delayed-type hypersensitivity reaction [7]. Another possible mechanism is the production of antigen-antibody complexes induced by an infection or drug that activates the complement system, which in turn leads to neutrophil chemotaxis [8].

In recent years, a new concept called pharmacological interaction has been developed to explain drug-induced hypersensitivity reactions. This concept implies direct, reversible interactions of the drug with T-cell receptors and is classified as a T-cell mediated reaction. Previous drug exposure is not necessary [9].

In our patient, since the reaction occurred within a single day of taking the first bupropion tablet, we believe that the pathogenesis of AGEP involves a pharmacological interaction or an unknown mechanism.

The EuroSCAR group has developed a validated scale for determining causation of AGEP by a medication [2]. This scale suggests that our case was definitely caused by bupropion, while the Naranjo algorithm [10] suggests that it was probably caused by bupropion. These results were similar to those of Ray and Wall [11].

Although viral infections [5, 12] or hypersensitivity to mercury [13] has been reported in the etiology, Sidoroff et al. suggested that drugs are more likely to trigger AGEP, and they found no relationship between infection and the development of AGEP [14].

A high proportion of AGEP cases have been attributed to aminopenicillins or macrolides but, interestingly, not to sulfonamides, which have a higher potential for causing other cutaneous drug reactions. Some cases have been attributed to antimycotic drugs. Moreover, several nonantibiotics, especially calcium channel blockers, carbamazepine, and paracetamol, have been reported as the culprit agents in numerous cases [2].

To the best of our knowledge, 129 different drugs have been implicated in the etiology of AGEP [3]. Recently, tigecycline and labetalol and psychotropic drugs such as amoxapine, sertraline, and bupropion were added to this list [3, 15, 16]. When we searched the literature for an association between bupropion and AGEP, ours was the second reported case [11].

The differential diagnosis of AGEP includes generalized pustular psoriasis. Although the pustules in the two diseases cannot be distinguished clinically, histopathological examination shows widespread edema in the dermis, vasculitis, perivascular eosinophilic infiltration, and focal keratinocyte necrosis in AGEP, while the presence of regular acanthosis in the epidermis supports pustular psoriasis [17, 18]. In our case, the minimal irregular acanthosis, widespread dermal edema, and perivascular lymphocytic and eosinophilic infiltration were thought to favor a diagnosis of AGEP.

The treatment of AGEP involves stopping the causative drug and supportive treatment for the symptoms and local lesions. Systemic corticosteroids are not required in most cases [2].

Acute generalized exanthematous pustulosis should be included in the differential diagnosis of a patient with a sudden-onset widespread pustular eruption. In such patients, a history of psoriasis and drug use should also be investigated. We also need to consider bupropion as the cause of these cutaneous side effects.

Conflict of Interests

The authors declare that there is no conflict of interests regarding the publication of this paper.

References

[1] I. M. Freedberg, A. Z. Eisen, K. Wolf et al., *Fitzpatrick's Dermatology in General Medicine*, McGraw-Hill, New York, NY, USA, 6th edition, 2003.

[2] A. Sidoroff, S. Halevy, J. N. B. Bavinck, L. Vaillant, and J.-C. Roujeau, "Acute generalized exanthematous pustulosis (AGEP)—a clinical reaction pattern," *Journal of Cutaneous Pathology*, vol. 28, no. 3, pp. 113–119, 2001.

[3] J. Z. Litt, *Drug Eruptions & Reactions Manual*, Taylor & Francis, New York, NY, USA, 19th edition, 2013.

[4] C. Beylot, P. Bioulac, and M. S. Doutre, "Acute generalized exanthematic pustuloses," *Annales de Dermatologie et de Vénéréologie*, vol. 107, pp. 37–48, 1980.

[5] J.-C. Roujeau, P. Bioulac-Sage, C. Bourseau et al., "Acute generalized exanthematous pustulosis: analysis of 63 cases," *Archives of Dermatology*, vol. 127, no. 9, pp. 1333–1338, 1991.

[6] M. Britschgi, U. C. Steiner, S. Schmid et al., "T-cell involvement in drug-induced acute generalized exanthematous pustulosis," *The Journal of Clinical Investigation*, vol. 107, no. 11, pp. 1433–1441, 2001.

[7] A. Moreau, A. Dompmartin, B. Castel, B. Remond, and D. Leroy, "Drug-induced acute generalized exanthematous pustulosis with positive patch tests," *International Journal of Dermatology*, vol. 34, no. 4, pp. 263–266, 1995.

[8] C. Beylot, M.-S. Doutre, and M. Beylot-Barry, "Acute generalized exanthematous pustulosis," *Seminars in Cutaneous Medicine and Surgery*, vol. 15, no. 4, pp. 244–249, 1996.

[9] W. J. Pichler, "Pharmacological interaction of drugs with antigen-specific ımmune receptors: the p-i concept," *Current Opinion in Allergy & Clinical Immunology*, vol. 2, no. 4, pp. 301–305, 2002.

[10] C. A. Naranjo, U. Busto, E. M. Sellers et al., "A method for estimating the probability of adverse drug reactions," *Clinical Pharmacology & Therapeutics*, vol. 30, no. 2, pp. 239–245, 1981.

[11] A. K. Ray and G. C. Wall, "Bupropion-induced acute generalized exanthematous pustulosis," *Pharmacotherapy*, vol. 31, no. 6, article 621, 2011.

[12] B. Rouchouse, M. Bonnefoy, B. Pallot, L. Jacquelin, G. Dimoux-Dime, and A. L. Claudy, "Acute generalized exanthematous pustular dermatitis and viral infection," *Dermatologica*, vol. 173, no. 4, pp. 180–184, 1986.

[13] H. Belhadjali, S. Mandhouj, A. Moussa et al., "Mercury-induced acute generalized exanthematous pustulosis misdiagnosed as a drug-related case," *Contact Dermatitis*, vol. 59, no. 1, pp. 52–54, 2008.

[14] A. Sidoroff, A. Dunant, C. Viboud et al., "Risk factors for acute generalized exanthematous pustulosis (AGEP)-results of a multinational case-control study (EuroSCAR)," *British Journal of Dermatology*, vol. 157, no. 5, pp. 989–996, 2007.

[15] S. Ozturk, C. Ustun, S. Pehlivan, and H. Ucak, "Acute generalized exanthematous pustulosis associated with tigecycline," *Annals of Dermatology*, vol. 26, no. 2, pp. 246–249, 2014.

[16] E. Gómez Torrijos, C. García Rodríguez, M. P. Sánchez Caminero, A. Castro Jiménez, R. García Rodríguez, and F. Feo-Brito, "First case report of acute generalized exanthematous pustulosis due to labetalol," *Journal of Investigational Allergology & Clinical Immunology*, vol. 25, no. 2, pp. 148–149, 2015.

[17] C. Beylot, M.-S. Doutre, and M. Beylot-Barry, "Acute generalized exanthematous pustulosis," *Seminars in Cutaneous Medicine and Surgery*, vol. 15, no. 4, pp. 244–249, 1996.

[18] P. Auer-Grumbach, E. Pfaffenthaler, and H. P. Soyer, "Pustulosis acuta generalisata is a post-streptococcal disease and is distinct from acute generalized exanthematous pustulosis," *British Journal of Dermatology*, vol. 133, no. 1, pp. 135–139, 1995.

35

Type VI Aplasia Cutis Congenita: Bart's Syndrome

Ferit Kulalı,[1] Ahmet Yagmur Bas,[1] Yusuf Kale,[1] Istemi Han Celik,[1] Nihal Demirel,[1] and Sema Apaydın[2]

[1]*Division of Neonatology, Etlik Zübeyde Hanim Women's Health Teaching and Research Hospital, Ankara, Turkey*
[2]*Department of Pathology, Dr. Sami Ulus Maternity and Children Research and Training Hospital, Ankara, Turkey*

Correspondence should be addressed to Ferit Kulalı; fkulali@gazi.edu.tr

Academic Editor: Akimichi Morita

Bart's syndrome is characterized by aplasia cutis congenita and epidermolysis bullosa. We present the case of a newborn male who developed blisters on the mucous membranes and the skin following congenital localized absence of skin. Bart's syndrome (BS) is diagnosed clinically based on the disorder's unique signs and symptoms but histologic evaluation of the skin can help to confirm the final diagnosis. The patient was managed conservatively with topical antibacterial ointment and wet gauze dressing. Periodic follow-up examinations showed complete healing. We emphasized that it is important to use relatively simple methods for optimal healing without the need for complex surgical interventions.

1. Introduction

Bart's syndrome (BS) is characterized by aplasia cutis congenita (ACC) and epidermolysis bullosa (EB). It may be accompanied by nail abnormalities such as congenital absence, nail dystrophy, or further loss [1]. Its etiology and pathophysiology are still controversial although several hypotheses have been proposed [2].

Although the inheritance pattern appears to be autosomally dominant, isolated cases have been recognized. Lesions in BS are usually unilateral and involved the medial and/or dorsal surface of the limbs. They appear on extremities as sharply demarcated, glistening red ulceration that extend upward from the dorsal and the medial surface of the foot to the shin [3]. In this paper, the management of a sporadic case of Bart's syndrome is presented.

2. Case

A male infant was born to a 25-year-old gravida 2, para 2, mother via cesarean section at term. Labor and delivery were uncomplicated. Apgar scores were 8 and 9 at 1 and 5 minutes, respectively. The parents were not relatives, and the family history was unremarkable. They had a healthy, five-year-old girl. In their family there was no history of skin, connective tissue, or autoimmune disease.

He had normal weight, length, head circumference, and vital signs. On physical examination, he was found to have absence of skin over the anteromedial aspect of both lower legs, starting from the knees and extending to dorsal and medial plantar aspect of the feet. The lesions have sharply demarcated borders covered by a red ultrathin translucent membrane (Figure 1). On the second day, he developed blisters on the upper lip mucous membranes and on the left wrist (Figure 2). Results of his complete blood count, liver and renal function tests, electrolytes, ionized calcium, and magnesium were within normal limits. Serologic tests for TORCH were negative. Ophthalmological examination, abdominal and cranial ultrasound screening, and echocardiography revealed normal findings. Histopathological examination of the left wrist lesion demonstrated full or partial developed subepithelial vesicle formation (Figure 3). Direct immunofluorescent staining showed weak focal perivascular deposition of IgM, IgA, C3, and Fibrinogen but did not demonstrate IgG, C4, and C1q depositions that have suggested dystrophic epidermolysis bullosa. The combination of aplasia cutis congenital (ACC) and EB led to the diagnosis of Bart's Syndrome.

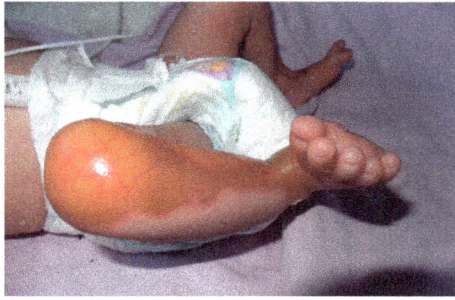

FIGURE 1: Sharply demarcated lesion margin.

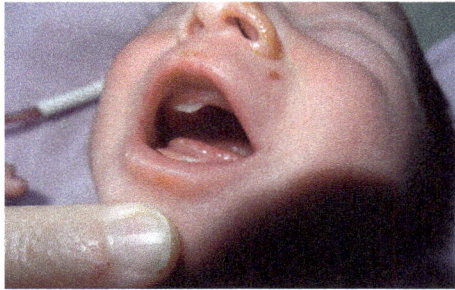

FIGURE 2: Blisters on the upper lip mucous membranes.

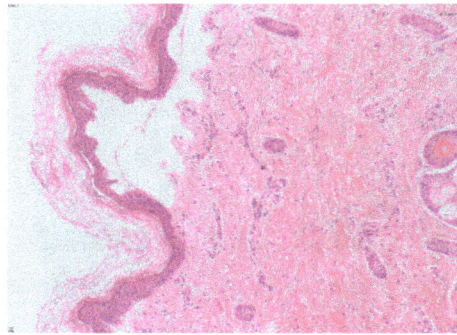

FIGURE 3: Subepithelial vesicle formation.

Patient was referred to dermatology. Physician recommended to allow the area to heal spontaneously by using conservative wound care such as topical antibacterial ointment and wet gauze dressing two to three times a day. The patient was treated by applying topical mupirocin (Bactroban) and wet gauze dressing (Bactigras) for 4 weeks and skin lesions had recovered substantially with appropriate therapy. The infant was discharged on the tenth day of hospital stay to continue local wound care by his mother.

3. Discussion

Bart's syndrome was originally described in a family with congenital absence of skin on the lower leg and widespread blistering of skin, mucous membrane, and nail dystrophy [3]. Previously, Frieden (1986) classified by location and presence of the other anomalies into nine groups. According to this classification, group 6 was defined as Bart's syndrome which is characterized by a combination of congenital localized absence of skin (CLAS) and EB [4]. Currently, however, we know that Bart's syndrome is characterized by EB with congenital absence of skin and is one of the subtypes of EB [5]. BS is sometimes accompanied by nail abnormalities which are not absolutely required for making the diagnosis. In our patient, there was involvement of congenital localized absence of skin and blistering lesions but there was no involvement of nail.

The scalp is the most frequent site of involvement, although trunk and extremities may also be involved [6]. ACC may be unilateral or less frequently bilateral. Our patient's lesions had symmetric involvement at both legs. BS

can also be associated with other anomalies as pyloric atresia, rudimentary ear development, flattened nose, broad nasal root, and wide-set eyes [7]. The present case had no associated anomalies.

BS is diagnosed clinically based on the disorder's unique signs and symptoms but histologic evaluation of the skin can help to confirm the final diagnosis [2]. Biopsy specimen revealed an increased inflammatory infiltrate in the dermis, probably because of capillary leakage.

Zelickson et al. demonstrated various abnormalities of anchoring fibrils, which are mainly composed of type VII collagen, at the dermal-epidermal junction in BS [8]. Duran-McKinster et al. proposed that congenital localized absence of skin in BS may follow the lines of Blaschko owing to physical trauma in utero [1].

Christiano et al. identified a mutation leading to a glycine-to-arginine substitution at type VII collagen [9]. The genetic abnormality has been associated with chromosome 3, with an autosomal pattern of inheritance. Molecular (DNA) analysis for the diagnosis could not be performed in the present case.

The predominant inheritance pattern is autosomally dominant, while some cases with unaffected parents are believed to occur due to sporadic mutation [10]. As shown in the study by Chiaverini et al. sporadic cases have been reported to be associated with mutations of the triple helix domain of collagen VII gene. This mutation that is correlated with synthesis of a thermolabile Col 7 may lead to BS. The present case had no family history of congenital localized absence of skin and blistering lesions; therefore he was a sporadic one. The different diagnosis of BS includes aplasia cutis congenita, epidermolysis bullosa, Adams-Oliver syndrome, and congenital bullous poikiloderma (Kindler syndrome).

The management of BS is usually conservative, preventing infection of affected area and allowing the affected portion to declare itself in order to optimize future reconstruction. The goal of treatment is to accelerate healing and reduce the risk of scarring [11]. Close follow-up for serious complications, such as hemorrhage, infection, hypothermia, and hypoglycemia, is important. Prognosis is good and depends on efficacy of treatment.

The use of prophylactic systemic antibiotics in therapy has not been recommended. We used topical antibacterial ointment and wet gauze dressing in our patient. Sterile dressings with Bactigras of the lesions were done twice daily.

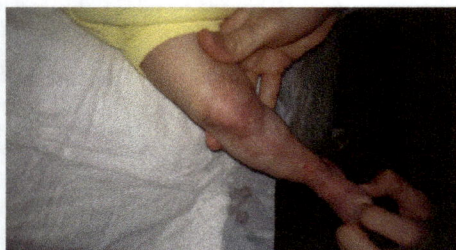

FIGURE 4: Healing of the lesions with conservative treatment.

Epithelialization process on the lesions was noted on the tenth day of hospital stay and the infant was discharged. As shown in Figure 4, the wound healing in this patient is rapid, efficient, and perfect.

We emphasized that it is important to use relatively simple methods for optimal healing without the need for complex surgical interventions.

Conflict of Interests

The authors declare no conflict of interests.

Authors' Contribution

Dr. Kulalı wrote the first draft of the paper. All of the authors collaborated on the second and subsequent drafts of the paper.

References

[1] C. Duran-McKinster, A. Rivera-Franco, L. Tamayo, M. De La Luz Orozco-Covarrubias, and R. Ruiz-Maldonado, "Bart syndrome: the congenital localized absence of skin may follow the lines of Blaschko. Report of six cases," *Pediatric Dermatology*, vol. 17, no. 3, pp. 179–182, 2000.

[2] C. Kothari, N. Doshi, A. Avila, and D. Martin, "Visual diagnosis: newborn with absence of skin," *Pediatrics in Review*, vol. 35, no. 10, pp. e49–e52, 2014.

[3] A. Rajpal, R. Mishra, K. Hajirnis, M. Shah, and N. Nagpur, "Bart's syndrome," *Indian Journal of Dermatology*, vol. 53, no. 2, pp. 88–90, 2008.

[4] I. J. Frieden, "Aplasia cutis congenita: a clinical review and proposal for classification," *Journal of the American Academy of Dermatology*, vol. 14, no. 4, pp. 646–660, 1986.

[5] J.-D. Fine, L. Bruckner-Tuderman, R. A. J. Eady et al., "Inherited epidermolysis bullosa: updated recommendations on diagnosis and classification," *Journal of the American Academy of Dermatology*, vol. 70, no. 6, pp. 1103–1126, 2014.

[6] G. Bharti, L. Groves, L. R. David, C. Sanger, and L. C. Argenta, "Aplasia cutis congenita: clinical management of a rare congenital anomaly," *Journal of Craniofacial Surgery*, vol. 22, no. 1, pp. 159–165, 2011.

[7] B. J. Bart and R. C. Lussky, "Bart syndrome with associated anomalies," *American Journal of Perinatology*, vol. 22, no. 7, pp. 365–369, 2005.

[8] B. Zelickson, K. Matsumura, D. Kist, E. H. Epstein Jr., and B. J. Bart, "Bart's syndrome: ultrastructure and genetic linkage," *Archives of Dermatology*, vol. 131, no. 6, pp. 663–668, 1995.

[9] A. M. Christiano, B. J. Bart, E. H. Epstein Jr., and J. Uitto, "Genetic basis of Bart's syndrome: a glycine substitution mutation in the type VII collagen gene," *Journal of Investigative Dermatology*, vol. 106, no. 6, pp. 1340–1342, 1996.

[10] C. Chiaverini, A. Charlesworth, A. Fernandez et al., "Aplasia cutis congenita with dystrophic epidermolysis bullosa: clinical and mutational study," *British Journal of Dermatology*, vol. 170, no. 4, pp. 901–906, 2014.

[11] A. D. Aygun, E. Yilmaz, A. N. Citak Kurt et al., "Aplasia cutis congenita and epidemolysis bullosa: bart syndrome," *International Journal of Dermatology*, vol. 49, no. 3, pp. 343–345, 2010.

36

A Rare Case of Zosteriform Cutaneous Metastases from a Nasopharyngeal Carcinoma

Andrés González García,[1] **Emiliano Grillo Fernández,**[2] **Ignacio Barbolla Díaz,**[1]
Asunción Ballester,[2] **Héctor Pian,**[3] **and Guadalupe Fraile**[1]

[1]*Department of Internal Medicine, University Hospital Ramón y Cajal, Madrid, Spain*
[2]*Department of Dermatology, University Hospital Ramón y Cajal, Madrid, Spain*
[3]*Department of Pathology, University Hospital Ramón y Cajal, Madrid, Spain*

Correspondence should be addressed to Andrés González García; andres_gonzalez_garcia@hotmail.com

Academic Editor: Jacek Cezary Szepietowski

From a clinical point of view, the most common presentations of cutaneous metastatic disease are papules and nodules. However, a wide morphological spectrum of lesions has been described, including erythematous patches or plaques, inflammatory erysipelas-like lesions, diffuse sclerodermiform lesions with induration of the skin, telangiectatic papulovesicles, purpuric plaques mimicking vasculitis, and alopecia areata like scalp lesions. The so-called zosteriform pattern has been described to be in few cases and to the best of our knowledge has never been described associated with a metastasis of a nasopharyngeal carcinoma. This case highlights the relevance of including cutaneous metastases in the differential diagnosis of patients with nonhealing herpes zoster-like lesions, especially in those with underlying neoplasm recently diagnosed.

1. Introduction

Nasopharyngeal carcinoma, although rare in western countries, is a common tumor arising in the nasopharyngeal region [1]. The lesions are mostly undifferentiated carcinomas and are associated with Epstein-Barr virus. On the other hand, the skin metastases are rarely reported [2]. Despite the infrequent skin involvement in these tumors, zosteriform pattern metastasis is a rare, not well-defined, entity, with only few cases published in literature in other kind of solid tumors [3].

We present a case of a zosteriform distribution of its cutaneous metastases, which has not been described previously.

2. Case Report

A 63-year-old man was referred for evaluation in Internal Medicine Department due to enlargement neck masses without any other symptomatology. Previously, he had been referred to an otorhinolaryngologist because of a mild hypoacusis. Several biopsies were undertaken from the neck masses and the histology revealed lesions with a necrotic background, a polymorphic lymphoid cell population, and poorly differentiated syncytial groups of atypical cells of epithelial lineage.

The complementary studies demonstrated osteolytic lesions in the vertebral column compatible with metastatic infiltration. At that moment there was no evidence of metastasis spread at any other location. A chemotherapy cycle was begun and provided a good clinical response.

Three months later, the patient was admitted to the Emergency Department because he had presented with asthenia and painful erythematous, papule-nodular lesions in the left side of the chest. The temperature was 36,2°C, the pulse 82 beats per minute, the blood pressure 100/66 mm Hg, and the respiratory rate 18 breaths per minute. There were erythematous papules following a metameric distribution on the chest and several lesions in the posterior neck area, one of which adhered to deeper underlying structures (Figure 1). This eruption was treated as a herpes zoster infection by his family physician with 3 weeks of valacyclovir without improvement. With the patient's background in mind, a biopsy from

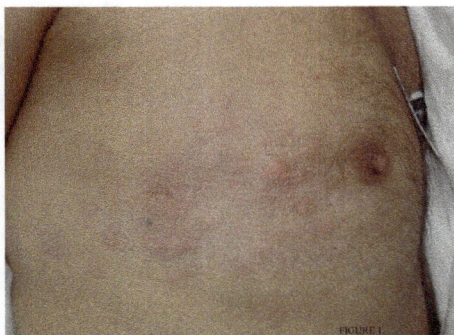

FIGURE 1: Erythematous nodules following a metameric distribution on the chest.

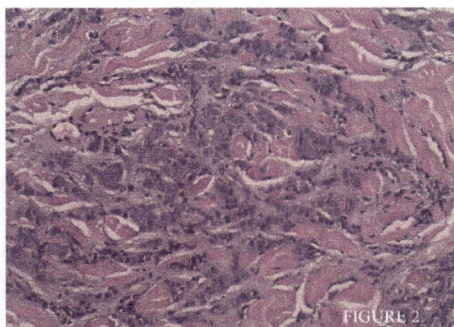

FIGURE 2: Infiltration of deep dermis syncytial groups of large cells with vacuolated clear cytoplasm and vesicular nuclei.

the lesions on the chest was performed and revealed infiltration of a nonkeratinizing lymphoepithelioma-like lesion (Figures 2 and 3). The patient was transferred to the Oncology Department in order to begin with a proper treatment for its condition. Unfortunately new computed tomographic (CT) scans showed evidence of metastatic disease, with new bone lesions and lung nodules. After 3 weeks, the bone lesions had progressed and pain developed, and palliative irradiation and pain medication were required. One month later he opted to pursue palliative care only before he dies.

3. Discussion

Lymphoepithelioma-like carcinoma consists of a proliferation of poorly differentiated epithelial tumor cells with large vesicular nuclei and prominent nucleoli surrounded and infiltrated by dense lymphoplasmocytic infiltrates, mainly T lymphocytes. This tumor is a distinctive subtype of nasopharyngeal carcinoma but may also affect other organs such as the salivary gland, thymus, lungs, and skin [4].

Despite the well described skin involvement with solid tumors, zosteriform metastases are a rare entity, with only few cases published in the literature. A recent meta-analysis reviewed 4,774 patients published in the English literature since 1970 with zosteriform pattern cutaneous involvement. There were eight (14%) lymphomas (1 Hodgkin's lymphoma, 2 non-Hodgkin's lymphomas, 3 cutaneous B-cell lymphomas,

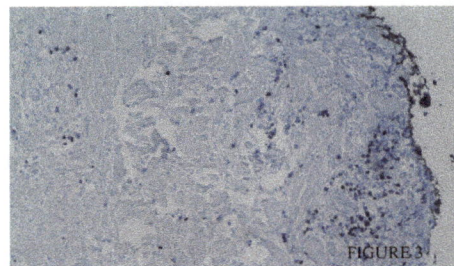

FIGURE 3: Dermis cell with Epstein-Barr virus- (EBV-) encoded RNA (EBER).

and 2 cutaneous T-cell lymphomas), seven (12%) breast cancers, seven (12%) squamous cell carcinomas (SCC), six (11%) digestive tumors (2 gastric tumors, 3 colon tumors, and 1 gallbladder tumor), six (11%) respiratory tumors (5 lung tumors and 1 larynx tumor), and four (7%) urinary tumors (2 kidney tumors, 1 bladder tumor, and 1 prostate tumor) [3]. Many of the dermatomal metastases have been initially diagnosed as herpes zoster which is a common finding in immunocompromised oncology patients [5].

Several hypotheses tried to explain the mechanism of these patterns, but none of these theories have been validated. In our biopsy Epstein-Barr virus (EBV) genome was detected and its association with nasopharyngeal carcinoma and lymphoepithelioma variant is well known [6].

As both the principal etiology agent zoster-varicella virus (ZVV) and EBV belong to the Herpesviridae genre it is not unreasonable to hypothesize that EBV could contribute to the neurotropic distribution of the metastases. Watabe et al. described one case with a zosteriform pattern on a T-cell skin lymphoma where high EBV copies were detected. They gave more importance to the viral role as principal head of the dermatology distribution and the genesis of the tumor [7].

To the best of our knowledge, nasopharyngeal carcinoma has not been described to be associated with a metastatic zosteriform pattern. We performed a search of the medical literature by using the Embase, MEDLINE, and Scopus databases. We used the following terms as subject headings: "nasopharyngeal carcinoma," "exanthema," "skin neoplasms, secondary," and "herpes zoster." In addition, we searched the following keyword terms in all possible combinations: rash, zosteriform, papule, and nasopharyngeal. All references of each relevant report of the above searches were examined. The search disclosed no prior reports of nasopharyngeal carcinoma that caused a zosteriform rash.

4. Conclusions

Because dermatome metastases can mimic herpes zoster, which is a common finding in the immunocompromised oncology patient [3, 8] many of the cases in the literature were initially diagnosed and treated with antiviral agents without improvement. It is important to establish an elevated grade of suspicion in these patients in order not to delay the diagnosis, particularly when there is a background.

The case presented highlights the relevance of including cutaneous metastases in the differential diagnosis of patients with nonhealing herpes zoster-like lesions, especially in those with underlying neoplasm recently diagnosed.

Conflict of Interests

The authors have no conflict of interests to declare in relation to this paper.

Acknowledgment

The authors would like to thank Dr. María Ahijón Lana for her support and help with the paper.

References

[1] A. R. A. Razak, L. L. Siu, F.-F. Liu, E. Ito, B. O'Sullivan, and K. Chan, "Nasopharyngeal carcinoma: the next challenges," *European Journal of Cancer*, vol. 46, no. 11, pp. 1967–1978, 2010.

[2] N. M. Luk, K. H. Yu, C. L. Choi, and W. K. Yeung, "Skin metastasis from nasopharyngeal carcinoma in four Chinese patients," *Clinical and Experimental Dermatology*, vol. 29, no. 1, pp. 28–31, 2004.

[3] P. Savoia, P. Fava, T. Deboli, P. Quaglino, and M. G. Bernengo, "Zosteriform cutaneous metastases: a literature meta-analysis and a clinical report of three melanoma cases," *Dermatologic Surgery*, vol. 35, no. 9, pp. 1355–1363, 2009.

[4] J. C. Iezzoni, M. J. Gaffey, and L. M. Weiss, "The role of Epstein-Barr virus in lymphoepithelioma-like carcinomas," *American Journal of Clinical Pathology*, vol. 103, no. 3, pp. 308–315, 1995.

[5] B. W. LeSueur, R. J. Abraham, D. J. DiCaudo, and W. J. O'Connor, "Zosteriform skin metastases," *International Journal of Dermatology*, vol. 43, no. 2, pp. 126–128, 2004.

[6] H.-D. Liu, H. Zheng, M. Li, D.-S. Hu, M. Tang, and Y. Cao, "Upregulated expression of kappa light chain by Epstein–Barr virus encoded latent membrane protein 1 in nasopharyngeal carcinoma cells via NF-κB and AP-1 pathways," *Cellular Signalling*, vol. 19, no. 2, pp. 419–427, 2007.

[7] H. Watabe, T. Kawakami, Y. Soma, T. Baba, and M. Mizoguchi, "Primary cutaneous T-cell-rich B-cell lymphoma in a zosteriform distribution associated with Epstein-Barr virus infection," *The Journal of Dermatology*, vol. 29, no. 11, pp. 748–753, 2002.

[8] S. Niiyama, K. Satoh, S. Kaneko, S. Aiba, M. Takahashi, and H. Mukai, "Zosteriform skin involvement of nodal T-cell lymphoma: a review of the published work of cutaneous malignancies mimicking herpes zoster," *The Journal of Dermatology*, vol. 34, no. 1, pp. 68–73, 2007.

37

Recurrent Thrombotic Vasculopathy in a Former Cocaine User

Preeti Jadhav,[1] **Hassan Tariq,**[1] **Masooma Niazi,**[2] **and Giovanni Franchin**[1]

[1]*Bronx Lebanon Hospital Center, Department of Medicine, 1650 Selwyn Avenue, Suite No. 10C, Bronx, NY 10457, USA*
[2]*Bronx Lebanon Hospital Center, Department of Pathology, 1650 Grand Concourse, Bronx, NY 10457, USA*

Correspondence should be addressed to Preeti Jadhav; pjadhav@bronxleb.org

Academic Editor: Thomas Berger

We report a case of a 35-year-old female who presented to the emergency room (ER) complaining of a pruritic rash involving multiple areas of the body. She had a significant history of cocaine use in the past. She had first developed a similar rash in 2013 when she was diagnosed with cocaine-induced vasculitis. Her urine toxicology had been positive for cocaine in the past until July 2013. She was incarcerated and attended a drug rehabilitation program after which she quit cocaine use, which was consistent with negative urine toxicology on subsequent admissions. Further workup did not reveal any other, autoimmune or infectious, etiology of this clinical presentation. The patient underwent biopsy of the skin lesion that was consistent with thrombotic vasculopathy likely secondary to levamisole.

1. Introduction

Levamisole is an anthelmintic and immunomodulator drug, which has been used in cancer therapy, to treat various immunological renal diseases and to treat a number of skin diseases, including Behçet's disease. It works as a nicotinic acetylcholine receptor agonist that causes continued stimulation of the parasitic worm muscles, leading to paralysis [1, 2]. However, the drug was withdrawn from the human market in 1999 because of serious side effects including leukopenia, agranulocytosis, and skin vasculitis [1–3]. This drug lately has been increasingly used as an adulterant in cocaine sold in the United States and Canada. According to one survey done in 2009, approximately 70% of cocaine in the USA is contaminated with levamisole [3, 4]. Small vessel cutaneous vasculitis may occur following the use of cocaine adulterated with levamisole [1]. Patients often present with tender purpura on the ears and necrotic reticuloform purpura on the trunk or extremities. Lab abnormalities usually detected are anti-neutrophil antibodies (ANCA), antiphospholipid antibodies, leukopenia, or neutropenia. Skin biopsy findings are often suggestive of leukocytoclastic vasculitis and small vessel thrombosis [3–6]. Urine toxicology testing can confirm cocaine use provided the patient utilized cocaine in the preceding two to three days. Testing for levamisole in serum or urine is difficult due to the short half-life (5.6 hours) of levamisole [3].

2. Case Presentation

A 35-year-old female was transferred to the emergency department (ED) of our hospital from a drug rehabilitation center for necrotic skin lesions. Two days before this presentation, the patient had noticed an itching sensation in her left ear. Later a reddish black rash appeared on the left ear. The rash was painful and progressively got worse, involving the right ear, hands, and lower back.

She denied fever, arthralgia, insect bite, or recent travel. Her medical history was significant for seizure disorder, asthma, bipolar disorder, and polysubstance abuse. She denied any recent use of recreational drugs and attested that she last used cocaine 8 months prior to being incarcerated.

On examination patient was afebrile. Vital signs were noted as blood pressure 135/73 mm of hg, pulse rate of 95/min, and respiratory rate of 17/min, saturating 98% on room air. She was alert and oriented to time, place, and self. Precordial examination revealed normal heart sounds without any murmur or gallops. Auscultation of lungs revealed

TABLE 1: Laboratory workup.

Labs (reference normal range)	Year 2011	Year 2015 (Jan.)
WBC (4.8–10.8 k/μL)	1.9	5.9
ANC (1.5–8 k/μL)	0.6	4.6
B2 microglobulin (0.8–2.2 mg/L)		1.3
Myeloperoxidase MPO (P-ANCA) (<1.0)	<1	<0.1
Proteinase PR3 (C-ANCA) (<1.0)	18	1.2
C3 level (90–150 mg/dL)		91
C4 level (16–47 mg/dL)		<7
ESR (0–30 mm/hr)	34	60
CRP (≤5.5 mg/L)		166
ANA	Negative	Negative
Neutrophil Ab	Detected	

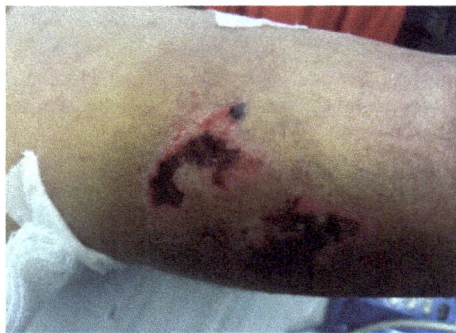

FIGURE 1: Multiple necrotic purple lesions on arms.

bilateral air entry without any adventitious sounds. There were multiple necrotic purple lesions on arms (Figure 1) bilateral pinnae, buttocks, and finger. All lesions had erythematous base, clear margins, no pus, or discharge.

The patient had a similar rash two years before this presentation and was diagnosed with levamisole-induced purpura as the workup to elucidate other etiologies that could have explained that the rash was unremarkable (Table 1). She had urine toxicology screening during each hospitalization that had been positive for cocaine and phenobarbital in the past (from 2011) but was subsequently negative since July 2014.

During the current admission the patient underwent biopsy of the skin lesion that showed several dermal vessels occluded by fibrin and platelet thrombi without signs of inflammation, consistent with thrombotic vasculopathy (Figure 2) likely secondary to levamisole.

She was treated with systemic steroids and discharged to rehabilitation center.

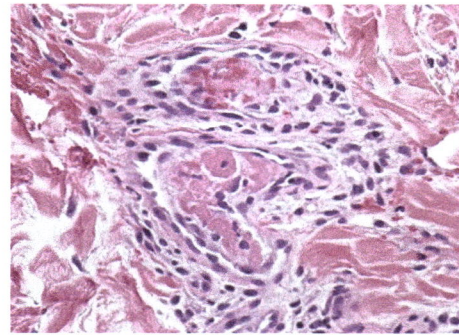

FIGURE 2: Thrombotic vasculopathy. High magnification showing occluded vessels with intraluminal fibrin and platelet thrombi (magnification 400x, H&E stain).

3. Discussion

Levamisole-induced vasculitis was first described in the 1970s [1]. This syndrome produces a characteristic clinical presentation of vasculitis in association with a variable pattern of immunologic disturbances. Cutaneous manifestations associated with levamisole use are varied and include nonspecific eruptions, lichenoid eruptions, fixed drug rash, and cutaneous vasculitis [4]. Lesions may appear suddenly and enlarge rapidly. Purpuric papules, plaques, hemorrhagic bullae, and even midline destruction have also been reported [7–9]. In the cocaine-levamisole cutaneous vasculopathy syndrome, lesions frequently have a distinctive morphology; they tend to be stellate with a bright erythematous border and necrotic appearing center [1, 2]. One of the most unique features of this syndrome is that the rash has a predilection for the ears, which may be due to the fact that the lower temperature of the ear may facilitate the deposition of immune complexes [10].

The syndrome has a very interesting spectrum of autoantibody findings. The immunological evidence is usually limited to presence of p-ANCA and sometimes c-ANCA antibodies [7, 8]. Anti-PR3 and anti-MPO are antibodies, respectively, associated with these ANCA patterns [1, 2].

The histology of cutaneous lesions typically shows thrombotic vasculitis or leukocytoclastic vasculitis with or without vascular occlusion [4–6]. The natural history of levamisole-induced vasculitis is spontaneous resolution without treatment when the levamisole is withdrawn. Immunologic abnormalities generally resolve within 2 to 14 months of withdrawal of the levamisole [2].

Detection of levamisole in both serum and urine must be performed using GC-MS or liquid chromatography-tandem mass spectrometry (LC-MS), as it is not detectable by routine toxicologic testing [11]. Clinical presentation and widespread adulteration of cocaine with levamisole are considered sufficient to make the diagnosis of this syndrome without any positive diagnostic test [10].

The important differential diagnosis to consider is Granulomatous Polyangiitis (GPA). In cocaine induced vasculitis, unlike GPA, granulomas and leukocytoclasia are not present histologically [9, 11–13]. In patients with cocaine-induced vasculitis, disease tends to be localized, whereas in patients with cutaneous GPA disease that was initially localized invariably progresses to be systemic, classically affecting organs such as the kidneys and lungs and the nasal cavity. Moreover, PR3 is more typical for vasculitis associated with cocaine use than GPA [9, 11–13].

Other most common causes of small- and medium-sized vasculitis like infectious, allergic, or drug related ones can be ruled out based on history and laboratory workup [11–14].

Review of articles from various sources showed that in cases reported to have cutaneous vasculitis associated with cocaine use, urine toxicology was positive for cocaine indicating active cocaine use. These lesions usually resolve spontaneously within a few weeks of drug discontinuation and recur with subsequent contaminated cocaine abuse.

We report a unique case where the patient presented with typical cutaneous vasculitis presumably from prior exposure to levamisole/cocaine however in abstinence for at least 8 months prior to current vasculitis flare. We propose that cocaine/levamisole use may trigger an abnormal immune response that may develop with clinical cutaneous vasculitis in the future even in the absence of new exposure to the drug.

Conflict of Interests

The authors of the paper do not have a direct financial relation with the commercial identities mentioned in the paper that might lead to a conflict of interests.

Authors' Contribution

All authors have made contribution to the paper and have reviewed it before submission.

References

[1] M. R. Carter and S. Amirhaeri, "p-ANCA-associated vasculitis caused by levamisole-adulterated cocaine: a case report," *Case Reports in Emergency Medicine*, vol. 2013, Article ID 878903, 4 pages, 2013.

[2] F. Rongioletti, L. Ghio, F. Ginevri et al., "Purpura of the ears: a distinctive vasculopathy with circulating autoantibodies complicating long-term treatment with levamisole in children," *British Journal of Dermatology*, vol. 140, no. 5, pp. 948–951, 1999.

[3] R. Abdul-Karim, C. Ryan, C. Rangel, and M. Emmett, "Levamisole-induced vasculitis," *Proceedings (Baylor University. Medical Center)*, vol. 26, no. 2, pp. 163–165, 2013.

[4] A. G. Verstraete, "Detection times of drugs of abuse in blood, urine, and oral fluid," *Therapeutic Drug Monitoring*, vol. 26, no. 2, pp. 200–205, 2004, Review.

[5] R. L. Gross, J. Brucker, A. Bahce-Altuntas et al., "A novel cutaneous vasculitis syndrome induced by levamisole-contaminated cocaine," *Clinical Rheumatology*, vol. 30, no. 10, pp. 1385–1392, 2011.

[6] C. Chung, P. C. Tumeh, R. Birnbaum et al., "Characteristic purpura of the ears, vasculitis, and neutropenia—a potential public health epidemic associated with levamisole-adulterated cocaine," *Journal of the American Academy of Dermatology*, vol. 65, no. 4, pp. 722–725.e2, 2011.

[7] M. M. McGrath, T. Isakova, H. G. Rennke, A. M. Mottola, K. A. Laliberte, and J. L. Niles, "Contaminated cocaine and antineutrophil cytoplasmic antibody-associated disease," *Clinical Journal of the American Society of Nephrology*, vol. 6, no. 12, pp. 2799–2805, 2011.

[8] R. L. Gross, J. Brucker, A. Bahce-Altuntas et al., "A novel cutaneous vasculitis syndrome induced by levamisole-contaminated cocaine," *Clinical Rheumatology*, vol. 30, no. 10, pp. 1385–1392, 2011.

[9] S. K. Bhinder and V. Majithia, "Cocaine use and its rheumatic manifestations: a case report and discussion," *Clinical Rheumatology*, vol. 26, no. 7, pp. 1192–1194, 2007.

[10] H. Tran, D. Tan, and T. P. Marnejon, "Cutaneous vasculopathy associated with levamisole-adulterated cocaine," *Clinical Medicine & Research*, vol. 11, no. 1, pp. 26–30, 2013.

[11] E. Kouassi, G. Caillé, L. Léry, L. Larivière, and M. Vézina, "Novel assay and pharmacokinetics of levamisole and p-hydroxylevamisole in human plasma and urine," *Biopharmaceutics and Drug Disposition*, vol. 7, no. 1, pp. 71–89, 1986.

[12] D. G. Macfarlane and P. A. Bacon, "Levamisole-induced vasculitis due to circulating immune complexes," *British Medical Journal*, vol. 1, no. 6110, pp. 407–408, 1978.

[13] X. Chevalier, G. Rostoker, B. Larget-Piet, and R. Gherardi, "Schoenlein-Henoch purpura with necrotizing vasculitis after cocaine snorting," *Clinical Nephrology*, vol. 43, no. 5, pp. 348–349, 1995.

[14] R. Grau, "Pseudovasculitis: mechanisms of vascular injury and clinical spectrum," *Current Rheumatology Reports*, vol. 4, no. 1, pp. 83–89, 2002.

38

Buschke-Löwenstein Tumour: Successful Treatment with Minimally Invasive Techniques

Estefânia Correia[1] and António Santos[2]

[1]*Family Practice Unit of Pedras Rubras, Rua Divino Salvador de Moreira 160, 4470-105 Maia, Portugal*
[2]*Department of Dermatology, Portuguese Institute of Oncology, Portugal*

Correspondence should be addressed to Estefânia Correia; estefaniascorreia@gmail.com

Academic Editor: Jaime A. Tschen

We report a case of an 80-year-old female who presented with a four-year history of a growing mass in the perianal area with pain and bleeding during defaecation. Clinical examination revealed a locally destructive, cauliflower-like, verrucous mass measuring 10 × 12 cm in diameter. Histologic findings revealed a moderate degree of dysplasia of the epithelium with koilocytosis atypia, acanthosis, and parakeratosis, features that are consistent with Buschke-Löwenstein tumour. Polymerase-chain-reaction assay for human papillomavirus (HPV) showed an infection with HPV type 11. Full-thickness excision of involved skin was undertaken by cryotherapy and electrocautery over five months. The entire wound was left open to heal by secondary intention. After 3 years of follow-up, the patient has not experienced a recurrence, with excellent functional results, but the cosmetic results were satisfactory. These minimally invasive techniques can be safer and more cost-effective than surgery and the General Practitioner can play a key role in diagnosis.

1. Introduction

Buschke-Löwenstein tumour (BLT), also known as giant condyloma acuminatum, is a very rare, sexually transmitted disease that affects the anogenital region [1–3].

The human papillomavirus (HPV) has been identified as an important contributory factor in the development of BLT [4].

Although this is a well-differentiated, benign lesion, its management is often challenging due to the size, probable local invasion, and elevated recurrence rates [4].

Without a well-defined treatment protocol for BLT, many medical and/or surgical treatment options can be found in the literature with very different results [5].

We present a case report from the Portuguese Institute of Oncology and a review of the literature.

2. Case Report

An 80-year-old female was referred to the department of dermatology with a four-year history of a growing mass in the perianal area with pain and bleeding during defaecation. She had not received any treatment previously. The patient's medical history was as follows: cervical cancer diagnosed 25 years before, treated successfully with radiotherapy, and a non-Hodgkin lymphoma diagnosed 11 years before, treated with chemotherapy for one year. She denied sexual promiscuity and alcohol or drugs abuse. On dermatological examination, there was a cauliflower-like growth on her anogenital area, which was fleshy, sessile, and slightly friable in areas with some bleeding and foul-smelling, purulent exudate on the surface. Grossly, the lesion measured 10 × 12 cm with a central thickness of 3.5 cm (Figure 1).

Anoscopy with a flexible endoscope, vaginal speculum examination, and inguinal lymph node palpation were normal. Routine laboratory examinations and serological tests for syphilis, HIV, hepatitis B, and hepatitis C were negative. A thoracic-abdominal-pelvic computed tomography (CT) scan showed no local invasion and HPV-11 was found on large and deep biopsy specimen with polymerase chain reaction (PCR). The biopsy also showed moderate degree of

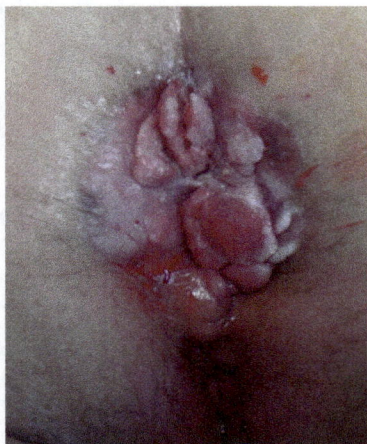

FIGURE 1: Large cauliflower-like giant condyloma acuminatum on the anogenital area.

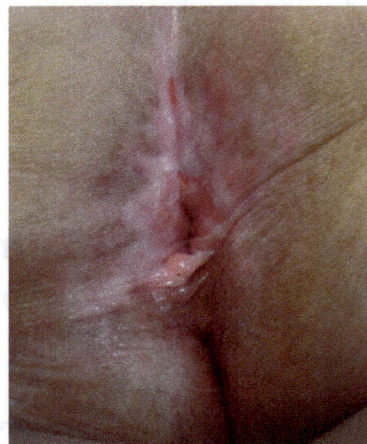

FIGURE 3: The perineal and perianal areas at 36 months postoperatively with a satisfactory appearance and no recurrence.

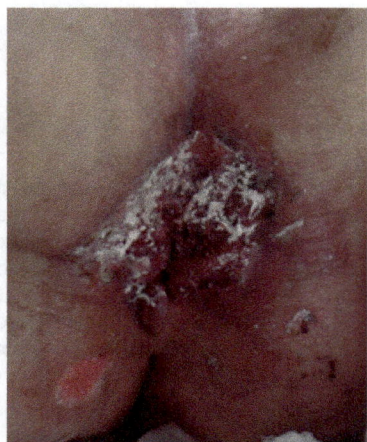

FIGURE 2: Perineum after electrocautery and cryotherapy.

3. Discussion

BLT is a slow-growing, expansive, cauliflower-like, destructive lesion [6, 7] that occurs very rarely in female population [8]. The location is chiefly the vulva (90%) and an anorectal location is less frequent [9]. Most patients are adults and present with long-standing symptoms, a finding noted in our patient with a median duration of symptoms of 5 years [2, 10–13]. The main differential diagnosis includes hemorrhoids so the General Practitioner should know this rare tumour. Furthermore, it is important to note the psychological influence of the disease on the patient, whose feeling of shame permitted the lesion to evolve to this point, despite pain and bleeding [14].

The exact origin and etiology are not completely understood yet. Common opinion is that it is a viral infection associated mostly with the presence of HPV types 6 and 11 and very rarely with the presence of HPV types 16 and 18 [8]. The pathogenesis of HPV infection is undoubtedly influenced by the host's immune lymphocytes and natural killer cells, whose activity is boosted by interferons [7]. Immunosuppression is a risk factor for the rapid growing of condylomas and their malignant transformation [15, 16]. The patient's immunological status must be checked including screening test serology for STDs (HIV, syphilis, hepatitis B virus (HBV), and hepatitis C virus (HVC)) [17]. Our patient has an infection with HPV serotype 11 and is not currently immunosuppressed, although she underwent radiotherapy and chemotherapy in the past.

The locoregional extension must be carefully assessed to establish the therapeutic strategy. In respect to this, abdominal and pelvic magnetic resonance imaging is useful [7].

The BLT diagnosis can be difficult due to the lack of malignant cytological characteristics, especially if the biopsy includes only the surface epithelium. Therefore, a large and deep biopsy with carefully performed sections and a detailed histopathological examination is required [14].

dysplasia of the epithelium with koilocytosis atypia, acanthosis, and parakeratosis. Although surgical excision was recommended, the patient refused this due to its cosmetic and functional disability. After obtaining written consent, she underwent local excision using electrosurgery (200–300 volts) and cryotherapy (−50°C; 30 seconds) with liquid nitrogen. Two cycles of electrosurgery and three cycles of cryotherapy were administered over five months (Figure 2).

The entire wound was left open to heal by secondary intention. These conservative therapies went without complications. She is now in the 36th month of follow-up (every 6 months) and presents no residual lesions or recurrence. Furthermore, the functional results were excellent with no evidence of anal canal or incontinence, and the cosmetic results were satisfactory because moderate depigmentation and a little superficial atrophic scar remained in the treated area (Figure 3).

Treatment of BLT can be classified into three types: topical therapy, tumour removal (surgery), and immunotherapy [18–20]. However, no gold standard currently exists for treating this rare disease. Treatment depends on the size of the lesion, how deep it is, its location, previous treatment, and also the physician's experience and skills [20]. In severe invasive cases, a surgical excision often plays a central role in the treatment of the BLT; however, surgical excision needs expert surgical technique, sophisticated anesthesia, and plastic reconstruction [21] and cannot avoid recurrence in more than 50% of patients [13, 18]. Furthermore, poor wound healing, fecal contamination of the operative site, fistulization, perineal abscesses, ulceration, difficulty in controlling hemorrhages, and extensive removal of soft tissue contribute to considerable postoperative morbidity and mortality [7, 13, 18, 22]. In addition, the emotional trauma associated with vulvar surgery, particularly in younger women, is considerable, and there is the risk of development of a phychosexual condition [23]. In light of these findings, cryotherapy and electrosurgery can be considered a good choice of treatment in noninvasive cases with a good response, and these techniques are considered minimally invasive surgery. In our case the CT scan excluded local invasion. It is very important to destroy the tissue to a depth of at least 5 to 8 mm because BLT infiltrates deeply into the underlying stroma [24]. In this case, the treatment was applied conveniently and economically with a bloodless field and minimal destruction to surrounding tissue. Unfortunately, the patient has a moderate depigmentation and a little superficial atrophic scar.

Chemotherapy and radiation therapy should be used only in case of disease recurrence because their effectiveness has not been fully documented [25].

A close follow-up is recommended in order to detect recurrence in an early phase. To date, there is no data in the literature in regard to the duration of follow-up. It seems that the recurrences are more frequent in the first months after surgery [26]. Currently our patient has been followed up every six months.

In conclusion, BLT is an infrequent and likely virulent infection with a challenging treatment because this tumour is characteristically locally very aggressive.

Therefore, prospective studies are necessary to further define the nature and treatment of this very rare disease.

Minimally invasive techniques such as cryotherapy and electrosurgery can be safer and more cost-effective than surgery. However, these techniques can only be applied in noninvasive cases.

As in a significant percentage of patients, the first manifestations of BLT are a growing mass with pain and bleeding; therefore the General Practitioner can play a key role in diagnosis.

When there is a BLT, a multidisciplinary team including dermatology should be involved in treatment and follow-up.

Finally, careful observation over a prolonged period of time is essential in order to detect recurrences and control potential complications related to the treatment.

Conflict of Interests

The authors declare that there is no conflict of interests regarding the publication of this paper.

References

[1] E. Balik, T. Eren, and D. Bugra, "A surgical approach to anogenital Buschke Loewenstein Tumours (giant condyloma acuminata)," *Acta Chirurgica Belgica*, vol. 109, no. 5, pp. 612–616, 2009.

[2] E. Erkek, H. Basar, O. Bozdogan, and M. C. Emeksiz, "Giant condyloma acuminata of Buschke-Löwenstein: successful treatment with a combination of surgical excision, oral acitretin and topical imiquimod," *Clinical and Experimental Dermatology*, vol. 34, no. 3, pp. 366–368, 2009.

[3] O. Miranda Aranzubía, J. García Rodríguez, R. C. González Alvarez, M. Alvarez Mújica, L. Rodríguez Robles, and J. Regadera Sejas, "Giant condyloma acuminatum (Buschke-Löwenstein tumor)," *Actas Urológicas Españolas*, vol. 32, no. 9, article 951, 2008.

[4] S. Agarwal, G. K. Nirwal, and H. Singh, "Buschke-lowenstein tumour of glans penis," *International Journal of Surgery Case Reports*, vol. 5, no. 5, pp. 215–218, 2014.

[5] Z. Radovanovic, D. Radovanovic, R. Semnic, Z. Nikin, T. Petrovic, and B. Kukic, "Highly aggressive Buschke-löwenstein tumor of the perineal region with fatal outcome," *Indian Journal of Dermatology, Venereology and Leprology*, vol. 78, no. 5, pp. 648–650, 2012.

[6] A. Lévy and C. Lebbe, "Buschke-Löwenstein tumour: diagnosis and treatment," *Annales d'Urologie*, vol. 40, no. 3, pp. 175–178, 2006.

[7] P. Parise, G. Sarzo, C. Finco, F. Marino, S. Savastano, and S. Merigliano, "Giant condyloma acuminatum of the anorectum (Buschke-Lowenstein tumour): a case report of conservative surgery," *Chirurgia Italiana*, vol. 56, no. 1, pp. 157–161, 2004.

[8] C. Yang, S. Liu, Z. Wang, and S. Yang, "Buschke-Löwenstein tumor in an old woman: Cryotherapy and holmium laser treatment," *Archives of Gynecology and Obstetrics*, vol. 288, no. 1, pp. 221–223, 2013.

[9] A. El Mejjad, M. El Amine, D. Mohamed et al., "Le condylome acuminé géant-tumeur de Buschke Loewenstein (à propos de 3 cas)," *Progrès en Urologie*, vol. 13, no. 3, pp. 513–517, 2003.

[10] M. G. Tytherleigh, A. J. Birtle, C. E. Cohen, R. Glynne-Jones, J. Livingstone, and J. Gilbert, "Combined surgery and chemoradiation as a treatment for the Buschke-Löwenstein tumour," *The Surgeon*, vol. 4, no. 6, pp. 378–383, 2006.

[11] G. De Toma, G. Cavallaro, A. Bitonti, A. Polistena, M. G. Onesti, and N. Scuderi, "Surgical management of perianal giant condyloma acuminatum (Buschke-Löwenstein tumor): report of three cases," *European Surgical Research*, vol. 38, no. 4, pp. 418–422, 2006.

[12] M. W. T. Chao and P. Gibbs, "Squamous cell carcinoma arising in a giant condyloma acuminatum (Buschke-Lowenstein tumour)," *Asian Journal of Surgery*, vol. 28, no. 3, pp. 238–240, 2005.

[13] Q. D. Chu, M. P. Vezeridis, N. P. Libbey, and H. J. Wanebo, "Giant condyloma acuminatum (Buschke-Lowenstein tumor) of the anorectal and perianal regions: analysis of 42 cases," *Diseases of the Colon and Rectum*, vol. 37, no. 9, pp. 950–957, 1994.

[14] A. M. Ciobanu, C. Popa, M. Marcu, and C. F. Ciobanu, "Psychotic depression due to giant condyloma Buschke-Löwenstein tumors," *Romanian Journal of Morphology and Embryology*, vol. 55, no. 1, pp. 189–195, 2014.

[15] H. P. Lorenz, W. Wilson, B. Leigh, T. Crombleholme, and W. Schecter, "Squamous cell carcinoma of the anus and HIV infection," *Diseases of the Colon & Rectum*, vol. 34, no. 4, pp. 336–338, 1991.

[16] A. Kibrité, N. C. Zeitouni, and R. Cloutier, "Aggressive giant condyloma acuminatum associated with oncogenic human papilloma virus: a case report," *Canadian Journal of Surgery*, vol. 40, no. 2, pp. 143–145, 1997.

[17] G. P. Mingolla, O. Potì, G. Carbotta, C. Marra, G. Borgia, and D. De Giorgi, "Reconstructive surgery in anal giant condyloma: report of two cases," *International Journal of Surgery Case Reports*, vol. 4, no. 12, pp. 1088–1090, 2013.

[18] K. I. Paraskevas, E. Kyriakos, E. E. Poulios, V. Stathopoulos, A. A. Tzovaras, and D. D. Briana, "Surgical management of giant condyloma acuminatum (Buschke-Löwenstein tumor) of the perianal region," *Dermatologic Surgery*, vol. 33, no. 5, pp. 638–644, 2007.

[19] S. B. Brown, "The role of light in the treatment of non-melanoma skin cancer using methyl aminolevulinate," *Journal of Dermatological Treatment*, vol. 14, supplement 3, pp. 11–14, 2003.

[20] B. Giomi, F. Pagnini, A. Cappuccini, B. Bianchi, L. Tiradritti, and G. Zuccati, "Immunological activity of photodynamic therapy for genital warts," *British Journal of Dermatology*, vol. 164, no. 2, pp. 448–451, 2011.

[21] P. Gholam, A. Enk, and W. Hartschuh, "Successful surgical management of giant condyloma acuminatum (Buschke-Löwenstein tumor) in the genitoanal region: a case report and evaluation of current therapies," *Dermatology*, vol. 218, no. 1, pp. 56–59, 2008.

[22] R. H. Gormley and C. L. Kovarik, "Human papillomavirus-related genital disease in the immunocompromised host: part II," *Journal of the American Academy of Dermatology*, vol. 66, no. 6, pp. 883.e1–883.e17, 2012.

[23] A. Geusau, G. Heinz-Peer, B. Volc-Platzer, G. Stingl, and R. Kirnbauer, "Regression of deeply infiltrating giant condyloma (Buschke-Löwenstein tumor) following long-term intralesional interferon alfa therapy," *Archives of Dermatology*, vol. 136, no. 6, pp. 707–710, 2000.

[24] P. Hillemanns, X. Wang, S. Staehle, W. Michels, and C. Dannecker, "Evaluation of different treatment modalities for vulvar intraepithelial neoplasia (VIN): CO_2 laser vaporization, photodynamic therapy, excision and vulvectomy," *Gynecologic Oncology*, vol. 100, no. 2, pp. 271–275, 2006.

[25] L. Battaglia, A. Vannelli, F. Belli et al., "Giant condyloma acuminatum of the anorectum: successful radical surgery with anal reconstruction," *Tumori*, vol. 97, no. 6, pp. 805–807, 2011.

[26] R. Patti, P. Aiello, G. L. Angelo, and G. Di Vita, "Giant condyloma acuminatum quickly growing: case report," *Il Giornale di Chirurgia*, vol. 33, no. 10, pp. 327–330, 2012.

39

Effectiveness of an Innovative Pulsed Electromagnetic Fields Stimulation in Healing of Untreatable Skin Ulcers in the Frail Elderly: Two Case Reports

Fabio Guerriero,[1,2,3] **Emanuele Botarelli,**[3] **Gianni Mele,**[3] **Lorenzo Polo,**[3]
Daniele Zoncu,[3] **Paolo Renati,**[3,4] **Carmelo Sgarlata,**[1] **Marco Rollone,**[2]
Giovannoi Ricevuti,[1,2] **Niccolò Maurizi,**[1] **Matthew Francis,**[1] **Mariangela Rondanelli,**[5]
Simone Perna,[5] **Davide Guido,**[2,6] **and Piero Mannu**[3]

[1]*Department of Internal Medicine and Medical Therapy, Section of Geriatrics, University of Pavia, 27100 Pavia, Italy*
[2]*Agency for Elderly People Services, Hospital Santa Margherita, 27100 Pavia, Italy*
[3]*Ambra Elektron, Associazione Italiana di Biofisica per lo Studio dei Campi Elettromagnetici in Medicina, 00186 Rome, Italy*
[4]*Alberto Sorti Research Institute, Medicine and Metamolecular Biology, 10122 Turin, Italy*
[5]*Department of Public Health, Experimental and Forensic Medicine, Section of Human Nutrition, Endocrinology and Nutrition Unit, University of Pavia, 27100 Pavia, Italy*
[6]*Department of Public Health, Experimental and Forensic Medicine, Biostatistics and Clinical Epidemiology Unit, University of Pavia, 27100 Pavia, Italy*

Correspondence should be addressed to Fabio Guerriero; fabio_guerriero@yahoo.it

Academic Editor: Jeung-Hoon Lee

Introduction. Recalcitrant skin ulcers are a major burden in elderly patients. Specifically, chronic wounds result in significant morbidity and mortality and have a profound economic impact. Pulsed electromagnetic fields (PEMFs) have proved to be a promising therapy for wound healing. Here we describe the first reported case of an innovative PEMF therapy, Emysimmetric Bilateral Stimulation (EBS), used to successfully treat refractory skin ulcers in two elderly and fragile patients. *Case Presentation*. Two elderly patients developed multiple chronic skin ulcerations. Despite appropriate treatment, the ulcers showed little improvement and the risk of amputation was high. Both patients underwent daily EBS therapy and standard dressing. After few weeks of treatment, major improvements were observed and all ulcers had healed. *Conclusion*. In patients with refractory ulceration, EBS therapy may be of real benefit in terms of faster healing. This case supports the supportive role for PEMFs in the treatment of skin ulceration in diabetes and is suggestive of a potential benefit of EBS in this clinical condition.

1. Introduction

Due to life expectancy increase and concomitant aging of the population, the prevalence of chronic cutaneous ulcers dramatically increased during the last decades, specifically when arising from atherosclerotic and microangiopathic processes [1, 2].

Several pathophysiological mechanisms related to aging counteract the healing process, such as the physiological loss of trophic dermoepidermal elasticity and concomitant alterations in skin microcirculation. Additionally, the broad spectrum of comorbidities, which often affect the subjects at risk, might further impair the healing process [3].

Wound healing is a complex process mediated by signals of molecular interaction involving the recruitment of mesenchymal cells, proliferation, and regeneration of the extracellular matrix. The healing process is a response of innate immunity for the restoration of tissue integrity. It is regulated by a pattern of events including coagulation, inflammation, granulation tissue formation, epithelialization, and tissue

TABLE 1: Clinical and biochemical data of the two patients.

	Patient 1		Patient 2	
	At admission	End EBS	At admission	End EBS
HbA1c (mmol/L)	38	41	51	48
RCP (mg/dL)	20.5	2.3	10.3	1.2
ESR (mm/h)	110	35	75	15
MMSE	26/30	28/30	29/30	29/30
Barthel Index	8/100	44/100	25/100	75/100
NRS	8	0	9	2

*HbA1c: glycosylated hemoglobin; RCP: C-reactive protein; ESR: erythrocytes sedimentation rate; MMSE: Mini Mental State Examination; NRS: Numeric Rating Scale.

FIGURE 1: EBS treatment performed at bedside.

remodeling. These events are mediated by cytokines and growth factors that modulate such cellular activities [4, 5].

Despite the modern advances in wound closure techniques and devices, there is a vital need for newer methods of enhancing the healing process to achieve optimal outcomes.

One of the promising but still debated therapeutic developments involves the use of electromagnetic fields (EMFs) for enhancing the healing process. It is hypothesized that electrical stimulation influences the migratory, proliferative, and synthetic functions of fibroblasts and also results in increased expression of growth factors [6].

This case report shows an innovative technique based on pulsed EMF (PEMF) stimulation, Emysimmetric Bilateral Stimulation (EBS), to enhance the healing of recalcitrant skin ulcers in two fragile elderly patients.

2. Cases Presentation

2.1. Materials and Methods. EBS therapy was carried out on two elderly patients, whose leg ulcers were chronic and healing was unsatisfactory. Both ulcers had not responded to conventional medication, including washing, disinfection, and advanced dressing for some months before coming to our attention.

We evaluated the effect of this innovative EMF stimulation, using EBS device, by the receding of leg ulcers and secondary biochemical and clinical changes in C-reactive protein (CRP), erythrocytes sedimentation rate (ESR), and comprehensive geriatric assessment (Table 1).

2.2. Experimental Protocol. Both elderly subjects received EBS stimulation daily after undressing and washing procedure. The intervention was conducted in a supine position with the knee fully extended. The lower leg and foot were supported with a foot stand so the ankle was kept in a neutral ankle position throughout the intervention. Each treatment session lasted for 25 minutes and was repeated daily until the wound healed (Figure 1).

2.3. Emysimmetric Bilateral Stimulation (EBS). Each EBS treatment (Elkmed© 2060) consists of a stimulation (about 20–25 minutes long) during which the patient is exposed to extremely weak EMF (powers in range 10–100 nW), emitted

by two sources: an in air-source placed in the front part of the machine and another consisting of a shaped aluminium conductor sheet placed directly on wounds, connected by 4 clamps that convey the signal from the machine. The in air-source at a distance of 1 meter generates electromagnetic power densities in the range of 50–100 nW/cm²; local emitters generate even lower power densities, between 0.5 and 50 nW/cm², depending on the terminal emitter used. Electromagnetic signals are pulsed at a frequency variable by preset programs. The carrier wave is peaked at 10.5 GHz. Pulsation consists of an amplitude modulation at total index ($m = 1$) and is square-shaped so that the carrier wave is switched on/off at a very high rate.

The purpose in designing EBS apparatus was to obtain the largest frequency band possible at extremely low powers in the emission. EBS's working principle is to introduce very weak electromagnetic fields noise in the range of radiomicrowave frequencies into the network of molecular chains interpenetrating the whole biological matter. The EMF noise is obtained creating many harmonics and interferences of electromagnetic weak signals within the exposed body. This is the ideal condition in order to obtain extremely low power electromagnetic noise spread over a wide frequency band, able to stimulate self-feeding and reenhance traveling wave-packets, whose role is involved in biocommunication, homeostasis, and regeneration [7–9].

3. Case Report 1

The patient, C. C., was a 91-year-old female, suffering from chronic heart failure and osteoarthrosis with subsequent functional impairment. She was a retired teacher and lived alone without any external caregiving support. She came to our department presenting painful skin ulcers of the lower extremities with inflammatory signs and alarming initial gangrene. They arose from accidental wounds 6 months before and increased in size despite wound care performed by the patient herself (washing, disinfection, dressing with topical silver sulfadiazine, etc.). No history of diabetes was reported.

At admission, she presented in poor general condition and was malnourished, while cognitive functions were intact. A skin examination was performed at the time of admission

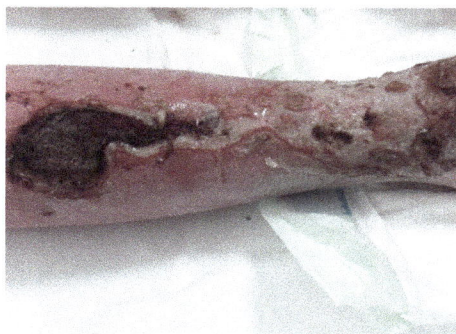

FIGURE 2: Initial gangrene of the lower limb at admission.

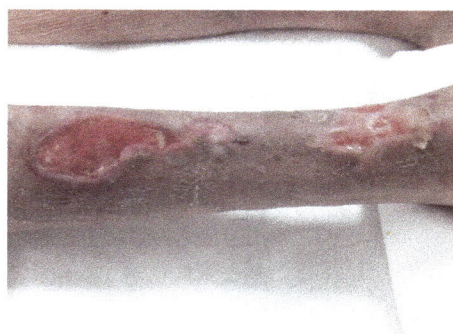

FIGURE 4: After 2 weeks of EBS treatment and standard dressing.

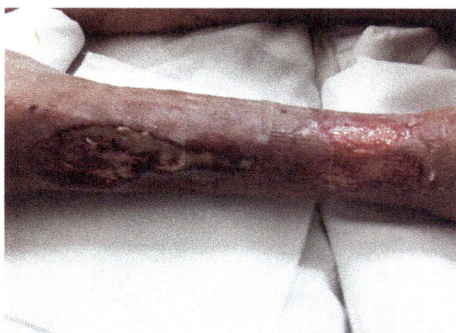

FIGURE 3: Seven days after EBS treatment and standard dressing.

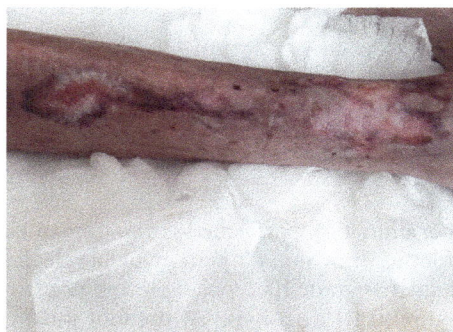

FIGURE 5: Skin ulcers completely heal after 5 weeks.

and showed extensive right leg ulcers. These lesions had a necrotic appearance, without granulation tissue, and were covered by purulent exudates (Figure 2).

Blood sample showed increased levels of CRP and ESR. Main clinical data are shown in Table 1. A Doppler ultrasound of the lower limbs showed distally an initial decrease of arterial signal with normal venous axis. The ankle brachial index was 0.9, so that arterial insufficiency was not causing or contributing to the nonhealing wound [10].

Consultation from the vascular surgery department proposed a demolitive surgical approach that was refused. Given the lack of response, risk of amputation, and general deterioration in the patient, EBS stimulation was proposed and started on a compassionate use basis, with informed consent, 2 days after her hospitalization. She parallel underwent standard medication with washing, enzymatic debridement, dressing, and parenteral antibiotics (amoxicillin/clavulanic acid 3 grams daily).

After 7 days of therapy, the wide ulcers of the lower limb started to present some granulation tissue with irregular edges and discrete fibrinous exudate (Figure 3). Following a two-week EBS treatment period, all wide ulcers of the lower limb had improved with remarkable reduction and marked granulation tissue was apparent on the wide ulcers (Figure 4). The patient's general condition improved in parallel.

Following 5 weeks of EBS treatment, the ulcers on the leg had completely healed (Figure 5) and the patient was able to walk using a walking aid. ESR and CRP consequently decreased to almost normal values.

At discharge ulcer healing was complete with no relapse observed up to now.

4. Case Report 2

An 83-year-old diabetic male patient, S. I., was admitted to our department as he was suffering from chronic foot diabetic ulcer that was present for 8 months. Concurrent comorbidities were chronic heart failure, chronic atrial fibrillation, and hyperuricemia.

Until admission, the old man had been for long an outpatient in a diabetic foot center. During this period, a 1 cm ulcer appeared on his right foot after a prolonged walk, and it increased in size despite appropriate wound care and glycemic control. As the ulcer was recalcitrant, tissue drainage surgery had been proposed.

On admission the patient presented in good clinical conditions. The glycemic control was stable with basal bolus scheme adopting rapid short-acting insulin analogue glulisine and long-acting glargine insulin. Glycosylated hemoglobin levels were 51 mmol/mol, and adjustments of his insulin dose and addition of on-demand fast-acting insulin were not required. The patient was treated with oral antibiotics (amoxicillin/clavulanic acid 2 grams/daily) from two weeks before admission. Clinical and biochemical data are shown in Table 1. Wound-related pain represented a relevant issue, as the consequent limitations in mobility with gradual immobilization syndrome.

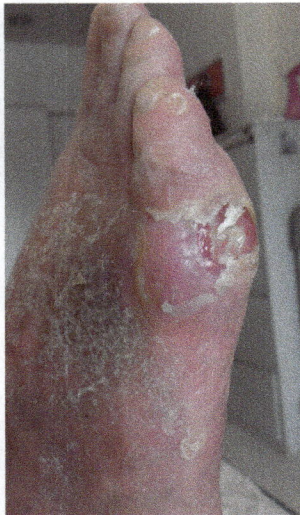

FIGURE 6: Foot diabetic ulcer at admission.

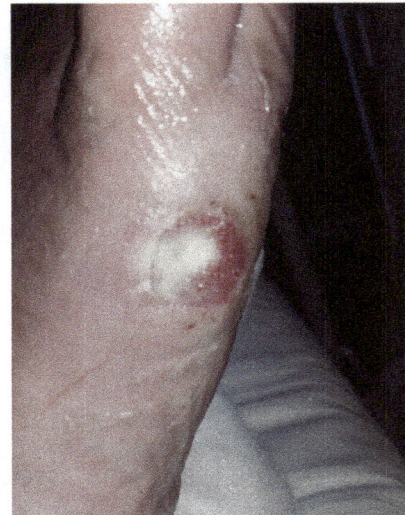

FIGURE 7: Wound epithelization after 10 days of EBS treatment.

A skin examination performed at the time of admission showed a foot ulcer of about 2.5 cm involving the fascia, and it was evaluated as grade II according to the Wagner grading system (Figure 6) [11]. An X-ray of the foot was performed and showed no occurrence of osteomyelitis.

Given unresponsiveness to conventional dressings until then and patient's awareness of the longtime expected healing after drainage surgery, EBS therapy was initiated with informed consent. Standard medication with washing, disinfection, l-lysine hyaluronate, and dressing was performed, while antibiotic therapy was administered endovenously.

Since the beginning of EBS stimulation, there was a noticeable improvement of the recalcitrant foot lesion, observed by the increase of granulation tissue, and wound borders receding corresponding to reepithelialization.

Figure 7 shows changes in the diabetic ulcer, respectively, after 10 days of treatment. As the foot ulcer clinically improved, antibiotics were discontinued, and pain became completely tolerated, making walking possible without any aid.

After 3 weeks of EMF stimulation the ulcer completely healed (Figure 8) and the patient was discharged to home.

5. Discussion

In spite of the advancements in cutaneous ulceration treatment, this common condition continues to devastate the community of patients, especially the elderly, who suffer from micro- and macrovascular afflictions. In this respect, the development of new techniques aimed to assist the process of skin healing and repair is of primary importance.

In the last two decades there has been an increasing interest in the PEMF for the management of ischemic, pressure, and venous ulcers. The basic mechanisms underlying EMF are not clear. PEMFs are low frequency fields with very specific shape and amplitude. They can be applied in

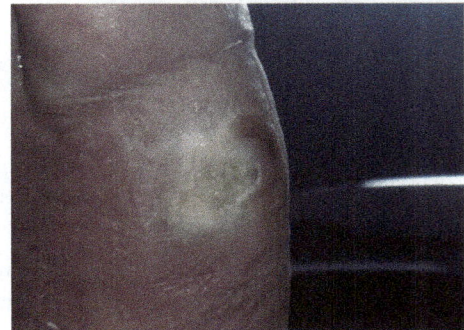

FIGURE 8: Complete diabetic ulcer healing at discharge.

the presence of a cast or wound dressing and the risk of infection is significantly low [12].

It has been suggested that PEMFs, by altering or augmenting preexisting endogenous electrical fields, may trigger specific, measurable cellular responses such as DNA synthesis, transcription, and protein synthesis [13]. Such cellular responses appear to occur within a window of PEMF parameters (frequency, amplitude, timing, and length of exposures). It has been reported that PEMFs decrease the doubling time of fibroblasts and induce differentiation of skin fibroblasts in culture. Increased collagen synthesis, angiogenesis, and bacteriostasis are some mechanism by which PEMFs may contribute to wound healing [14].

Some recent studies have showed that the treatment with PEMFs may result in shorter healing time and limb function recovery, enhancing the quality of life of the patient. In the treatment of pressure ulcers, three controlled clinical trials tried PEMF but findings were controversial [15–17]. A recent randomized controlled study on 13 diabetic patients confirmed the effectiveness of EMF for promoting the healing in terms of enhancing wound closure and facilitating microcirculation [18]. The authors' findings demonstrated that

EMF treatment can elicit vasodilation and increase peripheral blood flow. The increase in microcirculation has been already described to inhibit the inflammation and accelerate the cell proliferation [19].

In this regard a previous animal study showed that PEMFs accelerate time to wound closure, granulation, and cell proliferation in diabetic and normal mice, by upregulation of fibroblast growth factor-2 mediated angiogenesis. Besides in this study EMF was showed to prevent tissue necrosis in response to a standardized ischemic insult [20].

According to our case reports, the sequence of clinical events observed in our patients suggests a beneficial role for EBS stimulation, as no other new or relevant therapeutic intervention concomitant to treatment with EBS was initiated. The relevant issue regarding EBS efficacy was that both patients were suffering from chronic recalcitrant ulcers that were not healing under standard medications and had been proposed for demolitive surgery. EBS stimulation was started after consent of the patients for conservative and compassionate use basis.

EBS stands different than the conventional PEMF stimulation devices as it adopts low power stimulations to cover a wide range of frequency bands, shapes, and durations of pulses of the EMF. The core principle is the utilization of PEMF noise-like stimuli to trigger self-arrangements in the living system of treated subjects and improve wound regeneration. Recently, the group led by Montagnier has detected experimentally the presence of electromagnetic signals originating in the water surrounding biomolecules [21]. To us this should be the key-point of EBS stimulation technique: the stimuli involved in the interaction between human body and extremely weak electromagnetic signals are not energetic but potential and phase based actors, able to produce a phase shift in domains of coherent bound-water constituting cells.

However, as single case reports, several limitations warrant acknowledgement. Wound healing is influenced by multiple variables, and it was not possible to strictly control for all potential confounders in this case. There are many possible confounding variables in these reports, mainly regarding the different characteristics of patients and ulcers, thus the difficulty of conducting standardized studies. Actually studies with cell cultures are carrying on to clarify the biological and molecular effects of EBS on wound healing and cellular regeneration.

Based on literature and on our clinical experience, we conclude that the use of PEMFs and EBS in wound control, although recent, constitutes a very promising technique.

Larger studies should be conducted with lengthier follow-up periods and coverage of randomized population.

6. Conclusions

While the observations reported in our reports should be interpreted with caution and need to be confirmed in a controlled study, the sequence of events is suggestive of a beneficial role for EBS therapy in chronic skin ulcers healing. These findings are consistent with recent knowledge on the role of EMF in the treatment of wounds. EBS is a novel EMF stimulation, whose innovative working principle is promising for several clinical applications.

Consent

Written informed consent was obtained from the patients for publication of these case reports and any accompanying images.

Conflict of Interests

The authors report no conflict of interests in this work.

Authors' Contribution

All authors contributed toward data analysis and drafting and critically revising the paper and agree to be accountable for all aspects of the work.

References

[1] C. J. Moffatt, P. J. Franks, D. C. Doherty, R. Martin, R. Blewett, and F. Ross, "Prevalence of leg ulceration in a London population," *QJM*, vol. 97, no. 7, pp. 431–437, 2004.

[2] O. Nelzen, D. Bergqvist, and A. Lindhagen, "Venous and non-venous leg ulcers: clinical history and appearance in a population study," *British Journal of Surgery*, vol. 81, no. 2, pp. 182–187, 1994.

[3] M. Briggs and S. J. Closs, "Patients' perceptions of the impact of treatments and products on their experience of leg ulcer pain," *Journal of Wound Care*, vol. 15, no. 8, pp. 333–337, 2006.

[4] A. J. Singer and R. A. F. Clark, "Cutaneous wound healing," *The New England Journal of Medicine*, vol. 341, no. 10, pp. 738–746, 1999.

[5] G. C. Gurtner, S. Werner, Y. Barrandon, and M. T. Longaker, "Wound repair and regeneration," *Nature*, vol. 453, no. 7193, pp. 314–321, 2008.

[6] D. S. Weiss, R. Kirsner, and W. H. Eaglestein, "Electrical stimulation and wound healing," *Archives of Dermatology*, vol. 126, no. 2, pp. 222–225, 1990.

[7] L. Brizhik, E. Del Giudice, S. E. Jørgensen, N. Marchettini, and E. Tiezzi, "The role of electromagnetic potentials in the evolutionary dynamics of ecosystems," *Ecological Modelling*, vol. 220, no. 16, pp. 1865–1869, 2009.

[8] M. Bischof and E. Del Giudice, "Communication and the emergence of collective behavior in living organisms: a quantum approach," *Molecular Biology International*, vol. 2013, Article ID 987549, 19 pages, 2013.

[9] F. Guerriero, E. Botarelli, G. Mele et al., "An innovative intervention for the treatment of cognitive impairment-Emisymmetric bilateral stimulation improves cognitive functions in Alzheimer's disease and mild cognitive impairment: an open-label study," *Neuropsychiatric Disease and Treatment*, vol. 11, pp. 2391–2404, 2015.

[10] H. Brem, R. S. Kirsner, and V. Falanga, "Protocol for the successful treatment of venous ulcers," *The American Journal of Surgery*, vol. 188, no. 1, supplement 1, pp. 1–8, 2004.

[11] F. W. Wagner Jr., "The dysvascular foot: a system for diagnosis and treatment," *Foot and Ankle*, vol. 2, no. 2, pp. 64–122, 1981.

[12] M. S. Markov, "Magnetic and electromagnetic fields—a new frontier in clinical biology and medicine," in *Proceedings of the Millennium International Workshop on Biological Effects in Biology and Medicine*, pp. 363–372, Heraklion, Greece, October 2000.

[13] R. Goodman and A. S. Henderson, "Some biological effects of electromagnetic fields," *Bioelectrochemistry and Bioenergetics*, vol. 15, no. 1, pp. 39–55, 1986.

[14] H. P. Rodemann, K. Bayreuther, and G. Pfleiderer, "The differentiation of normal and transformed human fibroblasts in vitro is influenced by electromagnetic fields," *Experimental Cell Research*, vol. 182, no. 2, pp. 610–621, 1989.

[15] S. Comorosan, R. Vasilco, M. Arghiropol, L. Paslaru, V. Jieanu, and S. Stelea, "The effect of diapulse therapy on the healing of decubitus ulcer," *Romanian Journal of Physiology*, vol. 30, no. 1-2, pp. 41–45, 1993.

[16] C. A. Salzberg, S. A. Cooper-Vastola, F. Perez, M. G. Viehbeck, and D. W. Byrne, "The effects of non-thermal pulsed electromagnetic energy on wound healing of pressure ulcers in spinal cord-injured patients: a randomized, double-blind study," *Ostomy Wound Management*, vol. 41, no. 3, pp. 42–46, 1995.

[17] A. Gupta, A. B. Taly, A. Srivastava, S. Kumar, and M. Thyloth, "Efficacy of pulsed electromagnetic field therapy in healing of pressure ulcers: a randomized control trial," *Neurology India*, vol. 57, no. 5, pp. 622–626, 2009.

[18] R. L. Kwan, W. C. Wong, S. L. Yip, K. L. Chan, Y. P. Zheng, and G. L. Cheing, "Pulsed electromagnetic field therapy promotes healing and microcirculation of chronic diabetic foot ulcers: a pilot study," *Advances in Skin & Wound Care*, vol. 28, no. 5, pp. 212–219, 2015.

[19] E. Isakov, H. Ring, I. Mendelevich et al., "Electromagnetic stimulation of stump wounds in diabetic amputees," *Journal of Rehabilitation Sciences*, vol. 9, no. 2, pp. 46–48, 1996.

[20] M. J. Callaghan, E. I. Chang, N. Seiser et al., "Pulsed electromagnetic fields accelerate normal and diabetic wound healing by increasing endogenous FGF-2 release," *Plastic and Reconstructive Surgery*, vol. 121, no. 1, pp. 130–141, 2008.

[21] L. Montagnier, J. Aïssa, S. Ferris, J.-L. Montagnier, and C. Lavalléee, "Electromagnetic signals are produced by aqueous nanostructures derived from bacterial DNA sequences," *Interdisciplinary Sciences: Computational Life Sciences*, vol. 1, no. 2, pp. 81–90, 2009.

40

A Case of Onychomycosis Caused by *Rhodotorula glutinis*

Hatice Uludag Altun,[1] **Tuba Meral,**[1] **Emel Turk Aribas,**[1]
Canan Gorpelioglu,[2] **and Nilgun Karabicak**[3]

[1] *Department of Clinical Microbiology, Faculty of Medicine, Turgut Ozal University, Emek, 06510 Ankara, Turkey*
[2] *Department of Dermatology, Faculty of Medicine, Turgut Ozal University, Emek, 06510 Ankara, Turkey*
[3] *Mycology Reference Laboratory, Public Health Institution of Turkey, Sıhhıye, 06100 Ankara, Turkey*

Correspondence should be addressed to Hatice Uludag Altun; hualtun@turgutozal.edu.tr

Academic Editor: Alireza Firooz

Rhodotorula spp. have emerged as opportunistic pathogens, particularly in immunocompromised patients. The current study reports a case of onychomycosis caused by *Rhodotorula glutinis* in a 74-year-old immunocompetent female. The causative agent was identified as *R. glutinis* based on the pinkish-orange color; mucoid-appearing yeast colonies on Sabouraud Dextrose Agar at 25°C; morphological evaluation in the Corn Meal-Tween 80 agar; observed oval/round budding yeast at 25°C for 72 hours; no observed pseudohyphae; positive urease activity at 25°C for 4 days; and assimilation features detected by API ID 32C kit and automated Vitek Yeast Biochemical Card 2 system. Antifungal susceptibility test results were as follows: amphotericin B (MIC = 0.5 μg/mL), fluconazole (MIC = 128 μg/mL), itraconazole (MIC = 0.125 μg/mL), voriconazole (MIC = 1 μg/mL), posaconazole (MIC = 0.5 μg/mL), anidulafungin (MIC = 0.5 μg/mL), and caspofungin (MIC = 16 μg/mL). Antifungal therapy was initiated with oral itraconazole at a dose of 400 mg/day; seven-day pulse therapy was planned at intervals of three weeks. Clinical recovery was observed in the clinical evaluation of the patient before the start of the third cure. Although *R. glutinis* has rarely been reported as the causative agent of onychomycosis, it should be considered.

1. Introduction

Onychomycosis is the general name for a mycotic nail infection caused by dermatophytes, yeasts, and nondermatophyte molds. The prevalence of onychomycosis has been reported to be 2–30% and has increased in recent years [1]. Old age, toenail deformities, onychodystrophy, diabetes mellitus, psoriasis vulgaris, and psoriasis unguium, cellular immunity disorders, genetic predisposition, peripheral arterial circulatory disorder, other circulatory disorders, nail and nail fold microtrauma, heavy perspiration/hyperhidrosis pedum, and immunosuppression (HIV/AIDS) should be considered as risk factors for onychomycosis [2, 3].

Onychomycosis, which constitutes 50% of all nail diseases, is observed with clinical findings like onycholysis, subungual hyperkeratosis, discoloration, crumbly thick nails, or white patches on the nail surface [4]. Fungi that cause onychomycosis are categorized into three groups: dermatophytes, yeasts, and nondermatophyte molds [5]. Dermatophytes that cause onychomycosis according to asexual reproduction feature three groups (*Trichophyton*, *Epidermophyton*, and *Microsporum*) the most frequently observed species of which are *Trichophyton* and *Epidermophyton* [6]. The most common agents of onychomycosis among yeasts are *Candida albicans* and *Candida parapsilosis* [2, 7]. Onychomycosis, according to the state of the agent to penetrate the nail, can be classified into one of five types, which are distal-lateral subungual onychomycosis (DLSO), proximal subungual onychomycosis (PSO), superficial white onychomycosis (SWO), candidal onychomycosis (CO), and total dystrophic onychomycosis (TDO) [8]. The most common clinical form is DLSO [9]. Toenails are more frequently involved DLSO and *T. rubrum* is the most common pathogen [10].

Rhodotorula spp. are uncommon among the agents of onychomycosis in the literature. To date two cases have been reported as the causative agents of onychomycosis (*R. minuta* and *R. mucilaginosa*) [11, 12].

2. Case Report

A 74-year-old woman was admitted to the dermatology outpatient clinic of our hospital with complaints of deformity and thickening of the toenails that had continued for nearly three months. In the dermatological examination, of bilateral toenails, subungual hyperkeratosis in varying degrees, yellow-brown discoloration, and onycholysis were observed (Figure 1). The general physical examination was normal. Chronic diseases were absent, with the exception of hypertension. The patient did not have chronic or familial genetic diseases that could have caused nail disorders, malignancy, or previous trauma. The patient revealed that she had traveled to the Far East within the previous six months. The patient reported no use of systemic corticosteroid or broad-spectrum antibiotics. Other immunosuppressive conditions associated with *Rhodotorula* infection, such as AIDS, were absent. The patient's toenail samples were sent to the microbiology laboratory for fungal culture.

Clinically suspected of onychomycosis, according to nail culture results, the patient was diagnosed with DLSO caused by *R. glutinis*.

Antifungal therapy was initiated with 400 mg/day oral itraconazole; seven-day pulse therapy was planned at intervals of three weeks. The clinical evaluation of the patient before the start of the third cure, clinical recovery was detected. The patient's treatment is still underway; a fungal culture was planned again after six treatments.

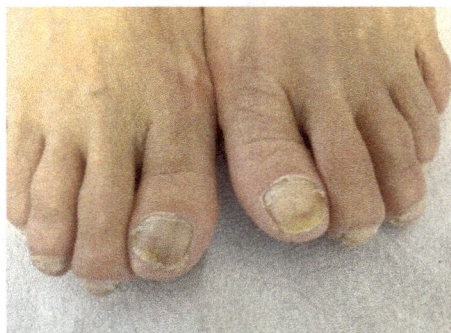

FIGURE 1: Discoloration and onycholysis image in bilateral toenail.

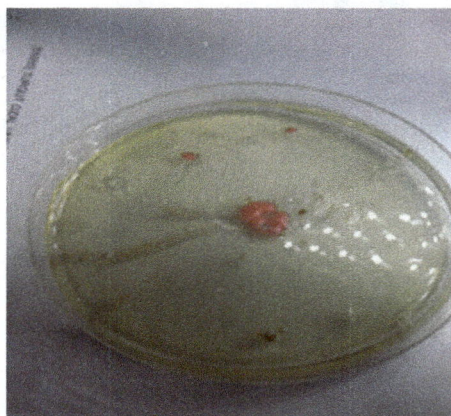

FIGURE 2: The yeast colonies on SDA at the first cultivation of the nail samples.

2.1. Fungal Identification.

The toenail samples were cultured on 2 Sabouraud Dextrose Agars (SDA; Salubris, Turkey) in the microbiology laboratory. One of SDA was incubated at 37°C and the other was incubated at 25°C. SDA, which was incubated at room temperature for four days, was observed to be a pinkish-orange pigmented colony (Figure 2). The pure passage of growing colonies was performed on the SDA medium (Figure 3). The Gram staining of these colonies was observed in the yeast cells forming blastospores. The yeast was thought to be *Rhodotorula*, due to its orange-pink pigmented appearance. The urease test was performed. The two strains of *C. albicans* (American Type Culture Collection (ATCC) 10231 and ATCC 24433) were used as a negative control, and *Cryptococcus neoformans* (ATCC 24067) was used as the positive control. Urease activity was positive.

The tested pathogen was indicated as *Rhodotorula glutinis/mucilaginosa* according to the Vitek automated identification system (bioMérieux, France) using Yeast Biochemical Card 2 (YCB). The species identification of the strains was performed at the Public Health Institution of Turkey-Mycology Reference Laboratory (PHIT-MRL). The pinkish-orange color, mucoid-appearing yeast colonies on SDA at 25°C, the morphological evaluation in the Corn Meal-Tween 80 agar, observed oval/round budding yeast at 25°C for 72

hours, no pseudohyphae, determination of positive urease activity at 25°C for four days, assimilation features detected by API ID 32C (bioMérieux, France) kit, evaluated together with conventional mycological methods identified the species as *Rhodotorula glutinis* [13].

2.2. In Vitro Susceptibility Test.

Susceptibility tests of the strain to amphotericin B, fluconazole, itraconazole, voriconazole, posaconazole, anidulafungin, and caspofungin were performed using the microdilution method (M27-A3), recommended CLSI in PHIT-MRL. Quality control (QC) was performed using *Candida parapsilosis* ATCC 22019 and *Candida krusei* ATCC 6258. Due to the fact that after 24 hours of incubation there was no bacterial growth in growth control well and poor growth after 48 hours, minimum inhibitory concentration (MIC) was determined, after a 72-hour incubation according to the CLSI-M27A3 recommended resistance limit values [14]. Antifungal susceptibility test results were as follows: amphotericin B (MIC = 0.5 μg/mL), fluconazole (MIC = 128 μg/mL), itraconazole (MIC = 0.125 μg/mL), voriconazole (MIC = 1 μg/mL), posaconazole (MIC = 0.5 μg/mL), anidulafungin (MIC = 0.5 μg/mL), and caspofungin (MIC = 16 μg/mL).

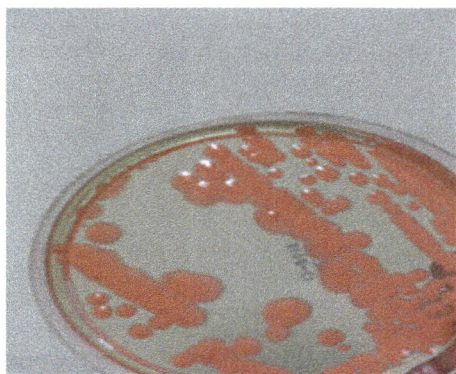

FIGURE 3: The yeast colonies on the SDA after subcultivation.

3. Discussion

Rhodotorula spp. are yeasts that are prevalent in nature. The *Rhodotorula* species are particularly found in soils, lakes, milk, fruit juices, and the resident flora of moist skin in humans. *Rhodotorula* infections are more frequently isolated in the Asia-Pacific region [15].

Infections that are caused by the *Rhodotorula* species are rare. *Rhodotorula* spp. are accepted as pathogen in recent years. Recently, catheter infections caused by *Rhodotorula* spp. are seen more frequently because of invasive procedures and, in particular, the increased use of central venous catheter [16]. *Rhodotorula mucilaginosa*, *R. glutinis*, and *R. minuta* are the species that cause disease in humans [16, 17]. *Rhodotorula* spp. were found to be the fourth most frequently observed species among non-*Candida* yeasts isolated from clinical specimens. The fact that invasive infections are reported less frequently in epidemiological studies should be taken into consideration [18].

Rhodotorula spp. are identified by the growth of the agent on cultures. Many morphological and physiological characteristics of the *Rhodotorula* species are similar to the *Cryptococcus* species in identification. Both types exhibit round-shaped, encapsulated yeast cells and urease activity, and fermenting carbohydrates specifications are determined to be positive. *Rhodotorula* species from *Cryptococcus* are separated by evident carotenoid pigments and not assimilating inositol. If there are visible capsules, they are typically thin different from *C. neoformans* [19].

The incidence of *Rhodotorula* spp. is 0.02% among fungal infections in patients with hematological malignancies [20]. Central venous catheters in patients with *Rhodotorula* fungemia are significant as both risk factor and prognostic factor [21, 22]. Another major risk factor is severe neutropenia. Steroid administration and the use of broad-spectrum antibiotics are also risk factors [15]. The cases of *Rhodotorula* infection reported in literature included fungemia, meningitis, endocarditis, skin lesions, eye infections, onychomycosis, and peritonitis [11, 12, 17, 23]. *Rhodotorula mucilaginosa* was the most common species of *Rhodotorula* fungemia,

followed by *Rhodotorula glutinis* [17]. According to a recent document, *R. glutinis* could be present in the skin of early systemic sclerosis patients at higher levels than in normal skin, raising the possibility that it could be triggering the inflammatory response found in systemic sclerosis [24].

Rhodotorula infections in immunocompetent patients are extremely rare. In the literature, *Rhodotorula* spp. were reported as a factor of onychomycosis in two cases. *Rhodotorula mucilaginosa* and *R. minuta* were found as the causative agent in those cases [11, 12]. One other case reported in the literature is nail psoriasis, masqueraded by secondary infection with *R. mucilaginosa* [25]. In these three cases, the patients were immunocompetent, as in the current case [11, 12, 25].

Treatment approaches against infections due to *Rhodotorula* are still controversial. In vitro susceptibility tests detected that amphotericin B, itraconazole, voriconazole, and 5-flucytosine are the most active antifungal agents, although voriconazole, particularly against *R. mucilaginosa* isolates, did not exhibit adequate activity [26]. In the literature, the low MICs to both posaconazole and ravuconazole were reported, though there is not sufficient clinical experience [27]. On the other hand, resistance to fluconazole, caspofungin, and micafungin was observed [21, 26, 28]. The mechanism of resistance to fluconazole is uncertain, but reported higher MIC values may indicate intrinsic resistance [12]. In the current case, according to the results of antifungal susceptibility tests, the MIC value for fluconazole was 128 μg/mL. High MIC values for fluconazole in the literature in patients with *Rhodotorula* onychomycosis ($\geq$128 = 16 μg/mL) were similar to the current results [11, 12]. MIC values determined for voriconazole (1 μg/mL) and posaconazole (0.5 μg/mL) were higher than those detected for itraconazole (0.125 μg/mL). Higher MIC values for caspofungin determined were similar to articles in the literature; the MIC value of anidulafungin was 0.5 μg/mL [21, 26, 28].

In the current case, according to the patient's clinical symptoms and the results of the antifungal susceptibility test, the patient was administered itraconazole therapy due to the sensitive results for this antifungal agent (itraconazole MIC = 0.125 μg/mL), which is effective on onychomycosis caused by *R. mucilaginosa*. In the literature, in one case of onychomycosis caused by *R. minuta*, following the administration of itraconazole treatment (itraconazole MIC value <0.125 μg/mL), it was reported that the patient fully recovered [12].

In conclusion, *Rhodotorula* spp. are rarely seen yeasts that can cause infection especially in immunosuppressed people. In the literature, *R. glutinis* is rarely reported as the causative agent of onychomycosis, although it should be considered as such.

Conflict of Interests

The authors have no conflict of interests in the submission of this paper.

References

[1] I. Effendy, M. Lecha, M. F. De Chauvin, N. Di Chiacchio, and R. Baran, "Epidemiology and clinical classification of onychomycosis," *Journal of the European Academy of Dermatology and Venereology*, vol. 19, no. 1, pp. 8–12, 2005.

[2] P. Nenoff, C. Krüger, G. Ginter-Hanselmayer, and H. J. Tietz, "Mycology—an update. Part 1: dermatomycoses: causative agents, epidemiology and pathogenesis," *Journal der Deutschen Dermatologischen Gesellschaft*, vol. 12, no. 3, pp. 188–210, 2014.

[3] L. Zisova, V. Valtchev, E. Sotiriou, D. Gospodinov, and G. Mateev, "Onychomycosis in patients with psoriasis—a multicentre study," *Mycoses*, vol. 55, no. 2, pp. 143–147, 2012.

[4] B. E. Elewski, "Onychomycosis: pathogenesis, diagnosis, and management," *Clinical Microbiology Reviews*, vol. 11, no. 3, pp. 415–442, 1998.

[5] P. R. Cohen and R. K. Scher, "Topical and surgical treatment of onychomycosis," *Journal of the American Academy of Dermatology*, vol. 31, no. 3, pp. 74–77, 1994.

[6] L. K. H. Souza, O. F. L. Fernandes, X. S. Passos, C. R. Costa, J. A. Lemos, and M. R. R. Silva, "Epidemiological and mycological data of onychomycosis in Goiania, Brazil," *Mycoses*, vol. 53, no. 1, pp. 68–71, 2010.

[7] C. Mügge, U.-F. Haustein, and P. Nenoff, "Causative agents of onychomycosis—a retrospective study," *Journal of the German Society of Dermatology*, vol. 4, no. 3, pp. 218–228, 2006.

[8] J. Faergemann and R. Baran, "Epidemiology, clinical presentation and diagnosis of onychomycosis," *British Journal of Dermatology*, vol. 149, no. 65, pp. 1–4, 2003.

[9] N. Zaias, B. Glick, and G. Rebell, "Diagnosing and treating onychomycosis," *The Journal of Family Practice*, vol. 42, no. 5, pp. 513–518, 1996.

[10] M. A. Bokhari, I. Hussain, M. Jahangir, T. S. Haroon, S. Aman, and K. Khurshid, "Onychomycosis in Lahore, Pakistan," *International Journal of Dermatology*, vol. 38, no. 8, pp. 591–595, 1999.

[11] M. M. L. da Cunha, L. P. B. dos Santos, M. Dornelas-Ribeiro, A. B. Vermelho, and S. Rozental, "Identification, antifungal susceptibility and scanning electron microscopy of a keratinolytic strain of Rhodotorula mucilaginosa: a primary causative agent of onychomycosis," *FEMS Immunology and Medical Microbiology*, vol. 55, no. 3, pp. 396–403, 2009.

[12] J. Zhou, M. Chen, H. Chen, W. Pan, and W. Liao, "Rhodotorula minuta as onychomycosis agent in a Chinese patient: first report and literature review," *Mycoses*, vol. 57, no. 3, pp. 191–195, 2014.

[13] D. H. Larone, *Medically Important Fungi: A Guide to Identification*, pp. 131-132, American Society for Microbiology Press, Washington, DC, USA, 4th edition, 2002.

[14] Clinical Laboratory Standards Institute, *Reference Method for Broth Dilution Antifungal Susceptibility Testing of Yeasts. M27-A3*, Clinical Laboratory Standards Institute (CLSI), Wayne, Pa, USA, 2008.

[15] M. H. Miceli, J. A. Díaz, and S. A. Lee, "Emerging opportunistic yeast infections," *The Lancet Infectious Diseases*, vol. 11, no. 2, pp. 142–151, 2011.

[16] J. García-Suárez, P. Gómez-Herruz, J. A. Cuadros, and C. Burgaleta, "Epidemiology and outcome of *Rhodotorula* infection in haematological patients," *Mycoses*, vol. 54, no. 4, pp. 318–324, 2011.

[17] F. F. Tuon and S. F. Costa, "*Rhodotorula* infection. A systematic review of 128 cases from literature," *Revista Iberoamericana de Micologia*, vol. 25, no. 3, pp. 135–140, 2008.

[18] M. A. Pfaller, D. J. Diekema, D. L. Gibbs et al., "Results from the ARTEMIS DISK global antifungal surveillance study, 1997 to 2007: 10.5-year analysis of susceptibilities of noncandidal yeast species to fluconazole and voriconazole determined by CLSI standardized disk diffusion testing," *Journal of Clinical Microbiology*, vol. 47, no. 1, pp. 117–123, 2009.

[19] P. R. Murray, E. J. Baron, J. H. Jorgensen, M. L. Landry, and M. A. Pfaller, "Mycology," in *Manuel of Clinical Microbiology*, A. Basustaoglu, A. Kubar, S. T. Yıldıran, and M. Tanyüksel, Eds., p. 1768, ASM Press, Washington, DC, USA, 1-2. 9th edition, 2009.

[20] L. Pagano, M. Caira, A. Candoni et al., "The epidemiology of fungal infections in patients with hematologic malignancies: the SEIFEM-2004 study," *Haematologica*, vol. 91, no. 8, pp. 1068–1075, 2006.

[21] A. K. Zaas, M. Boyce, W. Schell, B. A. Lodge, J. L. Miller, and J. R. Perfect, "Risk of fungemia due to *Rhodotorula* and antifungal susceptibility testing of *Rhodotorula* isolates," *Journal of Clinical Microbiology*, vol. 41, no. 11, pp. 5233–5235, 2003.

[22] T. E. Kiehn, E. Gorey, A. E. Brown, F. F. Edwards, and D. Armstrong, "Sepsis due to *Rhodotorula* related to use of indwelling central venous catheters," *Clinical Infectious Diseases*, vol. 14, no. 4, pp. 841–846, 1992.

[23] S. Menon, H. R. Gupta, R. Sequeira et al., "*Rhodotorula glutinis* meningitis: a case report and review of literature," *Mycoses*, vol. 57, no. 7, pp. 447–451, 2014.

[24] S. T. Arron, M. T. Dimon, Z. Li et al., "High *Rhodotorula* sequences in skin transcriptome of patients with diffuse systemic sclerosis," *Journal of Investigative Dermatology*, vol. 134, no. 8, pp. 2138–2145, 2014.

[25] K. Martini, H. Müller, H. P. Huemer, and R. Höpfl, "Nail psoriasis masqueraded by secondary infection with *Rhodotorula mucilaginosa*," *Mycoses*, vol. 56, no. 6, pp. 690–692, 2013.

[26] A. Gomez-Lopez, E. Mellado, J. L. Rodriguez-Tudela, and M. Cuenca-Estrella, "Susceptibility profile of 29 clinical isolates of *Rhodotorula* spp. and literature review," *Journal of Antimicrobial Chemotherapy*, vol. 55, no. 3, pp. 312–316, 2005.

[27] D. J. Diekema, B. Petroelje, S. A. Messer, R. J. Hollis, and M. A. Pfaller, "Activities of available and investigational antifungal agents against *Rhodotorula species*," *Journal of Clinical Microbiology*, vol. 43, no. 1, pp. 476–478, 2005.

[28] J. García-Suárez, P. Gómez-Herruz, J. A. Cuadros, H. Guillén, and C. Burgaleta, "*Rhodotorula mucilaginosa* catheter-related fungaemia in a patient with multiple myeloma," *Mycoses*, vol. 54, no. 4, pp. e214–e216, 2011.

41

Seborrheic Pemphigoid

Enzo Errichetti,[1] Giuseppe Stinco,[1] Enrico Pegolo,[2] Nicola di Meo,[3] Giusto Trevisan,[3] and Pasquale Patrone[1]

[1] *Institute of Dermatology, Department of Experimental and Clinical Medicine, University of Udine, San Michele Hospital, Piazza Rodolone 1, Gemona del Friuli, 33013 Udine, Italy*
[2] *Institute of Anatomic Pathology, Department of Medical and Biological Sciences, University of Udine, University Hospital of Santa Maria della Misericordia, Piazzale Santa Maria della Misericordia 15, 33100 Udine, Italy*
[3] *Institute of Dermatology and Venereology, University of Trieste, Maggiore Hospital, Piazza Ospedale 1, 34100 Trieste, Italy*

Correspondence should be addressed to Enzo Errichetti; enzoerri@yahoo.it

Academic Editor: Thomas Berger

Seborrheic pemphigoid (SP), first described in 1969 by Schnyder, is a peculiar variant of BP which clinically resembles pemphigus erythematosus, since it is characterized by ruptured bullae and erosions covered with crusts involving the seborrheic areas. To the best of our knowledge, from the first description only four other cases of SP have been reported, of which two are in the English literature. We report an additional case of SP in a 56-year-old man with cervical spondylogenic myelopathy with very impaired mobility.

1. Introduction

Bullous pemphigoid (BP) is a chronic, autoimmune, often pruritic, subepidermal, blistering dermatosis occurring mainly in elderly individuals aged 70 years and older. Classically, patients present with large tense bullae on apparently normal or erythematous skin, located at the sides of the neck, axillae, groins, upper inner aspects of the thighs, and abdomen. Not rarely, excoriated, eczematous, papular, or urticarial lesions may precede the onset of the blisters [1, 2]. In addition to the more classic findings, several atypical presentations of BP have been described, including forms confined to a particular cutaneous district (paralyzed extremity, pretibial area, umbilicus, vulva, and irradiated or peristomal sites) and variants presenting with vesicular, erythroderma, vegetating, dyshidrotic dermatitis-like, prurigo nodularis-like, toxic epidermal necrolysis-like, ecthyma-like, or pemphigus erythematosus-like lesions [2, 3].

The latter variant is known as "seborrheic pemphigoid" and is a very rare form of BP, since there are only a few cases reported in the literature. We report an additional case of seborrheic pemphigoid in a patient with cervical spondylogenic myelopathy with very impaired mobility.

2. Case Report

A 56-year-old man presented to our clinic with a three-month history of recurrent and mild itchy bullae quickly evolving in erosive lesions covered by crusts located on his scalp, forehead, auricular and periauricular regions, and interscapular area (seborrheic sites). The patient had been previously diagnosed as having impetigo and seborrheic dermatitis; however, specific therapies for these disorders were found to be completely ineffective. His medical history included an untreated progressive (during previous 4 years) slight bilateral age-related sensorineural hearing loss (presbycusis); bipolar disorder (since he was 35 years old) controlled from about 5 years with quetiapine, duloxetine, and lorazepam; and cervical spondylogenic myelopathy with very limited mobility (from about 2 years) which had worsened considerably in the last six months. The cervical problem has been treated only with physical therapies (but the patient is currently waiting for a surgical treatment). The man denied other drugs intake and health issues. Physical examination revealed very few flaccid blisters, several erosions (some of which with a peripheral epithelial collarette), and hematic and serous crusts on a slightly erythematous background

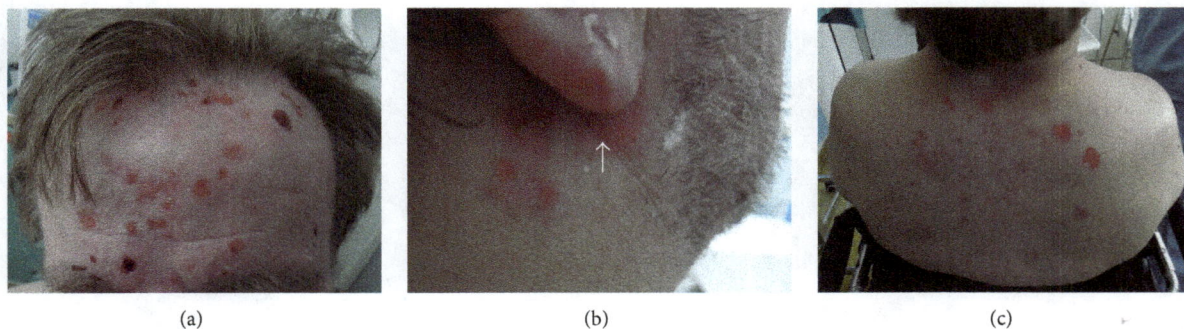

(a)   (b)   (c)

FIGURE 1: Several erosions (some of which with a peripheral epithelial collarette) and hematic and serous crusts on a slightly erythematous background on forehead (a), right periauricular region (b), and interscapular area (c); a flaccid blister (arrow) is visible under the right ear lobe (b).

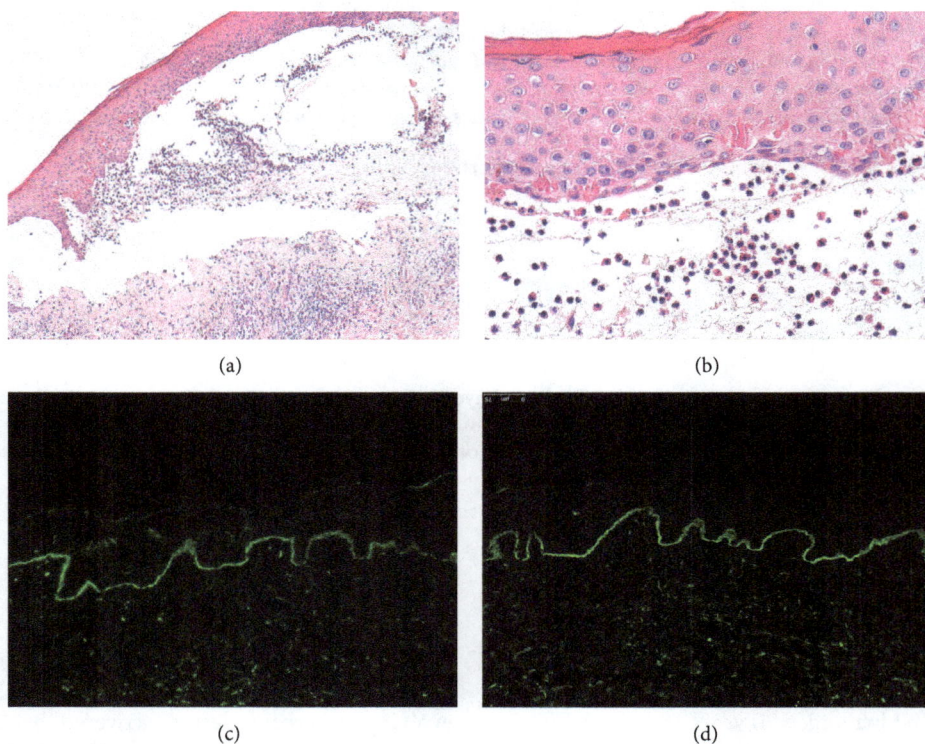

(a)   (b)

(c)   (d)

FIGURE 2: Subepidermal bulla containing eosinophils with an eosinophilic inflammatory cell infiltrate in the superficial dermis (H and E staining, magnification ×100) (a); detail of eosinophils in the subepidermal blister (H and E staining, magnification ×400) (b). Direct immunofluorescence tests show deposition of IgG (c) and C3 (d) at the basement membrane zone (200x).

(Figures 1(a), 1(b), and 1(c)); Nikolsky's sign was absent. No other significant skin or mucosal lesions were seen. A 6 mm punch biopsy specimen was taken from the edge of a blister of right periauricular region and submitted for histological examination, which showed subepidermal bulla containing eosinophils with an eosinophilic inflammatory cell infiltrate in the superficial dermis (Figures 2(a) and 2(b)). Direct immunofluorescence (IF) of perilesional skin detected IgG and C3 deposition at the basement membrane zone (Figures 2(c) and 2(d)). The result of immunoblotting showed IgG autoantibodies which reacted against BP230

in epidermal extracts; furthermore, the BP180 antibodies were also detected (value of 31.7 U/mL; cutoff value for positivity: 15.0 U/mL) by an enzyme-linked immunosorbent assay (ELISA) BP180-NC16a diagnosis kit. The detection of antinuclear and antiextractable nuclear antigens antibodies was negative. On the basis of clinical, histological, and laboratory findings, a diagnosis of seborrheic pemphigoid was made. Treatment with oral methylprednisolone at the dosage of 0.5 mg/kg/die mg produced a rapid improvement. After 5 weeks the patient achieved a complete remission and the steroid was gradually tapered during the subsequent 6 months up to dose of 0.1 mg/kg/die. The value of circulating anti-BP180-NC16a antibodies (ELISA test) was also progressively decreased (26.4 U/mL after 5 weeks, 21.6 U/mL after 3 months, and 18.1 U/mL after 6 months). Currently, after 9 months from the start of steroid therapy, the patient is free of disease and presents a value of circulating anti-BP180-NC16a antibodies under the cutoff value for positivity (13.2 U/mL) with a dose of methylprednisolone of 0.1 mg/kg/die.

3. Discussion

Seborrheic pemphigoid (SP) is a peculiar variant of BP which clinically resembles pemphigus erythematosus (known also as seborrheic pemphigus), since it is characterized by ruptured bullae and erosions covered with crusts involving the seborrheic areas [4]. The first instance of SP reported in the literature dates back to 1969, when Schnyder described a case in an elderly female [5]. It is important to underline that all cases [6–16] described as "SP" before Schnyder's report were actually instances of pemphigus erythematosus [5]. Such confusion was probably caused by the lack of availability of reliable serological tests and direct IF test of perilesional skin, which are very helpful particularly in the cases without detectable bullae [1, 17, 18]. To the best of our knowledge, since the first description four other instances of SP, similar to our case and original report of Schnyder, have been reported [1, 4, 17, 18], of which two are in English language in 1991 [18] and 2002 [1], respectively. Regarding the latter report, the authors emphasized a possible association between losartan intake and unleashing of the lesions in their patient [1].

When a blister is available, its histological examination shows a picture comparable to the classic form of BP, with a subepidermal cleavage [1]. Direct IF test of perilesional skin, which generally reveals linear deposition of IgG and C3 at the dermoepidermal junction [1], and detection of circulating IgG antibodies against basement membrane zone (indirect IF), BP230, and/or BP180 may be of aid in the diagnosis [1, 18].

The reasons underlying the peculiar location of the lesions in seborrheic areas in SP are not clear. It is well-known that the regional variability in the BP antigens skin expression may play a role in the distribution of the lesions of BP, given that the greatest concentration of BP antigens is in the skin of flexor surfaces of the arm, leg, and thigh, the most common sites involved in BP [19]. On the basis of this finding, it is possible to speculate that subjects with SP could present a higher expression of BP antigens in the seborrheic areas than the rest of the skin surface. Unfortunately, our patient denied further skin biopsies and therefore we have not been able to assess this hypothesis. We hope that future studies may evaluate this assumption. Another possible explanation for the peculiar localization of the lesion in SP could be that unknown factors typical of seborrheic areas may trigger or aggravate the disease in susceptible individuals. In this view, it is important to underline the ability of *Malassezia* yeast, which is notoriously localized to seborrheic sites, to activate the complement system, via either the alternative pathway or the classical pathway, with the possibility to amplify the complement-mediated inflammation which is characteristic of BP [20]. Considering that an increase of the static pool of already secreted sebum due to immobility and muscular paralysis plays a permissive role for growth of *Malassezia* yeast [21], the possible involvement of this microorganism could also explain a possible correlation between SP and cervical spondylogenic myelopathy with very limited mobility in our patients. In fact, albeit we can not exclude a coincidental association, there are three points that support a such link: the development of the disease after a relatively brief period from the significant worsening of the motor abilities, the age of onset lower than the average [3], and the well-known correlation between classical pemphigoid and neurodegenerative processes [22, 23].

Although SP may sometimes be confused with seborrheic dermatitis or impetigo, the main differential diagnosis is pemphigus erythematosus. In our opinion, the negativity of Nikolsky's sign, as described in the present case, may help to suspect a SP rather than pemphigus erythematosus, since in the latter it is almost always present [24]. Anyhow, only the histology, direct immunofluorescence examination, and serological studies allow us to definitely distinguish SP from pemphigus erythematosus and the other conditions mentioned above.

With regard to the therapy, according to other authors [3], our case confirms that relatively low dosages of systemic corticosteroids are effective in SP.

Conflict of Interests

The authors declare that there is no conflict of interests regarding the publication of this paper.

References

[1] E. Ruocco, A. Aurilia, G. Simonetti, E. Cozzani, A. Baroni, and G. Argenziano, "Bullous pemphigoid: three atypical cases," *Acta Dermato—Venereologica*, vol. 82, no. 3, pp. 222–223, 2002.

[2] G. Di Zenzo, R. della Torre, G. Zambruno, and L. Borradori, "Bullous pemphigoid: from the clinic to the bench," *Clinics in Dermatology*, vol. 30, no. 1, pp. 3–16, 2012.

[3] "Blistering diseases," in *Dermatology*, O. Braun-Falco, G. Plewig, H. H. Wolff, and W. H. C. Burgdorf, Eds., pp. 676–680, Springer, Berlin, Germany, 2nd edition, 2000.

[4] S. Welke, "Seborrheic pemphigoid (Schnyder)," *Hautarzt*, vol. 31, no. 1, pp. 18–20, 1980.

[5] M. U. Schnyder, "Seborrheic pemphigoid. A new nosologic entity?" *Bulletin de la Societe Francaise de Dermatologie et de Syphiligraphie*, vol. 76, no. 3, article 320, 1969.

[6] P. Pailheret, Courtin, and Testard, "Seborrheic pemphigoid," *Bulletin de la Société Française de Dermatologie et de Syphiligraphie*, vol. 5, pp. 772–773, 1959.

[7] S. Maissa and A. Relias, "Seborrheic pemphigoid developing into foliaceous pemphigus," *Bulletin de la Société Française de Dermatologie et de Syphiligraphie*, vol. 63, pp. 417–418, 1956.

[8] P. J. Michel and M. Blanchon, "Results obtained with cortisone in a case of generalized seborrheic pemphigoid," *Bulletin de la Société Française de Dermatologie et de Syphiligraphie*, vol. 59, no. 1, pp. 93–96, 1952.

[9] J. Watrin, P. Michon, C. Michon, J. Beurey, and R. Leduc, "Humoral study of a case of seborrheic pemphigoid and favorable therapy with ACTH and blood transfusions," *Bulletin de

la Société Française de Dermatologie et de Syphiligraphie, vol. 59, no. 1, pp. 39–41, 1952.

[10] C. Fassotte, "A case of seborrheic pemphigoid (Senear-Usher syndrome)," *Archives Belges de Dermatologie et de Syphiligraphie*, vol. 7, no. 3, pp. 208–213, 1951.

[11] R. Weille, "Case of seborrheic pemphigoid; monosymptomatic and benign evolution," *Bulletin de la Société Française de Dermatologie et de Syphiligraphie*, vol. 58, no. 4, pp. 353–356, 1951.

[12] P. Michel, M. Blanchon, and J. S. Paul, "Case of seborrheic pemphigoid with an implacable and fatal evolution in spite of quinacrine and cortisone," *Bulletin de la Société Française de Dermatologie et de Syphiligraphie*, vol. 58, no. 4, pp. 350–355, 1951.

[13] J. Watrin and P. Jeandidier, "Duhring's disease or seborrheic pemphigoid," *Bulletin de la Société Française de Dermatologie et de Syphiligraphie*, vol. 58, no. 4, pp. 347–349, 1951.

[14] A. Touraine, "Seborrheic pemphigoid (Senear-Usher syndrome, pemphigus erythematosus); general study; nosological situation," *Bulletin de la Société Française de Dermatologie et de Syphiligraphie*, vol. 58, no. 2, pp. 113–124, 1951.

[15] E. Griveaud and J. Duverne, "Seborrheic pemphigoid (Senear-Usher syndrome); evolution and treatment; histological and biological study," *Bulletin de la Société Française de Dermatologie et de Syphiligraphie*, vol. 58, no. 2, pp. 90–112, 1951.

[16] J. Margarot, P. Rimbaud, and P. Izarn, "Seborrheic pemphigoid; evolution toward pemphigus foliaceus," *Bulletin de la Société Française de Dermatologie et de Syphiligraphie*, vol. 57, no. 4, pp. 382–384, 1950.

[17] I. Schneider and S. Husz, "Seborrhoic pemphigoid," *Hautarzt*, vol. 37, no. 3, pp. 149–151, 1986.

[18] K. Tamaki, T. Furuya, Y. Kubota, A. Uno, and S. Shimada, "Seborrheic pemphigoid and polymorphic pemphigoid," *Journal of the American Academy of Dermatology*, vol. 25, no. 3, pp. 568–570, 1991.

[19] D. J. Goldberg, M. Sabolinski, and J. C. Bystryn, "Regional variation in the expression of bullous pemphigoid antigen and location of lesions in bullous pemphigoid," *Journal of Investigative Dermatology*, vol. 82, no. 4, pp. 326–328, 1984.

[20] H. R. Ashbee and E. G. V. Evans, "Immunology of diseases associated with *Malassezia* species," *Clinical Microbiology Reviews*, vol. 15, no. 1, pp. 21–57, 2002.

[21] M. Mastrolonardo, A. Diaferio, and G. Logroscino, "Seborrheic dermatitis, increased sebum excretion, and parkinson's disease: a survey of (im)possible links," *Medical Hypotheses*, vol. 60, no. 6, pp. 907–911, 2003.

[22] G. Stinco, P. Mattighello, M. Zanchi, and P. Patrone, "Multiple sclerosis and bullous pemphigoid: a casual association or a pathogenetic correlation?" *European Journal of Dermatology*, vol. 12, no. 2, pp. 186–188, 2002.

[23] G. Stinco, R. Codutti, M. Scarbolo, F. Valent, and P. Patrone, "A retrospective epidemiological study on the association of bullous pemphigoid and neurological diseases," *Acta Dermato-Venereologica*, vol. 85, no. 2, pp. 136–139, 2005.

[24] "Pemphigus," in *Dermatology*, J. L. Bolognia, J. L. Iorizzo, and R. P. Rapini, Eds., pp. 422–423, Mosby Elsevier, St. Louis, Mo, USA, 2nd edition, 2008.

42

Familial Kaposi's Sarcoma: A Report of Five Cases from Greece

Kalliopi Armyra, Anargyros Kouris, Arsinoi Xanthinaki, Alexandros Stratigos, and Irene Potouridou

Department of Dermatology and Venereology, Hospital "Andreas Sygros", Ionos Dragoumi 5, 16121 Athens, Greece

Correspondence should be addressed to Anargyros Kouris; kouris2007@yahoo.com

Academic Editor: Toshiyuki Yamamoto

Introduction. Familial cases of Kaposi's sarcoma have rarely been reported. Kaposi's sarcoma is not uncommon in Greece; its incidence is estimated at 0.20 per 100.000 habitants, showing an increased predominance in the Peloponnese, in Southern Greece. *Case Report.* We describe five cases of familial clustering of KS originating from Greece. *Discussion.* The pathogenesis of familial Kaposi's sarcoma is still far from being completely understood. Genetic, environmental, and infectious factors have been incriminated.

1. Introduction

Kaposi's sarcoma (KS) is a multifocal disease that was first described in 1872 by Moritz Kaposi. It has four principal clinical variants: (1) classic KS, (2) African endemic KS, (3) KS in iatrogenically immunocompromised patients, and (4) AIDS-related epidemic KS. Classic KS presents as blue-red to violet macules on the distal lower extremities that coalesce to form large plaques or develop into nodules or polypoid tumors. Initially, unilateral lesions may progress to a more widely disseminated multifocal pattern. Early lesions may regress, while others evolve and lead to lesions at different stages. Patients may also have lesions in the mouth and gastrointestinal tract that are usually asymptomatic.

Classic Kaposi's sarcoma mainly affects men over the age of 50 years, generally Jewish or of Mediterranean/Eastern Europe descent, and is also known as "Mediterranean KS." The highest incidence is observed in the Mediterranean area, especially in Sardinia and Southern Italy [1]. In Italy, the incidence is reported to be 0.98 per 100.000 men and 0.41 per 100.000 women [1]. In Greece, it is estimated at 0.20 per 100.000 habitants [2].

Although familial occurrence is rare, clustered occurrences within families have been reported in Sardinia and in the Peloponnese, in Southern Greece [3]. Familial clustering of classic KS suggests that infectious (viral), environmental, and genetic factors, either independently or in combination, contribute to the pathogenesis of the disease.

This is a retrospective study that reports five families, each of which had two members affected by KS. The patients were HIV-negative and had no recognized underlying immunodeficiency (Table 1). Four of the five familial occurrences originated from the Peloponnese and one from Central Greece who lived in Athens.

2. Case Reports

2.1. Family 1. A 78-year-old man, who originated from Southern Greece, was referred to "A. Sygros" Hospital exhibiting reddish-brown cutaneous lesions over different parts of his body that had manifested 18 years earlier. A biopsy specimen from lesional skin confirmed the clinical diagnosis of KS (Figure 1). The patient was treated with subcutaneous recombinant interferon alpha-2a (3×10^6 IU, 3 times per week). After one year, the dose was reduced to 3×10^6 IU once per month. At the last follow-up visit, all lesions displayed a marked decrease in the size.

A 36-year-old heterosexual man, son of the above mentioned patient, visited the outpatient clinic of "A. Sygros" Hospital with a red lesion that had appeared on his upper and lower extremities three years earlier. A skin biopsy indicated Kaposi's sarcoma (Figure 2). The patient was treated with alitretinoin gel 0.1%. At the scheduled follow-up visit, one month later, the improvement was visible.

TABLE 1: Characteristics of the patients with KS.

Family	Relationship	Age at the time of diagnosis	Age of onset	Type of KS	Location of the lesion	Duration (years)	Extracutaneous involvement	Risk factors	Treatment
1	Father	78	60	Reddish-brown macules and reddish-violaceous infiltrated plaques	Right thigh, calves, feet (including the toes), and hands	18	None	Diabetes mellitus type II	Interferon A-2a sc
	Son	36	33	Reddish-purple macules and irregular plaques	Thighs, knees, left forearm, the area of the right achilles tendon, and the middle finger of the left hand	3	None	None	Gel alitretinoin 0.1%
2	Mother	72	71	Reddish-violaceous papules, nodules, and infiltrated plaques	Chest, abdomen, back, and both arms and legs	1	None	None	Interferon A-2a sc
	Son	51	51	Reddish-brown papules and nodules	Abdominal area, right chest wall, left buttock, both thighs, both the medial malleoli areas, and the toes of both feet	1	None	Diabetes mellitus type II	Gel alitretinoin 0.1%, doxorubicin pegylated 20 mg/m^2
3	Sister	72	69	Reddish-violaceous papules and nodules	Right lateral, medial malleolus area	3	None	None	Radiotherapy
	Sister	51	51	Reddish-purple nodules and infiltrating plaques	Both hands, knees, calves, and feet	3 months	None	None	Gel alitretinoin 0.1%
4	Brother	65	65	Reddish-purple macules and irregular plaques	Both thighs, knees, and the right forearm	8 months	None	None	Cryosurgery, gel alitretinoin 0.1%
	Brother	79	79	Reddish-purple macules	Lower extremities	7 months	None	Diabetes mellitus type II, hypertension	Interferon A-2a sc
5	Father	75	73	Reddish-purple macules and irregular plaques	Both legs	2	None	Diabetes mellitus type II	Gel alitretinoin 0.1%
	Son	57	57	Reddish-purple nodules and infiltrating plaques	Left hand and knees	3 months	None	None	Cryosurgery

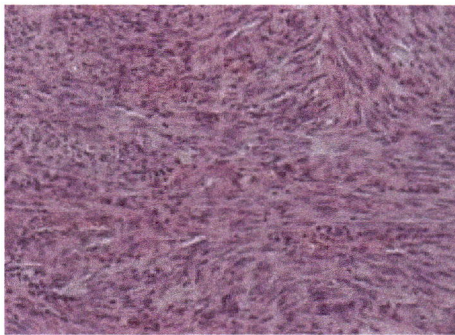

FIGURE 1: Spindle shaped forming numerous vascular slit-like spaces filled by red blood cells. (H+E ×250).

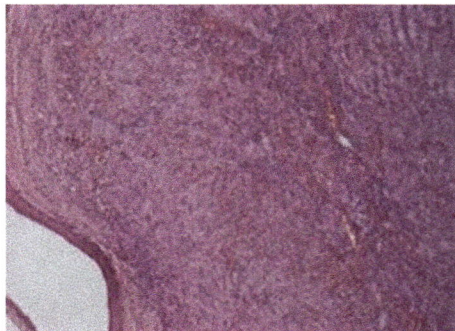

FIGURE 2: Blood filled vascular spaces-slits closely associated with interwearing spindle cells. (H+E ×40).

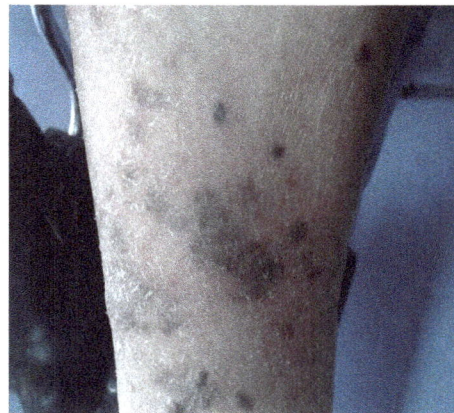

FIGURE 3: Reddish-violaceous papules, nodules, and infiltrated plaques on the legs.

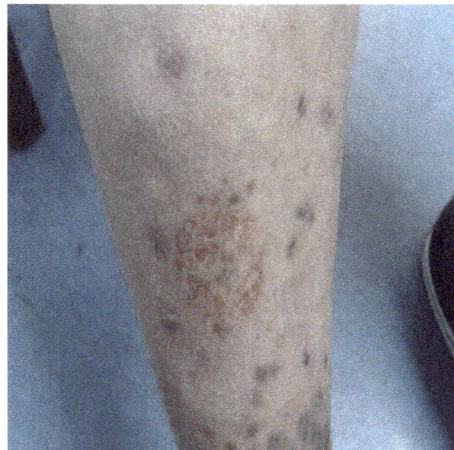

FIGURE 4: Reddish-purple lesions on the legs.

2.2. Family 2. A 72-year-old woman was admitted to "A. Sygros" Hospital with multiple violaceous cutaneous lesions all over her body (Figure 3). The disease had started one year earlier, with the appearance of a few purple macules and papules on her knees. The biopsy revealed Kaposi's sarcoma. The patient was treated with subcutaneous recombinant interferon alpha-2a (3×10^6 IU three times per week). Partial remission was observed 6 months later.

The son of the above patient, at the age of 51, was referred to "A. Sygros" Hospital with reddish cutaneous lesions in his left abdominal area. Biopsy specimens demonstrated Kaposi's sarcoma. Alitretinoin gel 0.1% was administered. The patient returned two years later with disseminated cutaneous KS. The patient was treated with doxorubicin pegylated 20 mg/m². After 6 cycles, almost complete remission of the disease was achieved. Both patients came from the Peloponnese, Southern Greece.

2.3. Family 3. A 72-year-old female, who originated from Central Greece, was admitted to our hospital for treatment of recurrent Kaposi's sarcoma. The disease had started 3 years earlier, at the age of 69, with the appearance of a few violaceous macules and papules on the right lateral malleolus area. The lesions were diagnosed as KS and treated with radiotherapy. Six months before admission to our hospital, she displayed a recurrence of the disease. Localized radiotherapy

resulted in remission of the lesions. At the scheduled follow-up visit, six months later, the lesions displayed noticeable improvement.

Her sister, aged 51, visited the outpatient clinic of "A. Sygros" Hospital with reddish-purple lesions on her hands and on the legs (Figure 4). Topical alitretinoin gel 0.1% was administered. At the last follow-up visit, all lesions showed a marked decrease in size.

2.4. Family 4. A 65-year-old man was referred to "A. Sygros" Hospital with reddish-brown cutaneous lesions over different parts of his body. The lesions had developed 8 months earlier, first appearing on his left thigh and gradually spreading to other parts of his body. The lesions were treated with cryosurgery. At the scheduled follow-up visit, three months later, the patient displayed a relapse and was treated with alitretinoin gel 0.1%. By the last follow-up visit, there was a marked decrease in five of seven lesions.

His brother, aged 79, visited the outpatient clinic of "A. Sygros" Hospital with a few purple macules and papules on his lower extremities. Clinical examination revealed several reddish-purple macules and a biopsy indicated Kaposi's sarcoma. The patient was treated with subcutaneous recombinant interferon alpha-2a (3×10^6 IU, 3 times a week) for one year. After two months of follow-up, lesions were markedly decreased. Both patients originated from the Peloponnese, Southern Greece.

2.5. Family 5. A 75-year-old man, who originated from the Peloponnese, was referred to "A. Sygros" Hospital with reddish-brown cutaneous lesions on his legs. The lesions had developed two years earlier, first appearing on his left thigh and right knee. The lesions were treated with alitretinoin gel 0.1%. At the last follow-up visit, there was a marked decrease in all lesions.

His son, aged 57, visited the outpatient clinic of "A. Sygros" Hospital with reddish-purple lesions on his left hand and on the legs. The lesions were treated with cryosurgery. Partial remission was observed 5 months later.

3. Discussion

Classic Kaposi's sarcoma is not uncommon in Greece. There are sporadic cases all over the country; endemic clustering has been observed in southern regions. A study from January 1990 to December 1994 estimated an incidence of 2.11 cases of KS per 100000 habitants, representing 1.35% of all malignancies [4]. In the Peloponnese, the incidence is estimated to be 0.8 per 100000 while, in more restricted areas of the Southern Peloponnese, it is 3-4 times higher, approximating that of African Kaposi's sarcoma [2]. Familial cases of KS have been reported in Greece previously [4, 5]. This is the third report of familial Kaposi sarcoma in Greece to be documented.

The first familial case was reported in 1909 by Radaeli [6]; since then, only a few cases have been published in the literature [5–10]. Finlay and Marks described a case of Kaposi's sarcoma in a mother and son of Italian origin [7]. Perniciaro et al. reported a case of a brother and sister, who were of German/English descent and suffered from KS on the lower extremity [8]. Cottoni et al. cited four families with KS, occurring in uncle and nephew, father and son, and two pairs of brothers, originating from Sardinia [9]. Guttman-Yassky et al. described a rare case of four Jewish siblings suffering from classic Kaposi's sarcoma [10].

Familial cases suggest that hereditary factors are involved in the pathogenesis of Kaposi's sarcoma. Different HLA antigens could affect individual susceptibility to the disease. Immunogenetic studies have shown an increased incidence of HLA DR5 antigen in familial Kaposi's sarcoma [9]. Guttmann-Yassky et al. analyzed 8 family members and demonstrated that 7 of them shared the HLA DRB1*11 antigen [10]. In a study of 32 Greek patients, an increased frequency of HLA-B18 and HLA-DR5 was demonstrated [11].

Classic Kaposi's sarcoma seems to be associated with human herpes virus 8 (HHV8) or Kaposi's sarcoma-associated herpes virus (KSHV). The prevalence of KSHV varies among geographic regions from 2% to 7% in Western Europe and North America, from 10% to 20% in the Mediterranean, and up to 100% in Sub-Saharan African countries [12]. KSHV infection is asymptomatic in most infected individuals. Nevertheless, it can provoke KS, albeit its progression is very slow. Classic KS develops in 0.03%–0.05% of individuals infected by KSHV aged over 50 years [13]. It is similarly observed that KSHV infection is higher among family members of cKS patients than that observed in control studies, which indicates intrafamiliar transmission of KSHV [1, 14]. In our retrospective study, some patients have passed away, while others are not followed up by our department anymore. This is the reason why we could not test KSHV.

Familial clustering of KS is rare and this fact argues against simple Mendelian inheritance. Nevertheless, the possibility that complex predisposing factors are involved cannot be excluded [10]. We presented five families, each having two members presenting with classic Kaposi's sarcoma. An interaction between a malignancy-linked virus, KSHV, genetic host factors, and altered immunity could possibly cause this disease. Further genetic investigation in larger studies is needed to elucidate whether there is a predisposition to infection or tumor formation within families of classic KS patients. Identifying risk factors of familial KS has important implications in the prevention and therapeutic approaches of this tumor.

Conflict of Interests

The authors declare that there is no conflict of interests regarding the publication of this paper.

References

[1] R. Mancuso, L. Brambilla, S. Agostini et al., "Intrafamiliar transmission of Kaposi's sarcomaassociated herpesvirus and seronegative infection in family members of classic Kaposi's sarcoma patients," *Journal of General Virology*, vol. 92, no. 4, pp. 744–751, 2011.

[2] A. Kaloterakis, *Kaposi's sarcoma in Greece. Mediterranean Kaposi's sarcoma [PhD. Thesis]*, University of Athens, Athens, Greece, 1984.

[3] K. Rappersberger, E. Tschachler, E. Zonzits et al., "Endemic Kaposi's sarcoma in human immunodeficiency virus type 1-seronegative persons: Demonstration of retrovirus-like particles in cutaneous lesions," *Journal of Investigative Dermatology*, vol. 95, no. 4, pp. 371–381, 1990.

[4] J. D. Stratigos, I. Potouridou, A. C. Katoulis et al., "Classic Kaposi's sarcoma in Greece: a clinico-epidemiological profile," *International Journal of Dermatology*, vol. 36, no. 10, pp. 735–740, 1997.

[5] A. Kaloterakis, C. Papasteriades, A. Filiotou, J. Economidou, S. Hadjiyannis, and J. Stratigos, "HLA in familial and nonfamilial Mediterranean Kaposi's sarcoma in Greece," *Tissue Antigens*, vol. 45, no. 2, pp. 117–119, 1995.

[6] F. Radaeli, "Nuovo contributo alla conoscenza dell'angioendotelioma cutaneo (Sarcoma idiopatico multiplo) di Kaposi," *Giorn. Ital. della Mal. Ven. e della Pelle*, vol. 44, pp. 223–256, 1909.

[7] A. Y. Finlay and R. Marks, "Familial Kaposi's sarcoma," *British Journal of Dermatology*, vol. 100, pp. 323–326, 1979.

[8] C. Perniciaro, D. J. Gross, J. W. White Jr., and R. M. Adrian, "Familial Kaposi's sarcoma," *Cutis*, vol. 57, no. 4, pp. 220–222, 1996.

[9] F. Cottoni, I. M. Masia, M. V. Masala, M. Mulargia, and L. Contu, "Familial Kaposi's sarcoma: case reports and review of the literature," *Acta Dermato-Venereologica*, vol. 76, no. 1, pp. 59–61, 1996.

[10] E. Guttman-Yassky, A. Cohen, Z. Kra-Oz et al., "Familial clustering of classic Kaposi sarcoma," *The Journal of Infectious Diseases*, vol. 189, no. 11, pp. 2023–2026, 2004.

[11] C. Papasteriades, A. Kaloterakis, A. Filiotou et al., "Histocompatibility antigens HLA-A, -B, -DR in Greek patients with Kaposi's sarcoma," *Tissue Antigens*, vol. 24, no. 5, pp. 313–315, 1984.

[12] T. F. Schulz, "Epidemiology of Kaposi's sarcoma-associated herpesvirus/human herpesvirus 8," *Advances in Cancer Research*, vol. 76, pp. 121–160, 1999.

[13] F. Vitale, D. V. Briffa, D. Whitby et al., "Kaposi's sarcoma herpes virus and Kaposi's sarcoma in the elderly populations of 3 Mediterranean islands," *International Journal of Cancer*, vol. 91, no. 4, pp. 588–591, 2001.

[14] E. Guttman-Yassky, Z. Kra-Oz, J. Dubnov et al., "Infection with Kaposi's sarcoma-associated herpesvirus among families of patients with Classic Kaposi's sarcoma," *Archives of Dermatology*, vol. 141, no. 11, pp. 1429–1434, 2005.

43

Postural Hypotension Associated with Nonelastic Pantyhose during Lymphedema Treatment

Jose Maria Pereira de Godoy,[1] **Daniel Zucchi Libanore,**[2] **and Maria de Fatima Guerreiro Godoy**[3]

[1] *Cardiology and Cardiovascular Surgery Department, Medicine School in São José do Rio Preto (FAMERP), Avenida Constituição 1306, 15025120 São José do Rio Preto, SP, Brazil*
[2] *Research Group in Godoy Clinic, Avenida Constituição 1306, 15025120 São José do Rio Preto, SP, Brazil*
[3] *Medicine School in São José do Rio Preto (FAMERP) and Research Group in Godoy Clinic, Avenida Constituição 1306, 15025120 São José do Rio Preto, SP, Brazil*

Correspondence should be addressed to Jose Maria Pereira de Godoy; godoyjmp@riopreto.com.br

Academic Editor: Gérald E. Piérard

The case of a 72-year-old female patient with elephantiasis is reported. The patient was submitted to two surgeries to remove the edema. After surgery, the leg again evolved to elephantiasis and eventually she was referred to the Clinica Godoy for clinical treatment. Intensive treatment was carried out (6 to 8 hours per day) and the patient lost more than 70% of the limb volume within one week. After this loss, the volume was maintained using grosgrain compression pantyhose for 24 hours per day. During the return appointment, the patient suffered from systemic hypotension (a drop of more than 30 mmHg within three minutes) while she was standing after removing the stocking. A further investigation showed that the symptoms only appeared when the stocking was worn for 24 hours. Thus, the patient was advised to use the stocking only during the day thereby avoiding the symptoms of hypotension.

1. Introduction

Rapid cardiovascular adjustment is essential to avoid orthostatic hypotension in the passage from the decubitus to the standing position; a response is required within seconds [1, 2]. Orthostatic hypotension is defined as a drop of at least 20 mmHg of systolic pressure or 10 mmHg of diastolic pressure within three minutes when changing from the supine or sitting position to the standing position [3]. Dizziness, blurred vision, weakness, nausea, palpitations, headache, syncope, and chest pains are the most commonly reported symptoms. Ineffective adrenergic vasoconstriction provides an inadequate response to adjust the systemic arterial pressure [4].

Studies suggest that orthostatic stress evokes regional differences in cerebral blood flow with possible differences in the carotid dynamics between the two vascular brain regions leading to acute changes in blood pressure [5, 6]. Graduated compression stockings might affect the sympathoadrenergic variability and heart rate variability in response to rest and after strenuous exercise by individuals in wheelchairs with spinal cord injury [7].

Nonelastic compression mechanisms are recommended in the treatment of lymphedema. The daily clinical experience shows that the maintenance of compression at night in the initial stage of the treatment of severe lymphedema (grades II and III) allows maintenance of the volume reductions achieved during the day. Thus, the use of compression at night is frequently indicated. However, one patient started to suffer from postural hypotension. The aim of this study is to report on a case of postural hypotension after the continuous use (24 hours/day) of nonelastic pantyhose for the treatment of lymphedema.

2. Case Report

We report on the case of a 72-year-old female patient who since the age of 45 has had lymphedema that evolved to elephantiasis. She was submitted to two surgeries to remove tissue related to the elephantiasis, but the lymphedema again progressed to elephantiasis during the years that followed. Eventually, the patient was referred to the Clinica Godoy for intensive treatment including mechanical lymphatic therapy, cervical stimulation, nonelastic compression stocking (grosgrain), and manual lymphatic therapy (Pereira de Godoy and de Fatima Guerreiro Godoy [8], and Pereira de Godoy et al. [9]). This technique uses a hand-made low-stretch compression stocking of a cotton-polyester fabric (Grosgrain) [10]. The patient, with a height of 81 kg, had a body mass index (BMI) of 34.6 kg/m^2 before starting treatment which dropped to 32.6 kg/m^2 after treatment. There was a 70% reduction in the volume of the leg within five days of treatment after which the use of a grosgrain nonelastic stocking was prescribed for 24 hours per day. On the patient's return visit to the clinic after 15 days of using the pantyhose, she presented with postural hypotension after removing the stocking for a physical evaluation. The reduction in systemic blood pressure, assessed in the standing position with measurements at one-minute intervals, showed a reduction of more than 30 mmHg within three minutes. With the drop in blood pressure, the patient had symptoms of hypotension and was placed in the supine position with improvement of the symptoms and the pressure returning to normal. Blood pressure measurements were repeated in the standing position and the patient again had hypotensive symptoms. The patient was advised not to use pantyhose at night and when it was taken off at the next appointment the patient had no symptoms of hypotension. Again the use of the pantyhose was reintroduced for 24 hours per day and again on removing it the patient had symptoms of hypotension with a 30 mmHg drop in blood pressure in 3 minutes. Finally, the patient was advised not to wear the pantyhose at night and the postural hypotension was definitively cured. This study was approved by the Research Ethics Committee of the Medicine School in São José do Rio Preto (FAMERP) number 144.958/12.

3. Discussion

The current study reports on postural hypotension with the continuous use (24 hours per day) of nonelastic grosgrain pantyhose. This situation, associated with compression therapy, has not been described in the literature previously. However, one method described to treat postural hypotension uses elastic stockings [6] although there is no recommendation to use the stockings for 24 hours per day as in this case.

In this study, the age of the patient (72 years old) may have contributed to her condition. Other known causes of hypotension, including dehydration, blood loss, neurological disorders, other cardiovascular and endocrine causes, and certain classes of medicines, were not present in this patient. The improvement in the symptoms with the removal of the compression garment at night and worsening of the

hypotension when it was reintroduced strongly suggests that the pantyhose contributed to these symptoms. About three years ago, a 29-year-old patient had very similar symptoms, but at that time the drop in pressure was not thought to have been an effect of the treatment. Hence, this is the second case and serves as a warning about this danger.

Grosgrain stockings are nonelastic compression mechanisms with a resting pressure of between 10 and 30 mmHg and thus they provide a good continuous compression. This complication is not seen with knee-length grosgrain stockings or even with pantyhose when used only during the daytime. Thus, this study is a warning about the possibility of hypotension when pantyhose is used 24 hours per day.

Orthostatic capacity is an important index for evaluating cardiovascular regulation. Reduced orthostatic tolerance may be associated with cardiac dysrhythmias, myocardial injury with ischemia, diminished cardiac and vascular function that appear to include reductions in circulating blood volume, compromised hemodynamic responses to central hypovolemia, and decreased cerebral and muscle blood flow [11–13]. We speculate that changes in any of these parameters could have contributed to orthostatic changes upon standing of this patient. However, we did not measure any of these variables. Further research should be directed at examining the exact mechanism that contributes to the orthostatic intolerance in subjects with grosgrain compression pantyhose.

The hypothesis for the occurrence of hypotension in this case is interference in the sympathetic nervous mechanisms involving the vascular system. The continuous compression (24 hours per day) may inhibit sympathetic reflexes thereby interfering in the control of pressure.

Conflict of Interests

The authors declare that there is no conflict of interests regarding the publication of this paper.

References

[1] J. M. Stewart, "Mechanisms of sympathetic regulation in orthostatic intolerance," *Journal of Applied Physiology*, vol. 113, no. 10, pp. 1659–1668, 2012.

[2] E. M. Braun, P. V. Tomazic, T. Ropposch, U. Nemetz, A. Lackner, and C. Walch, "Misdiagnosis of acute peripheral vestibulopathy in central nervous system ischemic infarction," *Otology and Neurotology*, vol. 32, no. 9, pp. 1518–1521, 2011.

[3] J. B. Lanier, M. B. Mote, and E. C. Clay, "Evaluation and management of orthostatic hypotension," *The American Family Physician*, vol. 84, no. 5, pp. 527–536, 2011.

[4] A. Y. Gur, E. Auriel, A. D. Korczyn et al., "Vasomotor reactivity as a predictor for syncope in patients with orthostatism," *Acta Neurologica Scandinavica*, vol. 126, no. 1, pp. 32–36, 2012.

[5] N. Goswami, A. Roessler, H. Hinghofer-Szalkay, J. Montani, and A. Steptoe, "Delaying orthostatic syncope with mental challenge: a pilot study," *Physiology and Behavior*, vol. 106, no. 4, pp. 569–573, 2012.

[6] K. Sato, J. P. Fisher, T. Seifert, M. Overgaard, N. H. Secher, and S. Ogoh, "Blood flow in internal carotid and vertebral arteries during orthostatic stress," *Experimental Physiology*, vol. 97, no. 12, pp. 1272–1280, 2012.

[7]   D. Rimaud, P. Calmels, V. Pichot, F. Bethoux, and F. Roche, "Effects of compression stockings on sympathetic activity and heart rate variability in individuals with spinal cord injury," *Journal of Spinal Cord Medicine*, vol. 35, no. 2, pp. 81–88, 2012.

[8]   J. M. Pereira de Godoy and M. de Fatima Guerreiro Godoy, "Development and evaluation of a new apparatus for lymph drainage: preliminary results," *Lymphology*, vol. 37, no. 2, pp. 62–64, 2004.

[9]   J. M. Pereira de Godoy, P. Amador Franco Brigidio, E. Buzato, and M. Fátima Guerreiro de Godoy, "Intensive outpatient treatment of elephantiasis," *International Angiology*, vol. 31, no. 5, pp. 494–499, 2012.

[10] J. M. P. de Godoy, A. P. Sanchez, D. Z. Libanore, and M. de Fatima Guerreiro Godoy,, "Adaptations in the treatment of congenital lymphedema centered on the quality of life," *Case Reports in Medicine*, vol. 2014, Article ID 456060, 3 pages, 2014.

[11] D. Xu, J. K. Shoemaker, A. P. Blaber, P. Arbeille, K. Fraser, and R. L. Hughson, "Reduced heart rate variability during sleep in long-duration spaceflight," *The American Journal of Physiology: Regulatory Integrative and Comparative Physiology*, vol. 305, no. 2, pp. R164–R170, 2013.

[12] J. J. Batzel, N. Goswami, H. K. Lackner et al., "Patterns of cardiovascular control during repeated tests of orthostatic loading," *Cardiovascular Engineering*, vol. 9, no. 4, pp. 134–143, 2009.

[13] N. Goswami, H. K. Lackner, E. K. Grasser, and H. G. Hinghofer-Szalkay, "Individual stability of orthostatic tolerance response," *Acta Physiologica Hungarica*, vol. 96, no. 2, pp. 157–166, 2009.

44

Staphylococcal Scalded Skin Syndrome in Neonate

K. Kouakou,[1] M. E. Dainguy,[1] and K. Kassi[2]

[1]*Department of Pediatrics, Training and Research Unit of Medical Sciences,*
Felix Houphouët Boigny University of Abidjan, Côte d'Ivoire
[2]*Department of Dermatology and Infectiology, Training and Research Unit of Medical Sciences,*
Felix Houphouët Boigny University of Abidjan, BP 5151, Abidjan 21, Côte d'Ivoire

Correspondence should be addressed to K. Kassi; siskakomlo@yahoo.fr

Academic Editor: Gérald E. Piérard

We described a case of Staphylococcal Scalded Skin Syndrome in infant age of 21 days by discussing clinical and management issues. This newborn presented large erythematous, eroded, and oozing areas covered by epidermal skin flap. The average surface of cutaneous unsticking on admission was 31.35% of body surface area corresponding to lesions of superficial second-degree burns. An important biological inflammatory syndrome including positive C-reactive protein was found. Under treatment, erythroderma decreased within 7 to 10 days and the newborn was completely healed after 3 weeks of followup, with the disappearance of the inflammatory syndrome and total body surface restored. This clinical case report showed that SSSS remains a major dermatological problem in neonates. Therefore, its diagnosis should be made without doubt and its care should start earlier in a neonate emergency unit in order to have good prognosis. And the rigorous "search and destroy" policy based on screening of staff and patients and isolation of identified patients advocated in the United Kingdom should be applied in neonate units in Côte d'Ivoire.

1. Introduction

Staphylococcal Scalded Skin Syndrome (SSSS) or acute staphylococcal epidermolysis is an exfoliative skin disease and a toxin mediated staphylococcal infections affecting mostly neonates and adolescents and it is rare in adults [1, 2]. Currently, the incidence of this disease is increasing in all ages. Its resistance to conventional antibiotic treatment is also a new reality. Prognosis is mostly favourable and skin lesions healed without scarring [3]. We describe a case of a newborn of 21 days of age with SSSS and discuss relevant pathology, clinical issue, and management.

2. Case Report

A newborn was hospitalized for erythroderma. The disease started with a sore throat and conjunctivitis. Within 48 hours, the newborn developed a fever and tender erythema which progresses to generalized erythematous skin lesions mostly seen in the axillary and groin areas. It was associated with formation of large fragile-roofed superficial blisters which rupture on the slightest pressure leading to extended areas of denuded and eroded skin. The Nikolski (easy separation of skin layers upon application of horizontal, tangential pressure to the skin) sign was present.

The medical history showed that her mother got pregnant two times. Her blood group was AB positive. The clinical examination during mother's pregnancy was normal out of the hemoglobin type which was abnormal (type AC). HIV test was negative. Vaccination for tetanus and hepatitis B was up to date. Her mother had not any blistering disease history. Drugs taken during mother's pregnancy were "Tanakan, Folifer, and Fansidar tablets," used at the 26th and the 32nd weeks of pregnancy according to the national program for malaria control in Côte d'Ivoire.

We found a history of traditional medicines use from the 3rd month of pregnancy to vaginal delivery. This delivery was normal under epidural anesthesia with marcaine at the 40th week of pregnancy. There was no family history of similar skin lesions.

In the birth, it was a female newborn weighing 3.7 kilograms (Kg) and of the size 45 centimeters (cm). Cranial

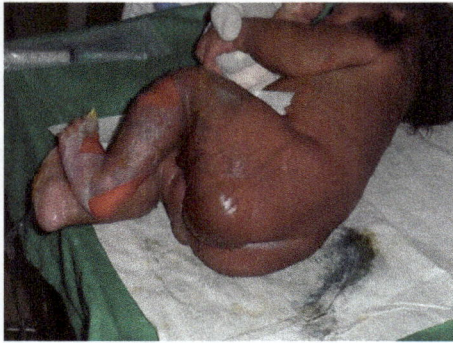

FIGURE 1: Staphylococcal Scalded Skin Syndrome in a newborn with generalized bullous epidermolysis.

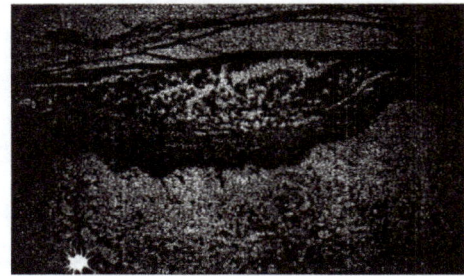

FIGURE 2: Superficial epidermolysis of the granular layer.

perimeter was estimated to be 33 cm and the APGAR score was estimated to be 8 at the first minute and 9 at the 5th minute.

Its clinical examination on admission revealed no fever with 36,2°C of temperature, and the respiratory frequency was 45 cycles/minute. The heart rate was 120 beatings/minute, and integuments were colored.

The examination of the skin and the mucous membranes highlighted the skin peeling and widespread blisters prevailing in the anterior and posterior parts of the lower limb relying on an erythematous basis. The epidermal necrolysis has quickly extended to the bottom and to the trunk during hospitalization. There appear large erythematous, eroded, and oozing areas covered by epidermal skin flap (Figure 1). Mucous membranes were intact. The genital examination showed unsticking lesions on the big and small lips of the vagina which bled when in contact. Other body system examinations were normal. The average surface of cutaneous unsticking on admission was 31.35% of the body surface area corresponding to the lesions of superficial second-degree burns.

We found an important biological inflammatory syndrome including positive C-reactive protein.

Three differential diagnoses were evoked with these clinical manifestations: (1) toxic epidermal necrosis drug induced (Lyell syndrome), (2) Staphylococcal Scalded Skin Syndrome (SSSS), and (3) Staphylococcal Shock.

The skin biopsy has shown superficial intraepidermal split into the granular layer (Figure 2) associated with little inflammatory infiltrate in the superficial dermal layer and no necrosis. This aspect characterizes SSSS.

Bacteriological examinations of urine, skin, and vaginal swabs were negative. The conjunctivae and nasopharyngeal cultures and the blood culture were positive to *Staphylococcus aureus*. In some, the diagnosis is done, based on (1) clinical finding of superficial blisters, (2) intraepidermal split on histology, and (3) demonstration of staphylococcal infection. In addition, the biological blood check did not find any abnormalities such as anemia and renal impairment. Immunofluorescence was not performed due to the lack of material in our setting.

The newborn was treated by a double antibiotic therapy combining ceftriaxone and aminoside at the neonate emergency unit. We added an important rehydration, antipain, and skin care with eosin liquid 1%. The treatment was effective and the outcome was rapidly favourable. The erythroderma decreased within 7 to 10 days and the newborn was completely healed after 3 weeks of followup, with disappearance of the inflammatory syndrome and total body surface restored.

3. Discussion

Generally, SSSS is regarded as mild disease, but in neonate and immunocompromised patient it is serious and occasionally fatal and the exfoliative toxins produced by *Staphylococcus aureus* are considered to be the pathogenetic agent in SSSS [4]. These exfoliative toxins are also responsible for causing bullous impetigo. It appears to be a relationship between the disease extent, the amount of toxin produced, and whether the toxin is released locally or systemically [3]. There are two exfoliative toxins that are identified, exotoxin A, the most produced one, and the exotoxin B. Most strains of *Staphylococcus aureus* isolated from patient suffering from SSSS belong to phage group II (about 80%) [3, 5]. These toxins have exquisite specificity in causing loss of desmosome-mediated cell adhesion within the superficial epidermis only [6]. When the toxins are released into the blood stream, the lack of protective antitoxin antibody in neonates allows the toxins to reach the epidermis where they act locally to produce the characteristic skin lesions [7]. These human exfoliative toxin antibodies which have neutralizing properties decrease from 0 to 3 months [8]. This could explain the severity of our case who is 21 days of age, and, unfortunately, we could not identify exfoliative toxin secretion and its type.

These toxins cause histopathologically a subcorneal split along the granular cell layer, resulting from intra-epidermal acantholysis, as we observed in our case where we found little dermal inflammatory cell and no cell necrosis.

This is similar to that found in bullous impetigo, but in bullous impetigo there is pronounced inflammatory cell infiltrate consisting mostly in neutrophils [3].

Thus, in our case, 2 risk factors were identified, the lack of the newborn's immune system and the use of traditional products during the pregnancy and delivery periods by her mother, which might favour the occurrence of the disease.

All these pathogenesis characteristics allow us to understand the clinical manifestations of SSSS particularly in neonate.

SSSS has usually a swift onset of painful, tender, and red skin accentuated in flexural and periorificial areas. After 24 to 48 hours, flaccid blisters and erosions develop and large areas of the overlying epidermis loosen and peel like a scald which can be extended [9]. In our case, the disease starts with the inflammation of the conjunctivae (conjunctivitis) which is a *Staphylococcus* commensal site like umbilicus and axilla.

The diagnosis is usually made on clinical ground [9]; it relies mainly on the recognition of the characteristic appearance of the rash with fever. But it is important to swab the skin, the orificial areas, and the mucus membranes for bacterial confirmation and to identify the primary focus infection and screening for *Staphylococcus aureus* carriage, as we performed in our case. The skin biopsy often shows a superficial intraepidermal split into the granular layer associated with little inflammatory infiltrate in the superficial dermal layer without necrosis as we found in our case. This diagnosis is made in our case based on (1) clinical finding of superficial blisters, (2) intraepidermal split on histology, and (3) demonstration of staphylococcal infection.

3.1. Treatment. Antistaphylococcal antibiotics, temperature regulation, maintaining fluid and electrolyte balance, nutritional management, and skin care form the basics of treatment [3].

These antibiotics represent one of the main pillars of SSSS treatment, but the growing concerns of the resistant strains of staphylococci anti-ETA and anti-ETB might be the future challenges.

In fact, resistance was observed for some antibiotics: 5% for gentamicin, 7% for tetracycline, and 2% for chloramphenicol, whereas there were no strains resistant to methicillin, cephalothin, cephalexin, and vancomycin [4].

In practice, blisters should be left intact because it helps to reduce further trauma to the skin. Topical antibiotics or antiseptic eye ointment is also helpful to manage the conjunctivitis. In the best case, patients should be managed in the pediatric intensive care unit and consideration needs to be given to mattress requirement, pain management, temperature regulation, fluid management (rehydration), nutrition, and skin care. Corticosteroids are contraindicated with the worsening of the disease [3]. Appropriate intravenous antibiotics against penicillin-resistant staphylococci should be used such as methicillin and flucloxacillin and the use of intravenous fluid management and analgesia in case of oral intake is reduced because of the perioral lesions [7]. In our case, we used a double antibiotic therapy combining ceftriaxone and aminoside at the neonate emergency unit. We added important rehydration, antipain, and skin care with eosin liquid of 1%. The treatment was effective and the newborn was completely healed after 3 weeks of followup, with the disappearance of the inflammatory syndrome and total body surface restored.

3.2. Followup. The prognosis of SSSS in childhood is mostly favourable. The mortality rate is approximately 4% and it is associated with extensive skin involvement [3]. In our case, under treatment, erythroderma decreased within 7 to 10 days and the newborn was completely healed after 3 weeks of followup, with the disappearance of the inflammatory syndrome and total body surface restored.

3.3. Prevention. As asymptomatic nasal carriage of staphylococci aureus is an important source of infection in neonates, strict control measures should be taken such as isolation of infected patients, barrier nursing, and antiseptic hand washing by both staff and visitor to the unit. The rigorous "search and destroy" policy based on screening of staff and patients and isolation of identified patients that is now being increasingly advocated in United Kingdom [9] should be applied in neonate units in Côte d'Ivoire.

4. Conclusion

While most cases of SSSS are easily treated, it remains an emergency case and a potential fatal condition in neonate. Its diagnosis should be made without doubt and its care should start early in neonate emergency unit in order to have good prognosis.

Conflict of Interests

The authors declare that there is no conflict of interests regarding the publication of this paper.

References

[1] J. C. Coleman and N. R. Dobson, "Diagnostic dilemma: extremely low birth weight baby with staphylococcal scalded-skin syndrome or toxic epidermal necrolysis," *Journal of Perinatology*, vol. 26, no. 11, pp. 714–716, 2006.

[2] S. Kadam, A. Tagare, J. Deodhar, Y. Tawade, and A. Pandit, "Staphylococcal scalded skin syndrome in a neonate," *Indian Journal of Pediatrics*, vol. 76, no. 10, p. 1074, 2009.

[3] G. K. Patel and A. Y. Finlay, "Staphylococcal scalded skin syndrome: diagnosis and management," *The American Journal of Clinical Dermatology*, vol. 4, no. 3, pp. 165–175, 2003.

[4] K. Murono, K. Fujita, and H. Yoshioka, "Microbiologic characteristics of exfoliative toxin-producing *Staphylococcus aureus*," *The Pediatric Infectious Disease Journal*, vol. 7, no. 5, pp. 313–315, 1988.

[5] E. Rieger-Fackeldey, L. R. W. Plano, A. Kramer, and A. Schulze, "Staphylococcal scalded skin syndrome related to an exfoliative toxin A- and B-producing strain in preterm infants," *European Journal of Pediatrics*, vol. 161, no. 12, pp. 649–652, 2002.

[6] C. B. Lillibridge, M. E. Melish, and L. A. Glasgow, "Site of action of exfoliative toxin in the staphylococcal scalded skin syndrome," *Pediatrics*, vol. 50, pp. 728–738, 1972.

[7] S. Ladhani, "Understanding the mechanism of action of the exfoliative toxins of *Staphylococcus aureus*," *FEMS Immunology and Medical Microbiology*, vol. 39, no. 2, pp. 181–189, 2003.

[8] T. Hubiche, M. Bes, L. Roudiere, F. Langlaude, J. Etienne, and P. del Giudice, "Mild staphylococcal scalded skin syndrome: an

underdiagnosed clinical disorder," *British Journal of Dermatology*, vol. 166, no. 1, pp. 213–215, 2012.

[9] G. A. Johnston, "Treatment of bullous impetigo and the staphylococcal scalded skin syndrome in infants," *Expert Review of Anti-Infective Therapy*, vol. 2, no. 3, pp. 439–446, 2004.

45

Harmful Effects of Synthetic Surface-Active Detergents against Atopic Dermatitis

Hajime Deguchi,[1,2] **Riho Aoyama,**[1,2] **Hideaki Takahashi,**[1,2]
Yoshinari Isobe,[3] **and Yutaka Tsutsumi**[2]

[1]*Fujita Health University School of Medicine, Toyoake, Aichi 470-1192, Japan*
[2]*Department of Pathology, Fujita Health University School of Medicine, Toyoake, Aichi 470-1192, Japan*
[3]*Isobe Clinic, Anjo, Aichi 446-0026, Japan*

Correspondence should be addressed to Yutaka Tsutsumi; tsutsumi@fujita-hu.ac.jp

Academic Editor: Jeung-Hoon Lee

We report herein two cases of intractable atopic dermatitis successfully treated by simply avoiding the contact with surface-active detergents in the daily life and living. The detergents were closely related to the exacerbation and remission of the disease. Steroid ointment was no longer used. We discuss that the removal of horny layer lipids by surface-active detergents accelerates the transepidermal water loss and disturbs the barrier function of the epidermis and thus is intimately involved in the pathogenesis of atopic dermatitis.

1. Introduction

Atopic dermatitis is etiologically related to abnormalities in physiologic functions of the skin, resulting in chronic persistent and irritating inflammation of type I and/or type IV allergic reactions: atopic dermatitis is a disease of altered epidermal barrier [1–4]. Allergens are usually not specified. Infants aged below 2 years show the lowest epidermal barrier function and are susceptible to atopic dermatitis [1–3]. The main victims are thus infants and young children, but the long-lasting disease is also seen in the adulthood. The treatment strategy against atopic dermatitis includes the external use of steroids or tacrolimus ointment, in addition to moisturizing and protective skin cares [5]. Internal use of antihistamines and antiallergic drugs and the elimination of exacerbating factors are also employed.

Dry skin is one of the major symptoms in atopic dermatitis. The abnormality of the epidermis, especially the horny layer (stratum corneum), is closely linked to loss of the barrier function. The transepidermal water loss is caused by reduced lipids in the horny layer. The lipid bilayers intermit between the horny keratinocytes (corneocytes). When the corneocytes are thought of as bricks, the lipids filling the spaces between the cells are the mortar or cement (brick and mortar model) [2, 4]. The lipid bilayers consist of ceramides, cholesterol and long-chained fatty acids, and impede penetration of lipophilic as well as hydrophilic substances [6–9]. Soap and detergents acting as surfactants may provoke skin damage such as scaling, dryness, tightness, roughness, erythema, and swelling. An itch-scratch cycle accelerates damaging the epidermal barrier [1–4].

We report herein two representative adult patients who showed exacerbation of atopic dermatitis after the contact with surface-active detergents and the disuse led to the remission. We propose that the removal of horny layer lipids by surface-active detergents is intimately involved in the pathogenesis of atopic dermatitis, as one of the authors have published Japanese-written books for promoting the general public and dermatitis patients to avoid using soap and detergents [10, 11].

2. Case Presentation

Case 1. Case 1 is a 50-year-old male, an office worker in a gas station. After a 10-month history of chronic prurigo treated with steroid ointment, he visited Isobe Clinic in Anjo, Aichi,

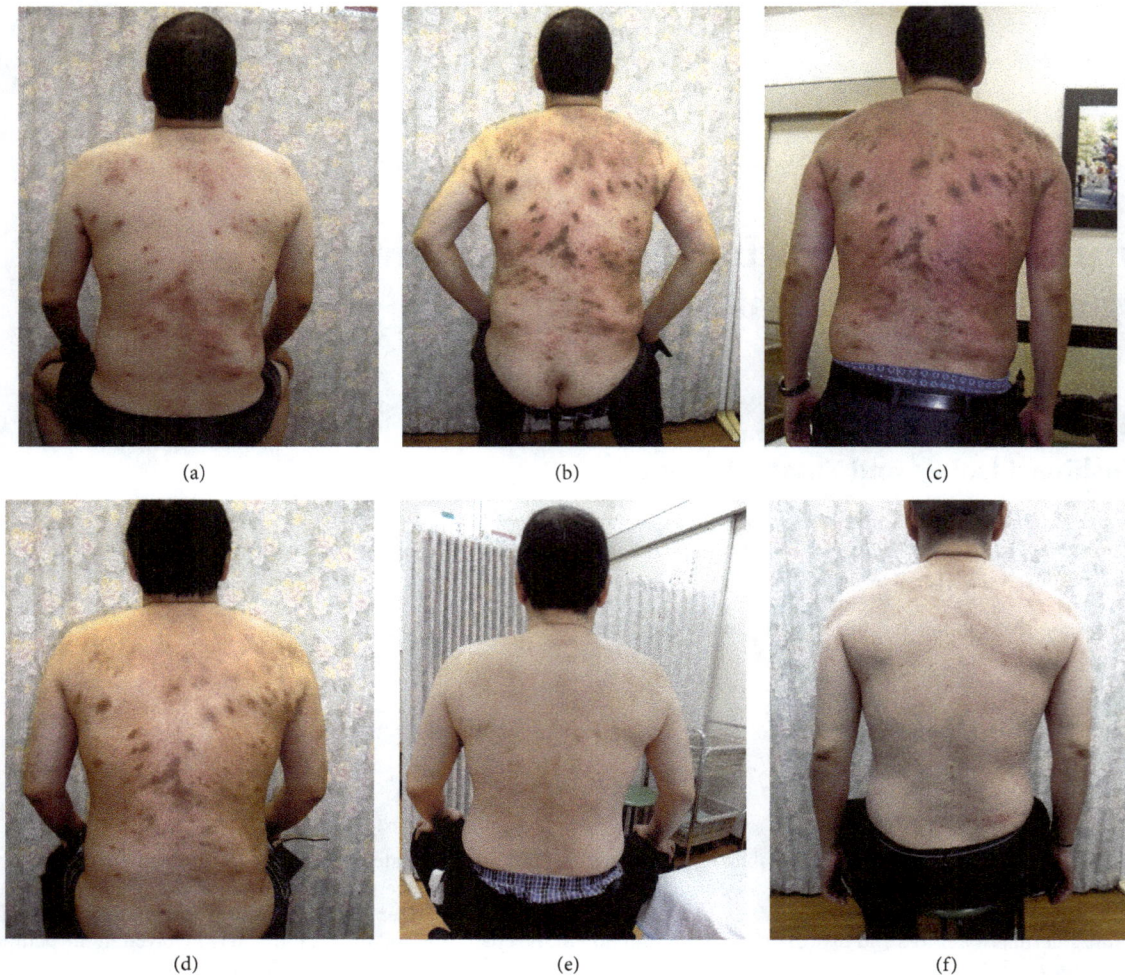

FIGURE 1: Clinical features of skin rash on the back in case 1 (a 50-year-old male). (a) December 4, 2010 (the first medical inspection), (b) January 12, 2011 (exacerbation), (c) January 26, 2011 (the worst state with erythematous reaction), (d) March 16, 2011 (alleviation), (e) July 17, 2012 (remission), and (f) March 11, 2014 (recurrence). Strict avoidance of the detergent-containing material and usage of cleansing soap without detergents were quite effective to control atopic dermatitis.

Japan, in November, 2010. He complained of itchiness all over his body, resulting in difficulty in sleeping. Based on the chronic and repetitive rash with itchy sensation, the diagnosis of atopic dermatitis was made (Figure 1(a)).

With the radioimmunosorbent assay for allergens in January, 2011, no specific antiallergens were identified in the serum. A total of 12 allergens were evaluated, including Japanese mugwort, house dust, house dust mite (*Dermatophagoides pteronyssinus*), *Alternaria* (air-floating black fungus), egg white, pork, shrimp, mackerel, cone, rice, buckwheat, and peanut. The serum IgE level was not significantly high, 189 IU/mL (normal range: ~170 IU/mL). Repeated bacterial culture tests performed four times during November, 2010, through April, 2013, failed to detect any specific pathogens. The biopsy was performed from his right abdominal skin. The microscopic findings are illustrated in Figure 2. Reactive downward acanthosis with lymphocytic exocytosis and spongiotic reaction focally resulting in small vesicle formation is shown. An eosinophilic microabscess was formed in the parakeratotic horny layer. The granular

keratinocytes disappeared. Superficial perivascular infiltration of lymphocytes and eosinophils was associated.

The patient was asked to avoid using synthetic surface-active detergent-containing material such as cleansing soap, household synthetic detergents, shampoo and conditioner, and cosmetic cream and lotion. The use of natural soap was also avoided. When bathing, the hair and body were washed only with warm or tepid water. The skin was cared with an ointment consisting of a mixture of vaseline and urea (urea concentration: 0.12%). Concurrently, the following drugs were prescribed: (A) Celtect (Oxatomide), 2 tablets (antiallergic drug), (B) Nipolazin (Mequitazine), 2 tablets (antihistamine), (C) Tarivid (Ofloxacin), 2 tablets (new quinolone antibiotics), and (D) Terramycin ointment (Tetracycline antibiotics). When necessary, Amikacin (aminoglycoside antibiotics) was intramuscularly injected. The antibiotics were administered because of the clinical suspicion of coinfection of anaerobic bacteria.

His skin condition was not significantly improved soon, and the rash was exacerbated in January, 2011 (Figure 1(b)).

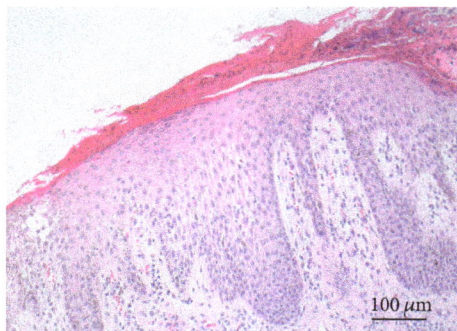

FIGURE 2: Microscopic features of the biopsied abdominal skin in case 1 (hematoxylin and eosin). The involved epidermis reveals reactive downward acanthosis with lymphocytic exocytosis and spongiotic reaction focally resulting in small vesicle formation. An eosinophilic microabscess is formed in the parakeratotic horny layer. The granular keratinocytes have disappeared. Superficial perivascular infiltration of lymphocytes and eosinophils is associated.

Figure 1(c) demonstrates the worst state of his erythematous rash on the back, photographed 10 days after Figure 1(b). One of the reasons for the exacerbation was considered to be linked to the fact that the cosmetic companies recently increased the concentration of synthetic surface-active agents in their products, including shampoo, hair conditioner, and synthetic cleaning soap. The patient was again advised to avoid strictly contacting with the detergent-containing material and using soap without detergents "Bajan" (soap prepared by electrolysis of sodium bicarbonate water, Kenbi, Iwate, Japan) for washing clothes. Two months later, the skin rash was improved with much less itchy sensation (Figure 1(d)). Thereafter, the avoidance strategy effectively alleviated the condition of his skin. One and half years later, the skin rash was controlled completely (Figure 1(e)), and his symptoms including itchy sensation disappeared and he became able to sleep well.

In March, 2014, itchy skin rash recurred, because his wife started to use the detergent-containing synthetic cleansing soap, which is widely used in Japan. On inspection, small-sized rash accompanied by itchy sensation was observed on his back (Figure 1(f)). For the symptomless two-year period, he and his wife believed that his atopic dermatitis has been cured completely. Reeducation of the patient of his wife was necessary to improve his skin condition. In March, 2014, his serum IgE level remains low as 59 IU/mL.

Case 2. Case 2 is a 48-year-old female, a housewife. The diagnosis of atopic dermatitis was made when she was a junior high school girl. In order to control the skin rash, steroid ointment was administered for some 40 years. The control status was not excellent, and she occasionally complained of itchiness all over the body. In June, 2007, she met one of the authors (Y. I.) who gave a lecture on how to treat and control atopic dermatitis. Y. I. personally delivered an ointment containing dibucaine and hydrophilic vaseline, which significantly relieved her itchy sensation.

When her skin rash was under control by the topical use of steroid subscribed from a university hospital, she happened to use shampoo and body soap equipped in a hotel. Thereafter, her face became markedly swollen by severe and itchy rash with secondary infection and scratch injury (Figure 3(a)). She thought that this event occurred as a rebound phenomenon of steroid therapy. Finally, the patient visited Isobe Clinic in October, 2007, and she was advised to avoid using synthetic surface-active detergent-containing material such as cleansing soap, household synthetic detergents, shampoo and conditioner, and cosmetic cream and lotion, and the skin was coated with an ointment containing a mixture of vaseline and urea. The use of natural soap was also avoided. Concurrently, the following drugs were prescribed: (A) Nipolazin (Mequitazine), 2 tablets (antihistamine), (B) Chloromycetin salve (antibiotics), (C) Tarivid (Ofloxacin), 2 tablets (antibiotics), (D) Cinal, 4 tablets (vitamin compounds), and (E) Depas05, 2 tablets (antianxiety drug). Azunol ointment (anti-inflammation drug) was also used when necessary.

By the end of November, 2007, her skin condition improved dramatically (Figure 3(b)). Thereafter, she continued to avoid thoroughly using the detergent and soap. In July, 2014, the condition of her skin was kept well without steroid therapy any longer.

3. Discussion

We report herein two representative adult cases of atopic dermatitis, against which the avoidance of synthetic surface-active detergent-containing materials such as cleansing soap, household synthetic detergents, shampoo and conditioner, and cosmetic cream and lotion was quite effective in relieving the symptoms and signs. The patients were also asked to avoid using natural soap. Activity of atopic dermatitis was histologically evident in the biopsied skin of case 1. Parakeratotic changes accompanied by disappearance of the granular keratinocytes directly represented epidermal barrier dysfunction. Reuse of the detergent-containing material exacerbated the skin condition. Supportive therapy included topical rubbing of an ointment containing a mixture of vaseline and 0.12% urea and administration of antihistamines, antiallergic drugs, and antibiotics. Steroid ointment was no longer used in these two cases. Such a cost-effective treatment strategy dramatically improved the condition of long-lasting and intractable atopic dermatitis. It is evident clinically that the synthetic surface-active detergent caused the exacerbation of atopic dermatitis.

One of the authors, Yoshinari Isobe, M.D., is a practical dermatologist in Anjo, Aichi, Japan, having long and deep experience of the cost-effective treatment against severe and refractory atopic dermatitis. He has promoted patients of atopic dermatitis and the general public not to use the material containing surface-active detergents in the daily life and living. Based on the clinical experience treating more than 400 adult cases of intractable atopic dermatitis, he published promoting books for the general public and dermatitis patients, written in Japanese [10, 11]. He insists that complete avoidance of the detergent results in complete remission of atopic dermatitis.

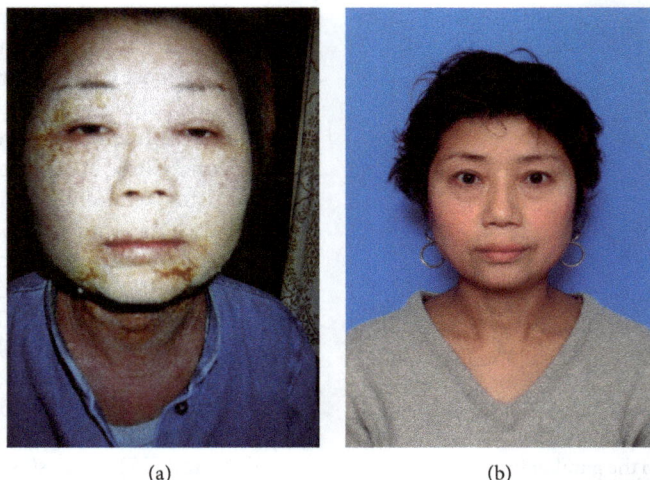

(a)   (b)

FIGURE 3: Clinical features of facial skin rash in case 2 (a 48-year-old female). (a) October, 2007 (severe rash), (b) June, 2014 (complete remission). After the patient happened to use shampoo and body soap equipped in a hotel, her face became markedly swollen by severe and itchy rash with secondary infection and scratch injury. Complete avoidance of the detergents and cleansing soap led to long-lasting complete remission without using steroid ointment. The patient allowed us to present her whole face.

We propose that the removal of horny layer lipids by the surface-active detergent is closely related to the pathogenesis of atopic dermatitis. The representative surface-active agent in the commercially available synthetic soap is polyoxyalkylene alkyl ether, an active emulsifier and detergent for cosmetics, general cleaner, emulsifier for emulsion polymerization. Polyoxyethylene lauryl ether, an emulsifier for cosmetics, is also commonly added (quoted from the ingredient labeling). The detergent takes the lipid component of the epidermal horny layer away and disturbs the barrier function of the epidermis. The transepidermal water loss is caused by the reduction of lipids in the horny layer. The horny keratinocytes (corneocytes) are known to be intermitted by the lipid bilayers, consisting of ceramides, cholesterol, and long-chained fatty acids. The lipid actively secreted from lamellar granules of the granular layer keratinocytes undergoes enzymatic processing to produce the lipid bilayers [6–8]. According to the brick and mortar model [2, 4], when the corneocytes are thought of as bricks, the lipids filling the spaces between the cells represent the mortar or cement.

The flattened corneocytes are interlocked by specially strengthened desmosomes with each other. The long chained ceramides ensure the cohesion of the lipid bilayers between the corneocytes. In other words, the corneocytes sealed in the lipid secretions form the insoluble and fluid impermeable surface coat. These structures give the physiologic stability of the horny layer [6–9]. The corneocytes are devoid of the cell organelles and nucleus but are still metabolically active. Hydrolases hydrolyze triglycerides into di- and monoglycerides, and proteases ensure the supply of amino acids in order to maintain the natural moisturizing factor from proteins [2, 4, 12]. It is known that the use of soap and detergents results in the elevation of horny layer pH and that the sustained increase in pH enhances the activity of degradatory proteases and decreases the activity of lipid-synthesizing enzymes [2, 4]. Normal flora may contribute

to skin surface homeostasis, and this sensitive balance is disturbed by the external use of inappropriate hygienic material and cosmetic products [3, 13].

Filaggrin, the key superficial epidermal component of keratinization and lipid secretion, is cleaved from profilaggrin, a major basic protein of keratohyalin granules of the granular layer keratinocytes. Filaggrin binds to and condenses keratin cytoskeleton in the corneocytes and is citrullinated to function as a natural moisturizing factor [14]. Abnormalities of the filaggrin gene are seen in some patients with atopic dermatitis [2, 4, 15, 16]. The importance of the lipid bilayers in the epidermal frontline should again be emphasized.

The transepidermal water loss is especially important in the barrier damage. Not only natural soap, household synthetic detergents, shampoo, and conditioner but also emulsifiers in creams or lotions and tensides in cleansing products contain surface-active substances and damage or even destroy the intercellular lipid bilayers. Loss of the lipophilic component out of the lipid bilayers increases transepidermal water loss, resulting in skin dehydration (dryness). The dysfunction of the lipid bilayers accelerates the diffusion and permeation of irritable water soluble substances into the deeper part of the epidermis. Topically applied occlusive substances such as urea-containing vaseline prevent the transepidermal water loss. Recently, barrier-restoring or ceramide-replacing therapies have been proposed for atopic dermatitis [17, 18].

We would like to emphasize the possibility of cost-effective and steroid-free therapy of intractable atopic dermatitis simply by avoiding the contact with the surface-active detergent in the daily life and living.

Consent

The patients described in the case report gave their informed consent for the case report to be published.

Conflict of Interests

The authors declare that there is no conflict of interests regarding the publication of this paper.

References

[1] T. Bieber, "Atopic dermatitis," *The New England Journal of Medicine*, vol. 358, no. 14, pp. 1483–1494, 2008.

[2] M. J. Cork, S. G. Danby, Y. Vasilopoulos et al., "Epidermal barrier dysfunction in atopic dermatitis," *Journal of Investigative Dermatology*, vol. 129, no. 8, pp. 1892–1908, 2009.

[3] M. Boguniewicz and D. Y. M. Leung, "Atopic dermatitis: a disease of altered skin barrier and immune dysregulation," *Immunological Reviews*, vol. 242, no. 1, pp. 233–246, 2011.

[4] F. Thawer-Esmail, "Skin barrier function and atopic eczema," *Current Allergy and Clinical Immunology*, vol. 24, no. 4, pp. 193–198, 2011.

[5] H. Saeki, M. Furue, F. Furukawa et al., "Guidelines for management of atopic dermatitis," *The Journal of Dermatology*, vol. 36, no. 10, pp. 563–577, 2009.

[6] T. Doering, W. M. Holleran, A. Potratzt et al., "Sphingolipid activator proteins are required for epidermal permeability barrier formation," *The Journal of Biological Chemistry*, vol. 274, no. 16, pp. 11038–11045, 1999.

[7] P. W. Wertz, "Lipids and barrier function of the skin," *Acta Dermato-Venereologica*, vol. 208, pp. 7–11, 2000.

[8] D. Tsuruta, K. J. Green, S. Getsios, and J. C. R. Jones, "The barrier function of skin: how to keep a tight lid on water loss," *Trends in Cell Biology*, vol. 12, no. 8, pp. 355–357, 2002.

[9] J. Segre, "Complex redundancy to build a simple epidermal permeability barrier," *Current Opinion in Cell Biology*, vol. 15, no. 6, pp. 776–782, 2003.

[10] Y. Isobe, *Atopic Dermatitis. You Can Cure without Steroid Therapy*, Waseda Publishing, Tokyo, Japan, 2001, (Japanese).

[11] Y. Isobe, *No Washing and No Atopic Dermatitis*, Kodansha Publishing, Tokyo, Japan, 2011, (Japanese).

[12] H. Lautenschläger, "Nitrosamine in Kosmetika-Haut in Gefahr?" *Kosmetische Praxis*, vol. 6, pp. 14–15, 2006.

[13] M. Boguniewicz and D. Y. M. Leung, "Recent insights into atopic dermatitis and implications for management of infectious complications," *The Journal of Allergy and Clinical Immunology*, vol. 125, no. 1–3, pp. 4–13, 2010.

[14] A. Sandilands, C. Sutherland, A. D. Irvine, and W. H. I. McLean, "Filaggrin in the frontline: role in skin barrier function and disease," *Journal of Cell Science*, vol. 122, no. 9, pp. 1285–1294, 2009.

[15] I. Nemoto-Hasebe, M. Akiyama, T. Nomura, A. Sandilands, W. H. I. McLean, and H. Shimizu, "*FLG* mutation p.Lys4021X in the C-terminal imperfect filaggrin repeat in Japanese patients with atopic eczema," *British Journal of Dermatology*, vol. 161, no. 6, pp. 1387–1390, 2009.

[16] M. Akiyama, "*FLG* mutations in ichthyosis vulgaris and atopic eczema: spectrum of mutations and population genetics," *British Journal of Dermatology*, vol. 162, no. 3, pp. 472–477, 2010.

[17] D. Sajić, R. Asiniwasis, and S. Skotnicki-Grant, "A look at epidermal barrier function in atopic dermatitis: physiologic lipid replacement and the role of ceramides," *Skin Therapy Letter*, vol. 17, no. 7, pp. 6–9, 2012.

[18] Y. Valdman-Grinshpoun, D. Ben-Amitai, and A. Zvulunov, "Barrier-restoring therapies in atopic dermatitis: current approaches and future perspectives," *Dermatology Research and Practice*, vol. 2012, Article ID 923134, 6 pages, 2012.

46

Drug Reaction with Eosinophilia and Systemic Symptoms: DRESS following Initiation of Oxcarbazepine with Elevated Human Herpesvirus-6 Titer

Seth L. Cornell,[1] Daniel DiBlasi,[2] and Navin S. Arora[2]

[1] Department of Medicine, Tripler Army Medical Center, Honolulu, HI 96859, USA
[2] Dermatology Service, Tripler Army Medical Center, Honolulu, HI 96859, USA

Correspondence should be addressed to Seth L. Cornell; seth.l.cornell.mil@mail.mil

Academic Editors: X.-H. Gao, S. Kawara, and I. Kurokawa

Drug reaction with eosinophilia and systemic symptoms (DRESS) is a rare and potentially fatal severe cutaneous reaction, which has a delayed onset after the initiation of an inciting medication. After recognition and withdrawal of the causative agent, along with aggressive management, a majority of patients will have complete recovery over several months. We present a rare case of DRESS secondary to oxcarbazepine with an elevated human herpesvirus-6 titer.

1. Introduction

Drug reaction with eosinophilia and systemic symptoms (DRESS) is a rare, severe, cutaneous reaction that was prototypically associated with aromatic anticonvulsant medications; however, it is now recognized that it can be caused by a variety of pharmacologic agents. Although no consensus has been reached regarding its pathogenesis, reactivation of human herpesvirus-6 (HHV-6) has been associated with DRESS. Presentation typically occurs within six to eight weeks after initiation of an offending medication and often resolves with prompt discontinuation; however, fatal cases have been reported. Here, we present a rare case of DRESS secondary to oxcarbazepine and associated with elevated HHV-6 titer.

2. Case Report

A 29-year-old Asian female presented to the emergency department for a progressively worsening rash over the prior week. The eruption originated as a solitary pruritic plaque on her left arm, which over the next two days spread to her trunk and legs. Her family physician initially prescribed a course of valacyclovir for presumed varicella zoster virus infection. She returned to the same provider three days later and the rash was noted to now involve the interdigital aspects of her hands and feet. Permethrin cream was prescribed due to concern for scabies. The lesions continued to worsen and the patient developed a fever and sore throat eight days after the eruption onset. She was subsequently instructed by her primary care provider to go to the emergency department for further evaluation.

In the emergency department, she complained of severe pruritis and painful oral lesions but denied having any painful skin lesions, skin sloughing, or any anogenital lesions. On exam, she was tachycardic to 131 bpm but was afebrile, normotensive, and in no acute distress. Cardiovascular and pulmonary examinations were unremarkable. Cutaneous examination revealed numerous erythematous discrete papules and minimal blanching on the bilaterally distal extremities, face, and neck (Figure 1). There were also discrete papules coalescing into nonblanching, erythematous plaques on her trunk and proximal extremities (Figures 2 and 3). The soft palate did exhibit petechiae, without any erosions or ulcerations. Cervical lymphadenopathy was also appreciated.

The patient had a history of Hodgkin lymphoma diagnosed, in 2007, at the age of 25, which was treated with chemotherapy and electron beam radiotherapy, and has been

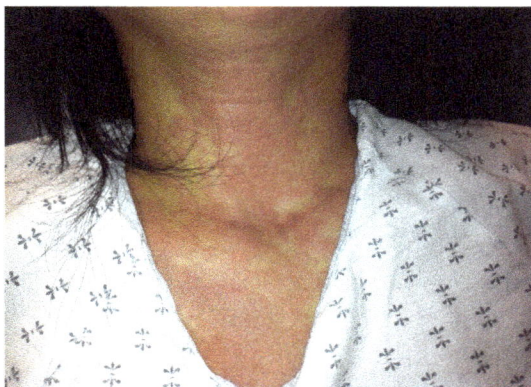

FIGURE 1: Anterior neck and upper chest: discrete and coalescing, slightly blanching, planar plaques.

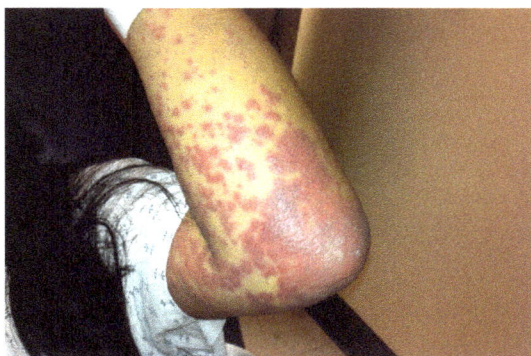

FIGURE 3: Bilateral wrists/palms: tender, nonblanching red violaceous papules and plaques, some with early vesiculation.

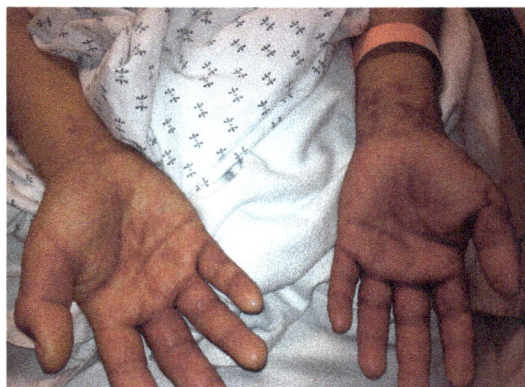

FIGURE 2: Left ventral arm/elbow: discrete and coalescing, nonblanching papules coalescing into plaques, most consistent with a palpable purpura.

in remission since then. Medications included venlafaxine for depression and oxcarbazepine for mood stabilization which was started approximately 2 months before. She endorsed allergies to latex and shellfish and admitted smoking less than one pack of cigarettes per day.

A cell blood count was notable for atypical lymphocytes at 9% (1.1×10^9/L) and elevated eosinophils of 7% (0.68×10^9/L). Liver enzymes were also elevated, with alanine aminotransferase at 130 units/L (15–46 units/L), aspartate aminotransferase at 108 units/L (13–69 units/L), and alkaline phosphatase of 267 units/L (38–126 units/L). Chemistry and coagulation studies were unremarkable. Despite a thorough discussion regarding the necessity of a skin biopsy, the patient declined.

The patient was diagnosed with DRESS based on a "definite" RegiSCAR score and subsequently admitted to the hospital. Oxcarbazepine was discontinued and prednisone was initiated at 1.5 mg/kg daily. During the hospitalization, liver enzymes downtrended, while the eosinophilia increased from 7% to 12% (1.55×10^9/L). An HHV-6 IgG level was checked 1 week after admission and was elevated at 7.96 IV (>1.11 indicates current or past infection).

The patient was discharged on hospital day three and was continued on prednisone 1.5 mg/kg daily, given the stabilization of her eruption. She was educated on the importance of avoiding aromatic epileptic drugs and to follow up with her psychiatrist for medication reevaluation.

One week after discharge, her eruption continued to improve and her lymphadenopathy had resolved. The lesions became blanchable on the trunk; however, her eosinophilia increased from 12% to 23% (4.68×10^9/L). On postdischarge day fifteen, there was a decrease in her edema with truncal desquamation. Prednisone dose was decreased to 1 mg/kg. On postdischarge day 27, the lesions had almost completely resolved, with residual postinflammatory hyperpigmentation observed on bilateral ankles. The prednisone was tapered off over the next month with total resolution of the rash and normalization of eosinophils (0.23×10^9/L).

3. Discussion

Adverse cutaneous reactions occur in approximately two to three percent of hospitalized patients [1]. Severe cutaneous reactions such as toxic epidermal necrolysis, Steven-Johnson Syndrome, angioedema, and serum sickness have been estimated to occur in about 1 out of every 1000 patients hospitalized [2].

The term DRESS was first proposed in 1996, though medical providers had likely been encountering this severe cutaneous adverse reaction (SCAR) since the advent of hydantoin derivatives for the treatment of convulsive disorders [3, 4]. First described in 1959, as a pseudolymphoma often accompanied by exanthem, eosinophilia, and fever, this potentially fatal SCAR has been known by a variety of names including drug-induced hypersensitivity syndrome, drug-induced delayed multiorgan hypersensitivity syndrome, anticonvulsant hypersensitivity syndrome, and phenytoin syndrome [5]. The lack of a standard nomenclature has caused considerable diagnostic confusion.

Originally described in 1996, the proposed diagnosis of DRESS required a cutaneous drug eruption with both hematologic abnormalities (eosinophilia or atypical lymphocytes) and systemic involvement (adenopathy, hepatitis, nephritis, pneumonitis, or carditis). More recently, a diagnostic scoring system has been proposed by the European Registry of Severe Cutaneous Adverse Reactions (RegiSCAR) that helps clinicians determine if DRESS is definite, probable, possible, or excluded [6]. According to this classification system, features consistent with DRESS include eosinophilia, fever, lymphadenopathy, atypical lymphocytes, leukopenia, diffuse rash, organ involvement, and disease duration greater than fifteen days. Determining the incidence of DRESS has been historically difficult given its discordant diagnostic denotation, though it has been estimated at between 1 in 1,000 and 1 in 10,000 drug exposures [7].

Although the exact pathogenesis of DRESS is not completely understood, proposed mechanisms include reactive drug metabolite formation with subsequent immunologic activation, slow acetylation, and reactivation of HHV-6 [8, 9]. DRESS has been strongly associated with aromatic anticonvulsant agents such as phenytoin, phenobarbital, and carbamazepine; however, several other classes of medications are also associated with DRESS.

The mainstay of treatment of DRESS is prompt diagnosis and removal of the offending agent. Corticosteroids are routinely used, though consensus regarding the dose and route of administration has not been established. Treatment with intravenous immune globulin has also been described [10]. After diagnosis, recovery typically occurs within six to nine weeks; however, mortality has been estimated at approximately 5% [11]. DRESS may also predispose affected patients to long-term autoimmune sequelae, most notably thyroid dysfunction, along with type 1 diabetes mellitus, and autoimmune hemolytic anemia [12].

Our case demonstrates typical symptoms of DRESS, such as the delayed onset of cutaneous lesions after the initiation of an aromatic anticonvulsant, peripheral eosinophilia, hepatitis, lymphadenopathy, and prolonged disease duration. The patient's symptoms slowly resolved with the removal of oxcarbazepine and the initiation of oral corticosteroid therapy. This case highlights a rarely described cause of DRESS with both oxcarbazepine and an elevated HHV-6 antibody likely implicated in disease development.

4. Conclusion

DRESS must be considered in all patients presenting with a cutaneous eruption and visceral organ involvement, with recent initiation of a new medication, especially aromatic anticonvulsants. The delayed onset of symptoms following initiation of a new medication and an elevated HHV-6 titer are suggestive of DRESS and may help differentiate it from other forms of severe cutaneous adverse reactions. Prompt recognition of DRESS, with immediate cessation of the offending medication, is paramount in treating this potentially fatal disease process.

Disclosure

This research received no specific grant from any funding agency in the public, commercial, or not-for-profit sectors.

Disclaimer

The views expressed in the paper are those of the authors and do not reflect the official policy or position of the Department of the Army, the Department of Defense, or the Unites States Government.

Conflict of Interests

All authors do not have any financial relationships to disclosse or any conflict of interests to declare.

Authors' Contribution

Drs. Seth L. Cornell, Daniel DiBlasi, and Navin S. Arora had full access to all of the data in the case report and take responsibility for the integrity of the data. Drs. Seth L. Cornell, Daniel DiBlasi, and Navin S. Arora all had equal and significant contributions to the drafting of the paper.

References

[1] M. Bigby, S. Jick, H. Jick, and K. Arndt, "Drug-induced cutaneous reactions. A report from the Boston collaborative drug surveillance program on 15,438 consecutive inpatients, 1975 to 1982," *The Journal of the American Medical Association*, vol. 256, no. 24, pp. 3358–3363, 1986.

[2] J. C. Roujeau and R. S. Stern, "Severe adverse cutaneous reactions to drugs," *The New England Journal of Medicine*, vol. 331, no. 19, pp. 1272–1285, 1994.

[3] H. Bocquet, M. Bagot, and J. C. Roujeau, "Drug-induced pseudolymphoma and drug hypersensitivity syndrome (Drug Rash with Eosinophilia and Systemic Symptoms: DRESS)," *Seminars in Cutaneous Medicine and Surgery*, vol. 15, no. 4, pp. 250–257, 1996.

[4] T. D. Jones and J. L. Jacobs, "Treatment of obstinate chorea with nirvanol," *The Journal of the American Medical Association*, vol. 99, pp. 18–21, 1932.

[5] S. Saltzstein and L. Ackerman, "Lymphadenopathy induced by anticonvulsant drugs mimicking clinically and pathologically malignant lymphomas," *Cancer*, vol. 12, pp. 164–182, 1959.

[6] S. H. Kardaun, A. Sidoroff, L. Valeyrie-Allanore et al., "Variability in the clinical pattern of cutaneous side-effects of drugs with systemic symptoms: does a DRESS syndrome really exist?" *British Journal of Dermatology*, vol. 156, no. 3, pp. 609–611, 2007.

[7] F. Fiszenson-Albala, V. Auzerie, E. Mahe et al., "A 6-month prospective survey of cutaneous drug reactions in a hospital setting," *British Journal of Dermatology*, vol. 149, no. 5, pp. 1018–1022, 2003.

[8] N. H. Shear and S. P. Spielberg, "Anticonvulsant hypersensitivity syndrome. *In vitro* assessment of risk," *Journal of Clinical Investigation*, vol. 82, no. 6, pp. 1826–1832, 1988.

[9] V. Descamps, A. Valance, C. Edlinger et al., "Association of human herpesvirus 6 infection with drug reaction with eosinophilia and systemic symptoms," *Archives of Dermatology*, vol. 157, pp. 934–940, 2007.

[10] K. S. Fields, M. J. Petersen, E. Chiao, and P. Tristani-Firouzi, "Case reports: treatment of nevirapine-associated dress syndrome with intravenous immune globulin (IVIG)," *Journal of Drugs in Dermatology*, vol. 4, no. 4, pp. 510–513, 2005.

[11] P. Cacoub, P. Musette, V. Descamps et al., "The DRESS syndrome: a literature review," *The American Journal of Medicine*, vol. 124, no. 7, pp. 588–597, 2011.

[12] Y. C. Chen, C. Y. Chang, Y. T. Cho et al., "Long-term sequelae of drug reaction with eosinophilia and systemic symptoms: a retrospective cohort study from Taiwan," *Journal of the American Academy of Dermatology*, vol. 68, pp. 459–465, 2013.

47

Pulmonary Tuberculosis and Lepromatous Leprosy Coinfection

F. A. Sendrasoa, I. M. Ranaivo, O. Raharolahy, M. Andrianarison, L. S. Ramarozatovo, and F. Rapelanoro Rabenja

Department of Dermatology, Joseph Raseta Befelatanana Hospital, 101 Antananarivo, Madagascar

Correspondence should be addressed to F. A. Sendrasoa; nasendrefa@yahoo.fr

Academic Editor: Bhushan Kumar

Simultaneous occurrence of leprosy and pulmonary tuberculosis is reported infrequently in the modern era. We report a case of pulmonary tuberculosis diagnosed in patient being treated with glucocorticoids for complications of leprosy (type II reaction). Physicians should recognize that the leprosy patients treated with glucocorticoid may develop tuberculosis.

1. Introduction

Leprosy and tuberculosis are two pathogens, which have been identified as infecting humans 9 000 and 4 000 years ago, respectively. They remain endemic in Madagascar, and the annual new case detection rates of leprosy and tuberculosis were 8 per 100 000 and 233 per 100 000, respectively. So, 2–6 cases of concomitant infection per 100 000 populations should be detected, in one year. However, no report of concomitant infection was identified in Madagascar. We aim to report a case of 49-year-old man who presented with pulmonary tuberculosis and lepromatous leprosy coinfection.

2. Case Presentation

A 49-year-old man, nonsmoker, was admitted to dermatology department and followed up for diffuse lepromatous leprosy. He was vaccinated with BCG and he had no past history of tuberculosis. Diagnosis of leprosy was documented based on histological and bacteriologic evidence: a slit skin smear from the ear lobe was positive for lepra bacilli (BI3+), histopathology from the lesion on the face showed granulomas consisting of epithelioid histiocytes and lymphocytes with central caseous surrounding vessels and nerves, and PCR of biopsy specimens were positive for *Mycobacterium leprae*. After successful treatment using dapsone (100 mg/day),

rifampicin (600 mg/month), and clofazimine (300 mg/month and 50 mg/day) during twelve months, hypopigmented skin lesions on the trunk and congestive rhinitis disappeared and the slit skin smear was negative. One month after the end of the treatment, he presented with diffuse papulonodular lesions on the face and trunk, fever, and alteration of general status. On the basis of his symptoms, diagnosis of leprosy reaction (type II) was made and the patient was treated using prednisone at a dose of 40 mg/kg/day. Outcome was unfavorable after two months of corticotherapy, and we had to wait for two supplementary months before we could get clofazimine to add corticoid. After 1 month of this treatment, he presented with fever, weight loss, and asthenia. Clinical examination revealed fever of 39°C, nodular lesions over face, trunk, forearms, and dorsum of hands (Figures 1(a), 1(b), and 1(c)). He presented no neurologic impairment. Biological examination showed inflammatory syndrome: CRP 393 mg/L, total leukocyte count $16,2 \times 10^9$/L, neutrophilia $15,3 \times 10^9$/L, and lymphopenia $0,48 \times 10^9$/L. Serum creatinine and alanine aminotransferase were normal. HIV status was negative. Two out of three sputum samples were positive for acid fast bacilli. Chest tomography showed alveolar-interstitial opacities at the left lower lobe (Figure 2). Bronchoscopy detected thickening of lower lobar bronchi, without malignancy in histopathology of biopsy specimens. The patient was treated by antitubercular treatment. One month

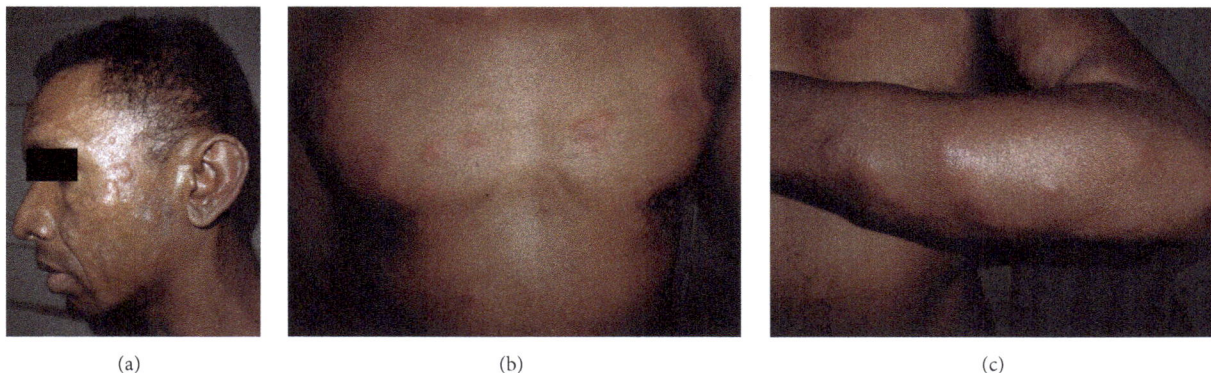

(a)   (b)   (c)

FIGURE 1: (a, b) Nodular lesions over face and trunk. (c) Nodular lesions over forearm.

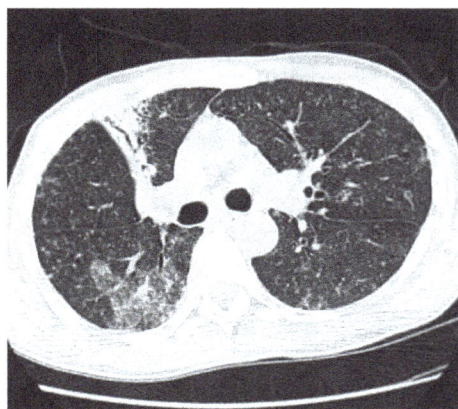

FIGURE 2: Alveolar-interstitial opacities at the left lower lobe.

after the onset of this treatment, there were only two nodular lesions on the trunk, fever disappeared, and general status improved.

3. Discussion

Concomitant pulmonary tuberculosis and leprosy case is uncommon, even in countries like Madagascar where both mycobacterial infections are endemic. On review of data from three leprosy referral centres in Hyderabad, India, from 2000 to 2013, three cases of this coinfection were identified [1]. To our knowledge, there have been no reported cases of concomitant pulmonary tuberculosis and leprosy in Madagascar.

Kumar et al. studied 117 patients of leprosy for evidence of concomitant tuberculosis. Nine patients (7,7%) showed evidence of active tuberculosis, bacteriologically and radiologically. Tuberculosis was found to occur throughout leprosy spectrum [2]. The interaction between leprosy and tuberculosis and their repercussions on the incidence of each other still remain a matter of debate [3].

The diagnosis of pulmonary tuberculosis was clinicoradiological and bacteriological in our patient. Mantoux test was not available because only one center had Mantoux test in Madagascar and it is very expensive.

The gap duration between the development of leprosy and tuberculosis ranged from 2 months to 10–15 years, and the study with largest data showed gap duration of about 10–15 years, where duration of tuberculosis in most of the cases was within six months (while in present case it was 17 months). Only two cases of tuberculosis were found to occur earlier than leprosy [4], as one study concluded that tuberculosis can occur during full spectrum of leprosy.

In case of leprosy, corticosteroids are used primarily in the treatment of type I and type II reactions and silent neuropathy. Rawson et al. reported development of pulmonary tuberculosis after corticosteroid intake in two cases of leprosy [1]. Prasad et al. reported also concomitant pulmonary tuberculosis and borderline leprosy with type II lepra reaction in a single patient who received corticosteroid for more than 3 months [5]. However, major trials of steroid treatment in multidrug therapy for leprosy, such as the TRIPOD studies, have failed to identify development of tuberculosis in some 300 patients who were followed up for over 24 months [6, 7]. This result may be correlated with low doses of prednisolone (around 20 mg/day). Dosing used in our case can be greater than this even if the duration of treatment was not long. Literature defined that steroid was for a minimum of 16 weeks to treat leprosy reactions.

Table 1 shows some cases of concomitant tuberculosis and leprosy reported in the literature.

4. Conclusion

Our patient's case illustrates an uncommon occurrence of concomitant pulmonary tuberculosis and leprosy, presumably the first reported case in Madagascar, and shows the increased risk of pulmonary tuberculosis in patients with leprosy treated with glucocorticoids. Therefore, it becomes imperative for physicians treating leprosy complications with

TABLE 1: Comparative analysis of some cases of leprosy-tuberculosis coinfection reported by various authors for last ten years.

	Sreeramareddy et al. [8]		Prasad et al. [5]	Trindade et al. [9]		Present author
Number of cases	2		1	2		1
	Case I	Case II	1	Case I	Case II	1
Age	65	50	34	31	46	49
Gap duration between leprosy and tuberculosis	3 M	2 Y	11 M	6 M	1 M	17 M
Types of leprosy	BL	LL	BL	BB-BT	BT-BB	LL
First infection	Leprosy	Leprosy	Leprosy	Tuberculosis	Leprosy	Leprosy
Past history of tuberculosis	No	NA	NA	NA	NA	No
Risk factors	Corticosteroids	Corticosteroids	Corticosteroids	NA	Corticosteroids	Corticosteroids
Types of tuberculosis	Pulmonary	Pulmonary	Pulmonary	Pleural TB	Pulmonary	Pulmonary
Chest radiographs // chest tomography	Pleural effusion + bilateral infiltrates	Cavitary lesion + bilateral infiltrates	Cavitation + fibroconsolidation	Pleural effusion	Parenchymal opacification	Alveolar-interstitial syndrome
Sputum	Positive	Positive	Positive	NA	Positive	Positive
Diagnosis of leprosy	NA	NA	Slit skin smear	Histopathology + Fite-Faraco	Histopathology	Histopathology
Lepra reaction	No	Type II	Type II	Type I	Type I	Type II

M: month; Y: year; NA: data not available; lepra reaction type I (reversal); lepra reaction type II (ENL).

steroids to have a high degree of suspicion to diagnose pulmonary tuberculosis.

Conflict of Interests

The authors declare that there is no conflict of interests regarding the publication of this paper.

References

[1] T. M. Rawson, V. Anjum, J. Hodgson et al., "Leprosy and tuberculosis concomitant infection: a poorly understood, age-old relationship," *Leprosy Review*, vol. 85, no. 4, pp. 288–295, 2014.

[2] B. Kumar, S. Kaur, S. Kataria, and S. N. Roy, "Concomitant occurrence of leprosy and tuberculosis—a clinical bacteriological and radiological evaluation," *Leprosy in India*, vol. 54, no. 4, pp. 671–676, 1982.

[3] G. R. Rao, S. Sandhya, M. Sridevi, A. Amareswar, B. L. Narayana, and Shantisri, "Lupus vulgaris and borderline tuberculoid leprosy: an interesting co-occurrence," *Indian Journal of Dermatology, Venereology and Leprology*, vol. 77, no. 1, p. 111, 2011.

[4] D. K. Agarwal, A. R. Mehta, A. P. Sharma et al., "Coinfection with leprosy and tuberculosis in a renal transplant recipient," *Nephrology Dialysis Transplantation*, vol. 15, no. 10, pp. 1720–1721, 2000.

[5] R. Prasad, S. K. Verma, R. Singh, and G. Hosmane, "Concomittant pulmonary tuberculosis and borderline leprosy with type-II lepra reaction in single patient," *Lung India*, vol. 27, no. 1, pp. 19–23, 2010.

[6] W. C. S. Smith, A. M. Anderson, S. G. Withington et al., "Steroid prophylaxis for prevention of nerve function impairment in leprosy: randomised placebo controlled trial (TRIPOD 1)," *British Medical Journal*, vol. 328, no. 7454, pp. 1459–1462, 2004.

[7] J. H. Richardus, S. G. Withington, A. M. Anderson et al., "Treatment with corticosteroids of long-standing nerve function impairment in leprosy: a randomized controlled trial (TRIPOD 3)," *Leprosy Review*, vol. 74, no. 4, pp. 311–318, 2003.

[8] C. T. Sreeramareddy, R. G. Menezes, and P. V. Kishore, "Concomitant age old infections of mankind-tuberculosis and leprosy: a case report," *Journal of Medical Case Reports*, vol. 5, no. 1, p. 43, 2007.

[9] M. Â. B. Trindade, D. Miyamoto, G. Benard, N. Y. Sakai-Valente, D. D. M. Vasconcelos, and B. Naafs, "Leprosy and tuberculosis co-infection: clinical and immunological report of two cases and review of the literature," *American Journal of Tropical Medicine and Hygiene*, vol. 88, no. 2, pp. 236–240, 2013.

48

Subcutaneous Emphysema Induced by Cryotherapy: A Complication due to Previous Punctures

Jared Martínez-Coronado, Bertha Torres-Álvarez, and Juan Pablo Castanedo-Cázares

Department of Dermatology, Hospital Central "Dr. Ignacio Morones Prieto", Universidad Autonoma de San Luis Potosí, 2395 Venustiano Carranza Avenue, 78210 San Luis Potosí, SLP, Mexico

Correspondence should be addressed to Juan Pablo Castanedo-Cázares; castanju@yahoo.com

Academic Editor: Mario Vaccaro

Cryosurgery is a common therapeutic modality used in dermatology; therefore we must be aware of its possible adverse effects. We report a case of a patient with subcutaneous emphysema which occurred following the application of cryotherapy after multiple punctures of local anesthetic and intralesional steroids in a chest keloid scar. Despite the fact that this condition was gradually resolved after expectant observation, we warn about this complication when sprayed cryotherapy is preceded by multiple punctures on cutaneous lesions above bony surfaces. In similar settings, cryotherapy must be first administered or a cotton-tip applicator should be used.

1. Introduction

Modern cutaneous cryosurgery was introduced in the 1960s [1], since then it is commonly used by most dermatologists around the world. It is recognized that this treatment was first applied in 1974 for keloidal scars by Pirece [2]. Cryotherapy induces vascular damage that leads to anoxia and tissue necrosis reducing the keloidal scar thickness [2, 3]. Thus, it is not an innocuous treatment and dermatologist must be aware of its side effects which can be immediate or delayed. Frequent short-term adverse features include pain, syncope, hemorrhage, edema, blistering, fever, infection, and pyogenic granuloma [1, 3]; long-term changes consist in permanent hypo- or hyperpigmentation, pseudoepitheliomatous hyperplasia, milia, nerve damage, alopecia, scar formation, and cartilage necrosis [1, 3]. We report a patient with keloid scar who presented subcutaneous emphysema after cryotherapy application, an uncommon complication finding in dermatologic literature [4–7].

2. Case Report

A 28-year-old woman presented with an 18-month history of 2 × 10 cm keloid scaring induced by acne vulgaris on the upper frontal thorax. Her lesion was first locally anesthetized with intralesional lidocaine and afterwards infiltrated with acetonide of triamcinolone, followed by two 40-second cycles of sprayed cryotherapy. The patient came back to our facilities 30 minutes after the procedure because the upper area of the treated zone started to bulk. Physical examination only revealed swelling and cutaneous crepitus on palpation. There was no erythema or pain, nor local increased temperature. Vital signs were normal and there were no systemic symptoms other than minor anxiety triggered by this outcome. We made clinical diagnosis of subcutaneous emphysema as a complication of cryotherapy due to the timeline of the clinical history: punctures followed by sprayed cryotherapy and then a prompt presence of local subcutaneous emphysema. The patient was retained in our facilities and after one hour of observation the skin became normal in appearance. However, subcutaneous crepitation continued upon complete resolution after three days. Clinical changes are shown in Figure 1.

3. Discussion

Subcutaneous emphysema (SE) is defined by the presence of air or other gases within the soft tissue compartment

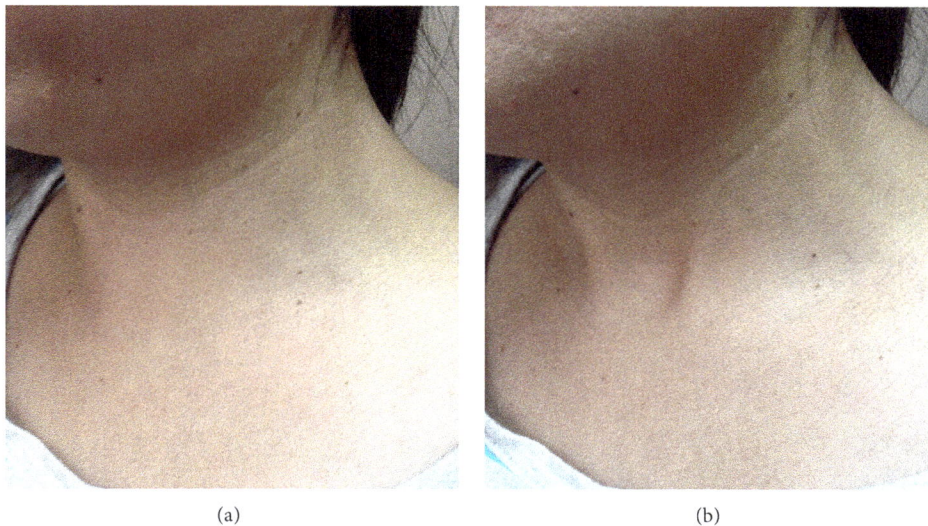

(a)   (b)

FIGURE 1: At (a) local subcutaneous augmented volume in the upper frontal chest and lower neck. (b) Normalization of the swelled area after one hour of conservative treatment.

[4, 5, 8]; it can be further divided as a result of infectious or noninfectious causes [5, 6]. There are several dermatologic conditions clustered within the second group such as irrigation of wounds with hydrogen peroxide, punch biopsy, or cryosurgery [6, 8]. During sprayed cryotherapy an opening on the skin surface acts as a one-way valve through which the positive pressure gas enters and spreads along the subcutaneous compartment [1, 4, 6]. Risk factors for SE secondary to cryotherapy are usually related to elderly patients. In these cases, atrophic skin is easier to be disrupted while applying positive pressure of a handheld spray device [5, 9]. This technique of cryotherapy on ulcerated skin after curettage procedures or freshly closed wounds has also been associated to this complication [4, 9]. Although this unfavorable event depends on the site where cryotherapy is applied, it is most likely to occur in areas of lax and thin skin, such as the periorbital area or on the dorsum of hands [1].

In our young patient, the SE was caused by the entrance of the sprayed liquid nitrogen through the disrupted skin, following the approximately 8 consecutive 27-gauge needle punctures performed on the treated area. The association between cryotherapy and subcutaneous emphysema in a previous punctured keloid scar has not been reported before. She presented sudden swelling of tissue around the treated site and cutaneous crepitus on palpation; those clinical characteristics are the main and almost pathognomonic of air accumulation in skin and subcutaneous tissue [1, 6–8]. This setting was similar to the classical SE clinical evolution secondary to cryotherapy, where clinical manifestations are evident within the first 24 hours [1, 9]. Other signs for this condition are erythema and bubbles mixed with serohematic exudate; those are consequence of the vasodilatation and inflammatory process [6, 7].

The clinical diagnosis in our patient was obvious because of the history of cryotherapy before the onset of symptoms. However, sometimes diagnosis of SE can be challenging because it could have an atypical presentation [4, 6, 7]. X-ray, ultrasonography, computed tomography scan, or magnetic resonance imaging can be used to confirm the diagnosis in patients. In these imaging studies, abnormal gas accumulation in soft tissues is seen [4, 7]. Histopathology of the dermatosis is characterized by the separation of collagen bundles in the dermis without mucin deposits or inflammation in the clear spaces and focal fragmentation of adipocyte cell membranes in the subcutaneous tissue. Nevertheless, skin biopsy is not required for diagnosis [7].

Because of its lethal condition, the most important differential diagnosis is SE caused by gas gangrene [7, 8], which is mainly caused by *Clostridium* species [8, 10]. It can be suspected by history of preceding trauma, extensive destruction of tissue with foul smell, local heat, pain, and systemic signs and symptoms such as fever and malaise [6–8, 10]. This condition shows no spontaneous recovery; thus culture from tissue material and blood must be done to synergize antibiotics and surgical treatment [6, 8, 10]. Other SE causes should also be excluded such as factitious subcutaneous emphysema, dental or endotracheal procedures, respiratory and gastrointestinal tract disease, and loosely sutured wounds [5, 9]. Angioedema and hematoma may look like SE; thus these conditions need to be excluded, too [7].

Our patient recovered spontaneously, so no extra treatment was necessary. This clinical evolution is similar to SE secondary to other dermatologic procedures, where manifestations used to disappear in the next 12 to 96 hours [6, 8, 9]. Sometimes conservative management with rest, support measures, and follow-up visits are the unique necessary treatment [7–9]. However, it has been described that insufflation may be manually forced out from the affected tissue by local and gentle pressure to the edematous area [1, 6]. There is not enough evidence to use low dose steroids and antibiotics [7].

Prognostic is excellent; no further complications of SE secondary to cryotherapy have been reported. It typically has self-limiting evolution, with prompt resolution and without permanent damage or relapses [1, 4, 6]. To prevent SE after cryotherapy we propose to use different cryosurgery techniques when cutaneous barrier is damaged, in atrophic skins and in thin cutaneous areas, especially in case of elderly patients. In those situations cotton swab technique may be preferred instead of spray nozzle.

Through this adverse experience we also confirm the importance of the order of combined therapies for dermatoses such as keloids. In the case of combined use of cryosurgery and other intralesional drugs, cryotherapy must be applied before the preceding interventions; in this way the risk of SE can be avoided.

Conflict of Interests

All authors declare no conflict of interests.

References

[1] G. F. Graham and K. L. Barham, "Cryosurgery," *Current Problems in Dermatology*, vol. 15, no. 6, pp. 223–250, 2003.

[2] J. J. Shaffer, S. C. Taylor, and F. Cook-Bolden, "Keloidal scars: a review with a critical look at therapeutic options," *Journal of the American Academy of Dermatology*, vol. 46, pp. S63–S97, 2002.

[3] S. Ud-Din and A. Bayat, "New insights on keloids, hypertrophic scars, and striae," *Dermatologic Clinics*, vol. 32, no. 2, pp. 193–209, 2014.

[4] P. Jensen, U. B. Johansen, and J. P. Thyssen, "Cryotherapy caused widespread subcutaneous emphysema mimicking angiooedema," *Acta Dermato-Venereologica*, vol. 94, article 241, 2014.

[5] S. Vano-Galvan, L. Bagazgoitia, B. Perez, and P. Jaen, "Subcutaneous emphysema caused by cryotherapy application over a corticosteroid-induced atrophic skin," *Journal of the European Academy of Dermatology and Venereology*, vol. 22, no. 4, pp. 508–509, 2008.

[6] J. Sánchez-Martín, F. Vázquez-López, S. Gómez-Díez, and N. Pérez-Oliva, "Benign subcutaneous emphysema after a skin biopsy," *Dermatologic Surgery*, vol. 34, no. 8, pp. 1141–1142, 2008.

[7] I. Fuertes, A. Guilabert, R. Salvador, and J. M. Mascaró Jr., "Atypical subcutaneous emphysema mimicking cellulitis," *Archives of Dermatology*, vol. 147, no. 2, pp. 253–255, 2011.

[8] A. Singal, P. Yadav, and D. Pandhi, "Benign subcutaneous emphysema following punch skin biopsy," *Journal of Cutaneous and Aesthetic Surgery*, vol. 6, no. 3, pp. 171–172, 2013.

[9] T. J. Lambert, M. J. Wells, and K. W. Wisniewski, "Subcutaneous emphysema resulting from liquid nitrogen spray," *Journal of the American Academy of Dermatology*, vol. 55, no. 5, supplement, pp. S95–S96, 2006.

[10] R. P. Jeavons, D. Dowen, P. R. P. Rushton, S. Chambers, and S. O'Brien, "Management of significant and widespread, acute subcutaneous emphysema: should we manage surgically or conservatively?" *Journal of Emergency Medicine*, vol. 46, no. 1, pp. 21–27, 2014.

49

Idiopathic Thrombocytopenic Purpura Misdiagnosed as Hereditary Angioedema

Michelle Fog Andersen[1] and Anette Bygum[2]

[1]Department of Otorhinolaryngology, Head and Neck Surgery, Køge Hospital, Lykkebaekvej 1, 4600 Køge, Denmark
[2]HAE Centre Denmark, Department of Dermatology and Allergy Centre, Odense University Hospital, Sdr. Boulevard 29, Entrance 142, 5000 Odense C, Denmark

Correspondence should be addressed to Michelle Fog Andersen; michellefog@yahoo.com

Academic Editor: Michihiro Hide

Hereditary angioedema is a rare, but potentially life-threatening genetic disorder that results from an autosomal dominant trait. It is characterized by acute, recurrent attacks of severe local edema, most commonly affecting the skin and mucosa. Swelling in hereditary angioedema patients does however not always have to be caused by angioedema but can relate to other concomitant disorders. In this report we are focusing on misdiagnosis in a patient with known hereditary angioedema, whose bleeding episode caused by idiopathic thrombocytopenic purpura was mistaken for an acute attack of hereditary angioedema. The case illustrates how clinicians can have difficulties in handling patients with rare diseases, especially in the emergency care setting.

1. Introduction

Hereditary angioedema (HAE), originally described by Quincke in 1882 [1], is a rare genetic disorder characterized by recurrent episodes of subcutaneous and submucosal swellings in any part of the skin, including the gastrointestinal tract and upper airway [2, 3]. The disease is caused by mutations in the gene encoding *SERPING1* causing deficiency of complement C1 inhibitor (C1-INH), a protein involved in the regulation of the complement, kinin-kallikrein, coagulation, and fibrinolytic systems [4]. The deficiency results in uncontrolled activation and release of bradykinin, which causes increased vascular permeability and dilatation with a resulting edema at the affected site [5, 6]. HAE is inherited in an autosomal dominant pattern and is estimated to affect 1 in 50,000 individuals, with no clear sex or ethnic variation [7, 8].

There are two classical types of HAE having identical clinical presentations. HAE type I represents 85% of patients with C1-INH deficiency and is characterized by a decreased production of circulating C1-INH. Patients with HAE type II, approximately 15% of cases, have normal concentrations of C1-INH but a dysfunctional protein, meaning a low functional level to be measured [4]. More rarely seen is a third type of HAE, primarily discovered in women, with normal fully functional C1-INH levels presenting with the typical clinical features of C1-INH deficiency. This type has been associated with mutations in F12, the gene encoding the plasma protease factor XII (FXII) [9].

For many health care professionals, HAE present an ongoing challenge due to the rarity and complexity of the clinical presentations, which may involve most organ systems. In this report we are focusing on misdiagnosis in a patient with known HAE who had a swelling caused by bleeding attributed to idiopathic thrombocytopenic purpura (ITP).

2. Case Presentation

A 74-year-old man had recurrent episodic attacks of abdominal pain and swelling involving the upper airways, extremities, and genitals from the age of three, leading to both unnecessary appendectomy and later tracheotomy because of laryngeal edema. However, he was not diagnosed with hereditary angioedema, before the age of 33 years, when he was admitted to the emergency unit with a severe swelling of his face. Biochemical analyses were consistent with HAE

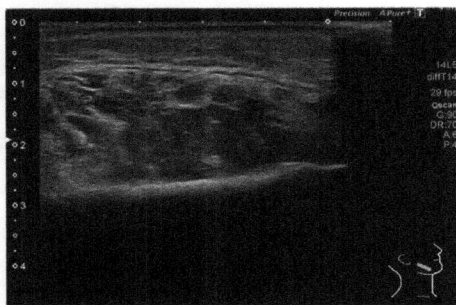

FIGURE 1: Ultrasound scan of the face shows a subcutaneous haematoma around the right masseter muscle measuring 2 cm in depth. No other pathology was found.

type I and later a family investigation disclosed a splice site mutation in the *SERPING1* gene (c. 1250-1G>A), a mutation also found in his son and some of his grandchildren. Since the diagnosis, he has been treated with Danazol and he is currently followed up at the National HAE Centre once yearly. After reducing Danazol to the minimum effective dose (200 mg o.d.), he has an average of three relatively mild attacks per year. The patient is monitored every six months with liver enzymes, lipid profile, complete blood cell count, urinalysis, and liver spleen ultrasound. His breakthrough attacks are treated with injections of C1-INH concentrate (Berinert).

In 2014 the patient presented at the local emergency room (ER) with a severe swelling in the lower part of his face associated with difficulty in swallowing, abdominal pain, and a few red spots on his extremities. He had no stridor or voice changes and there were no signs or symptoms of viral infection before the attack. Apart from the limited purpuric spots, the clinical presentation imitated HAE swelling, which was suggested to be the diagnosis. He was treated with C1-INH concentrate 1000 units intravenously and discharged from the ER. However petechiae evolved over most of his body and suddenly a large haematoma presented spontaneously on his right jaw. He was once again seen at the ER and the clinical examination revealed edema of the right side of his face and lips and inside the mouth and throat. Severe swelling over the right mandibular condyle was found with a palpable, soft, nonfluctuant discolored mass measuring 3 cm in diameter. Multiple small petechiae were detected on the extremities and thorax and in the facial area including mucosal bleeding inside the mouth. Abdominal examination revealed no hepatosplenomegaly or abdominal tenderness and normal bowel sounds were present. Examination of the urine was remarkable for microscopic haematuria. An ultrasound scan was performed showing a subcutaneous haematoma around the right masseter muscle (Figure 1). A computerised tomography (CT) of the neck, thorax, abdomen, and pelvis obtained no pathology besides the haematoma identified on the ultrasound scan. Laboratory tests presented normal white blood cell count and hemoglobin level. His platelet count was significantly low at 3×10^9/L [normal count: $150–450 \times 10^9$/L]. Bone marrow aspiration was performed and revealed trilinear marrow hyperplasia with megakaryopoiesis, compatible

with idiopathic thrombocytopenic purpura (ITP). It came out that the patient was diagnosed with ITP 10 years earlier, but he had forgot about this former diagnosis and seemingly it was not looked up in the ER. He was referred to a medical department and the tentative diagnosis of HAE was ruled out and treatment with prednisolone 50 mg o.d. was initiated. He responded well to therapy and was discharged 9 days later with normal platelet count. The patient tapered prednisolone over 4 months and today, 1.5 years after the incidence, he has normal blood counts and is not specifically treated for ITP. He still receives Danazol 200 mg o.d. for HAE, which in fact may stabilize his ITP as well.

3. Discussion

In most cases, the attacks of HAE follow a predictable course. Many episodes are preceded by prodromal symptoms including a tingling or burning sensation in the affected area. In two-thirds of the patients, a nonpruritic serpiginous erythematous rash on the trunk, arms, or legs referred to as erythema marginatum may appear as part of the prodrome [10, 11]. Our patient did not experience any kind of prodromal symptoms other than a general discomfort. Swelling attacks in HAE manifest as recurrent local nonpitting, nonpruritic subcutaneous or submucosal edema [2, 12, 13]. Classically, the swelling develops gradually over a period of 12–24 hours and then slowly subsides within 72 hours. Severe attacks may last up to 5 days.

Any individual part of the integument can be affected but is most common in the extremities, abdomen, genitourinary system, and upper respiratory tract. Approximately 50% of the attacks involve the abdomen with severe abdominal pain, nausea, vomiting, and diarrhea as dominant symptoms [2]. Our patient complained about severe abdominal pain, but there was no pathology in routine laboratory test or at the abdominal CT. Episodes of swelling may also involve the upper respiratory tract, including the tongue, pharynx, and larynx. Our patient's main complaint was however swelling in the lower part of his face associated with difficulty in swallowing and development of a large haematoma of the jaw associated with multiple small petechiae on the extremities. These manifestations are not consistent with HAE and should lead the clinician to consider other differential diagnoses than angioedema swelling.

There are numerous inciting factors known to the attacks of HAE. Episodes may be triggered by minor trauma, surgery, dental treatment, psychological stress, or the use of certain medications. In many cases however, the attacks occur without any identifiable trigger [7]. *Helicobacter pylori* infection is also considered among the causative factors [14].

The role of *Helicobacter pylori* is strongly proven and an association between chronic *Helicobacter pylori* infection and the occurrence of ITP has been found [15, 16]. Whether this Gram-negative bacterium plays a pathophysiological link with a key role in the pathogenesis could be speculated. We would recommend our patient to be tested in nearest future.

The classical complement pathway is an important driver in the pathogenesis of HAE. Increasing evidence suggests a contribution of complement activation in ITP [17, 18], the additional diagnosis for our patient. It could be considered that the disturbance of the coagulation system might increase the consumption of C1 and C1-INH and hereby act as a contributing cause in the development of HAE attacks. A correlation between ITP and angioedema has however not yet been described in the literature.

As illustrated in the disease history of our patient, onset of symptoms in HAE typically occurs in childhood and accelerates during adolescence. Despite the early onset in life, some patients are not diagnosed until adulthood, as there often is a significant diagnostic delay [3, 19].

The diagnosis of HAE should be suspected based on a history of recurrent attacks of angioedema or abdominal pain without associated urticaria [20]. Often the patient reports a family history of the condition but as 25% of the cases are caused by spontaneous mutations, having no family history does not rule out the diagnosis [13]. Laboratory testing is essential and required to confirm the diagnosis [4, 13]. It is not necessary to make an extensive paraclinical investigation every time the HAE patient is hospitalized, as most patients are self-administrating their attacks at home without any laboratory tests. Nevertheless, it is important to remain critical when something in the clinical demonstration does not agree with the overall picture. The diagnosis of ITP had already been demonstrated in the patient a decade earlier but it was not before the laboratory test had been performed that the diagnosis was reconsidered.

The therapeutic treatment of HAE can be divided into two regimens: the management of acute attacks and long-term prophylaxis [20, 21]. The treatment of choice in an acute attack consists of replacement with C1-INH concentrate (plasma-derived: Berinert, Cinryze or recombinant: Ruconest) and bradykinin B2 receptor antagonist (Firazyr) or, if those are unavailable, fresh-frozen plasma (contains C1-INH) [20–22]. Future attacks can be prevented by the use of attenuated androgens and the drug most frequently used is Danazol [21]. Although long-term prophylaxis with attenuated androgen is effective, it must be regarded critically due to a severe profile of side effects. Therapy with Danazol can be hepatotoxic and affect serum lipid levels. Hypertension, weight gain, acne, virilization, menstrual irregularities, and depression are also common [20, 21, 23]. More rare side effects as haematuria have been demonstrated [24]. Therefore, the microscopic haematuria found in this patient could be a result of the treatment although his low platelet count is more likely the cause. Due to the adverse event profile, all patients treated with Danazol must be monitored every six months with blood tests, urinalysis, and liver spleen ultrasound [23] as performed in our patient. Danazol is not only effective as long-term prophylaxis in HAE but also a good alternative therapeutic approach as treatment in ITP [25, 26]. This may explain why the patient did not have any symptoms of ITP for a long period of time as it turns out that he was possibly treated for both diseases. The side effects of Danazol are known to be dose dependent and therefore the dose had cautiously been reduced a few years earlier to achieve the lowest recommended effective dose at 200 mg daily [21].

When we tried a further dose reduction, he experienced the reported incident and had a relapse of ITP.

The diagnosis of HAE is often overlooked, as many of its symptoms mimic those of several other common conditions which is demonstrating diffuse swelling and abdominal discomfort [27, 28]. However, the clinical challenge is also seen the other way around. Swellings in HAE patients do not always have to be caused by angioedema but can relate to other concomitant disorders as demonstrated in this case. In fact, it is commonly seen that less experienced clinicians can have difficulties in looking beyond a rare initial diagnosis as they are concentrating too much on making the symptoms fit the original diagnosis. A thoroughly clinical examination in HAE patients is therefore essential like in other patients, giving the physicians the opportunity of looking outside the box and avoiding mental shortcuts [29]. If the clinical picture does not fit, it is most likely not the right diagnosis.

Conflict of Interests

The authors declare that there is no conflict of interests regarding the publication of this paper.

Acknowledgment

The authors thank Aalborg University Hospital for allowing the use of the ultrasound images.

References

[1] H. I. Quincke, "Über akutes umschriebenes hautödem," *Monatschrift Praktische Dermatologie*, vol. 1, no. 1, pp. 129–131, 1882.

[2] K. Bork, G. Meng, P. Staubach, and J. Hardt, "Hereditary angioedema: new findings concerning symptoms, affected organs, and course," *The American Journal of Medicine*, vol. 119, no. 3, pp. 267–274, 2006.

[3] A. Bygum, "Hereditary angio-oedema in Denmark: a nationwide survey," *British Journal of Dermatology*, vol. 161, no. 5, pp. 1153–1158, 2009.

[4] A. Agostoni, E. Aygören-Pürsün, K. E. Binkley et al., "Hereditary and acquired angioedema: problems and progress: proceedings of the third C1 esterase inhibitor deficiency workshop and beyond," *The Journal of Allergy and Clinical Immunology*, vol. 114, no. 3, pp. S51–S131, 2004.

[5] A. E. Davis, "New treatments addressing the pathophysiology of hereditary angioedema," *Clinical and Molecular Allergy*, vol. 6, no. 2, 2008.

[6] A. E. Davis, "The pathogenesis of hereditary angioedema," *Transfusion and Apheresis Science*, vol. 29, no. 3, pp. 195–203, 2003.

[7] U. C. Nzeako, E. Frigas, and W. J. Tremaine, "Hereditary angioedema: a broad review for clinicians," *Archives of Internal Medicine*, vol. 161, no. 20, pp. 2417–2429, 2001.

[8] A. Zanichelli, F. Arcoleo, M. P. Barca et al., "A nationwide survey of hereditary angioedema due to C1 inhibitor deficiency in Italy," *Orphanet Journal of Rare Diseases*, vol. 10, article 11, 2015.

[9] J. Björkqvist, S. de Maat, U. Lewandrowski et al., "Defective glycosylation of coagulation factor XII underlies hereditary angioedema type III," *The Journal of Clinical Investigation*, vol. 125, no. 8, pp. 3132–3146, 2015.

[10] M. Magerl, G. Doumoulakis, I. Kalkounou et al., "Characterization of prodromal symptoms in a large population of patients with hereditary angio-oedema," *Clinical and Experimental Dermatology*, vol. 39, no. 3, pp. 298–303, 2014.

[11] A. Reshef, M. J. Prematta, and T. J. Craig, "Signs and symptoms preceding acute attacks of hereditary angioedema: results of three recent surveys," *Allergy and Asthma Proceedings*, vol. 34, no. 3, pp. 261–266, 2013.

[12] B. L. Zuraw, "Hereditary angioedema," *The New England Journal of Medicine*, vol. 359, no. 10, pp. 1027–1036, 2008.

[13] T. Bowen, M. Cicardi, H. Farkas et al., "2010 International consensus algorithm for the diagnosis, therapy and management of hereditary angioedema," *Allergy, Asthma & Clinical Immunology*, vol. 6, no. 1, article 24, 2010.

[14] B. Visy, G. Füst, A. Bygum et al., "Helicobacter pylori infection as a triggering factor of attacks in patients with hereditary angioedema," *Helicobacter*, vol. 12, no. 3, pp. 251–257, 2007.

[15] M. Franchini and D. Veneri, "Helicobacter pylori-associated immune thrombocytopenia," *Platelets*, vol. 17, no. 2, pp. 71–77, 2006.

[16] K. Hagymási and Z. Tulassay, "Helicobacter pylori infection: new pathogenetic and clinical aspects," *World Journal of Gastroenterology*, vol. 20, no. 21, pp. 6386–6399, 2014.

[17] E. I. B. Peerschke, B. Andemariam, W. Yin, and J. B. Bussel, "Complement activation on platelets correlates with a decrease in circulating immature platelets in patients with immune thrombocytopenic purpura," *British Journal of Haematology*, vol. 148, no. 4, pp. 638–645, 2010.

[18] E. I. Peerschke, S. Panicker, and J. Bussel, "Classical complement pathway activation in immune thrombocytopenia purpura: inhibition by a novel C1s inhibitor," *British Journal of Haematology*, 2015.

[19] A. Agostoni and M. Cicardi, "Hereditary and acquired C1-inhibitor deficiency: biological and clinical characteristics in 235 patients," *Medicine*, vol. 71, no. 4, pp. 206–215, 1992.

[20] T. Craig, E. A. Pürsün, K. Bork et al., "WAO guideline for the management of hereditary angioedema," *World Allergy Organization Journal*, vol. 5, no. 12, pp. 182–199, 2012.

[21] M. Cicardi, K. Bork, T. Caballero et al., "Evidence-based recommendations for the therapeutic management of angioedema owing to hereditary C1 inhibitor deficiency: consensus report of an International Working Group," *Allergy*, vol. 67, no. 2, pp. 147–157, 2012.

[22] H. J. Longhurst, H. Farkas, T. Craig et al., "HAE international home therapy consensus document," *Allergy, Asthma & Clinical Immunology*, vol. 6, no. 1, article 22, 2010.

[23] K. Bork, A. Bygum, and J. Hardt, "Benefits and risks of danazol in hereditary angioedema: a long-term survey of 118 patients," *Annals of Allergy, Asthma & Immunology*, vol. 100, no. 2, pp. 153–161, 2008.

[24] S. W. Hosea, M. L. Santaella, E. J. Brown, M. Berger, K. Katusha, and M. M. Frank, "Long-term therapy of hereditary angioedema with Danazol," *Annals of Internal Medicine*, vol. 93, no. 6, pp. 809–812, 1980.

[25] F. Maloisel, E. Andrès, J. Zimmer et al., "Danazol therapy in patients with chronic idiopathic thrombocytopenic purpura: long-term results," *The American Journal of Medicine*, vol. 116, no. 9, pp. 590–594, 2004.

[26] Y. S. Ahn, W. J. Harrington, S. R. Simon, R. Mylvaganam, L. M. Pall, and A. G. So, "Danazol for the treatment of idiopathic thrombocytopenic purpura," *The New England Journal of Medicine*, vol. 308, no. 23, pp. 1396–1399, 1983.

[27] M. M. Gompels, R. J. Lock, M. Abinun et al., "C1 inhibitor deficiency: consensus document," *Clinical and Experimental Immunology*, vol. 139, no. 3, pp. 379–394, 2005.

[28] U. C. Nzeako and H. J. Longhurst, "Many faces of angioedema: focus on the diagnosis and management of abdominal manifestations of hereditary angioedema," *European Journal of Gastroenterology & Hepatology*, vol. 24, no. 4, pp. 353–361, 2012.

[29] G. R. Norman and K. W. Eva, "Diagnostic error and clinical reasoning," *Medical Education*, vol. 44, no. 1, pp. 94–100, 2010.

Diffuse Cutaneous Mucinosis in Dermatomyositis: A Case Report and Review of the Literature

Alexandra Caitlin Perel-Winkler[1] and Chris T. Derk[2]

[1] *St. Luke's-Roosevelt Hospital Center, New York, NY 10025, USA*
[2] *Division of Rheumatology, University of Pennsylvania, One Convention Boulevard, 8th Floor Penn Tower, Philadelphia, PA 19104, USA*

Correspondence should be addressed to Chris T. Derk; chris.derk@uphs.upenn.edu

Academic Editor: Ravi Krishnan

We present the case of a patient with dermatomyositis and diffuse cutaneous mucinosis and give an up-to-date detailed review of all the published cases in the English literature describing the demographics, clinical picture, pathology management, and outcomes of this unique group of patients.

1. Introduction

Mucin (hyaluronic acid complex) is a protein normally found as part of the dermal connective tissues and it is produced by mast cells and fibroblasts. As hyaluronic acid holds water, in disease states where mucin production is increased, the dermal connective tissue becomes swollen and is described as myxedematous. It is not uncommon to have findings of microscopic cutaneous mucinosis in the setting of collagen vascular diseases and mucin deposition in the correct clinical setting can be considered as histologic evidence of dermatomyositis (DM) [1]. Clinically evident forms of mucinosis have been described in hypothyroidism, thyrotoxicosis, scleromyxedema associated with monoclonal gammopathies, scleredema related to diabetes, and lichen myxedematosus. Cases of secondary cutaneous mucinosis have been described in systemic lupus erythematosus, systemic sclerosis, and dermatomyositis, albeit infrequently [2–8]. We present a case of dermatomyositis with evidence of diffuse cutaneous mucinosis in a patient recently treated for nonsmall cell lung cancer (NSCLC) without evidence of recurrence.

2. Case

A 57-year-old man with chronic obstructive lung disease, hypothyroidism, gastroesophageal reflux disease, and a prior history of NSCLC developed a pruritic, confluent, violaceous rash after cancer treatment. The patient was diagnosed with NSCLC in 2011 and was treated with paclitaxel and carboplatin and adjunctive radiation, with a restaging PET/CT scan showing excellent response. Four months after the completion of chemotherapy and radiation therapy the patient presented complaining of a pruritic rash. The rash first appeared on his hands and was noted to be consistent with Gottron's papules. Over the next nine months the rash worsened, and the patient developed violaceous erythema on his upper chest and back. Erythematous patches with white macules then developed on his lower legs, thighs, and buttocks. Three years after the treatment of his cancer, the patient had a diffuse, scaly, and erythematous rash on his arms (Figure 1), legs, buttocks, abdomen, neck, and face (Figure 2) with evidence of white macules (Figure 3) most prominent on the upper and lower extremities. Initial concern was for recurrence of his cancer; however, full body PET-CT revealed no new or active cancer. Skin biopsies showed evidence of interface dermatitis with sections of hyperkeratosis, mild spongiosis, interface vacuolar change, and dermal mucinosis without involvement of the panniculus or fascia (Figures 4 and 5). Muscle enzyme tests showed a normal creatinine phosphokinase level but an elevated aldolase at 9.5 U/L. A later full thickness biopsy performed showed evidence of interface dermatitis with mucin deposition. Two muscle biopsies were

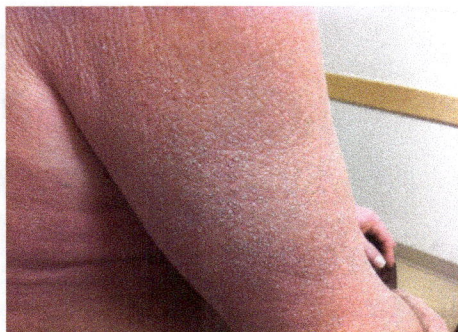

FIGURE 1: Cutaneous mucinosis: violaceous, scaly, and erythematous rash of the right arm.

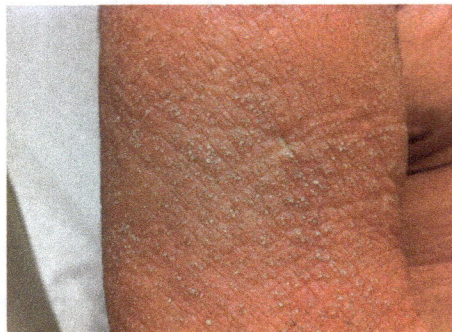

FIGURE 2: Cutaneous mucinosis: diffuse erythematous, violaceous rash of the face.

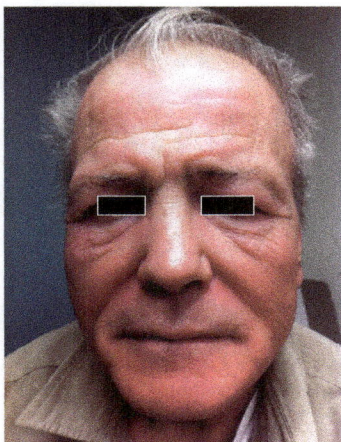

FIGURE 3: Cutaneous mucinosis: diffuse, scaly, and erythematous rash with white macules.

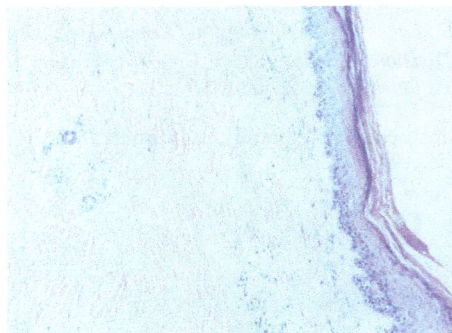

FIGURE 4: Skin biopsy: colloidal iron with hyaluronidase ×100. Dermal mucin deposition without fibroblast proliferation, with interface vacuolar changes.

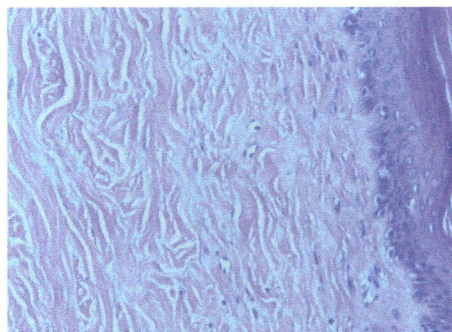

FIGURE 5: Skin biopsy: colloidal iron ×200: dermal mucin depositions without fibroblast proliferation.

performed and HLA1 staining showed diffuse labeling of the sampled myofibers. Only one necrotic myofiber was isolated; otherwise the specimens were largely normal without diffuse myofiber necrosis, inflammation, or definite vacuolation. An MRI of the patient's femurs showed hyperenhancement in the obturator internus and externus muscles bilaterally and the proximal hamstrings (right greater than left), indicating some degree of inflammation. Immunoserologic results included a positive ANA of 1 : 640 with a speckled pattern and a positive Smith antibody (Ab). Of the myositis autoantibody panel, anti-Ku and anti-U1RNP were found to be positive. Other labs included a normal TSH and a slightly elevated gamma-globulin fraction of 1.7 g/dL (reference range 0.7–1.2 g/dL) with a normal immunofixation.

Dermatomyositis with cutaneous mucinosis was diagnosed in light of the physical exam findings, MRI evidence of inflammation, evidence of interface dermatitis, and mucin deposition on the skin biopsies and positive serologies. The demonstration of mucinosis without fibroblastic proliferation or dermal thickening supported a diagnosis of cutaneous mucinosis as opposed to scleromyxedema or systemic sclerosis.

Prior to presentation at our clinic, 3 years after the initial symptoms began, the patient had tried multiple medical treatments. He was initially treated with 5 mg of oral prednisone, which was quickly increased to 20 mg without success. Methotrexate was initiated at 7.5 mg weekly and then titrated to 15 mg weekly without response. Plaquenil 200 mg was tried for 2 months but the patient discontinued the treatment as he felt it had no effect. Once we diagnosed the patient with dermatomyositis and diffuse cutaneous mucinosis, we initiated 60 mg of prednisone per day which was tapered to 40 mg daily two weeks later due to side effects.

Intravenous Immunoglobulin was initiated at 20 grams for 3 consecutive days every 6 weeks. At 3-month follow-up, the patient reported significant improvement in the amount of erythema and induration especially in the upper extremities and a decrease in the white macular lesions.

3. Discussion

3.1. Dermatomyositis and Cutaneous Mucinosis. Dermatomyositis is an inflammatory myopathy, which affects striated muscle and has cutaneous features. Typically a heliotropic rash, Gottron's papules, shawl sign, and erythematous plaques are some of the dermatologic manifestations; however, atypical cutaneous features, including plaque like mucinosis, have also been described [1]. The pathophysiology of dermatomyositis includes the expression of autoantibodies which target protein synthesis or translational particles in the muscle cell which triggers a humoral immune response. Activation of proinflammatory cytokines and chemokines leads to the migration of lymphoid cells to the perimysial and endomysial spaces; complement activation leads to the formation and deposition of membranolytic attack complexes onto endomysial capillaries. The result is microangiopathy and necrosis of endothelial cells leading to perivascular inflammation, muscle ischemia, and muscle fiber destruction [8, 13].

Mucin is a mucopolysaccharide produced by fibroblasts and consists of hyaluronic acid and sulfated glycosaminoglycans. Cutaneous mucinosis is subdivided into primary and secondary types; in primary, mucin deposition is the primary histologic feature and secondary, where mucin deposition is an additional finding to a primary clinicopathologic setting. Cutaneous manifestations of mucin can be focal or diffuse and are described as dermal or epidermal (follicular) [9, 14]. The pathophysiology of increased mucin deposition in connective tissue diseases is not completely understood and it is a rare finding. It is postulated that substances circulating in the serum, such as immunoglobulins, autoantibodies, or cytokines, stimulate glycosaminoglycan synthesis by fibroblasts leading to the production of mucin and its deposition in the skin [8, 12]. Pandya et al. linked the increased level of serum autoantibody titres with an increase in mucin lesions in patients with SLE [11, 15]. Interleukin-1 and interleukin-6 have also been shown to be elevated in patients with increased dermal mucin production in SLE and DM; however this is nonspecific as interleukins may be raised without evidence of mucinosis [2].

The concept of a hypoxic state contributing to the increased production of mucin has yet to be considered as part of the pathogenesis in DM. In cases of cutaneous mucinosis reported in the setting of venous insufficiency it has been hypothesized that reduced oxygen tension triggers chondrocytes to increase production of hyaluronic acid [16–18]. With perivascular inflammatory infiltrate, capillary obliteration, and myofiber necrosis as known sequelae of DM pathogenesis, it is conceivable that the biologic milieu of DM is hypoxic, and this may be a contributing factor towards mucin production.

Including our patient, there is a total of 12 cases in the English literature describing macroscopically evident cutaneous mucinosis in the setting of dermatomyositis (Table 1). Of these, three cases were associated with malignancy, and one patient had a history of autoimmune thyroiditis, inactive at the time of presentation.

Overall, clinical cutaneous manifestations of mucinous rashes are diverse: Chen, Requena, and Kaufmann describe plaque like skin changes, whereas Wang describes the rash as violaceous; Del Pozo and Johnson describe a distinctly papular rash. Most papers reported classic cutaneous findings of DM alongside the mucinous findings, with Gottron's papules and a heliotrope rash being common. Our patient had the most diffuse mucinous rash of the cases reported, involving the face, chest, back, and all extremities.

In the majority of cases, cutaneous symptoms preceded or occurred simultaneous to muscle weakness. Del Pozo et al. describe mucinous skin changes occurring four years after presentation and treatment of DM, and this is one of two cases where the mucinous skin changes did not resolve [2, 3]. In general, cutaneous lesions of mucinosis in the setting of DM seem to respond well to treatment when they appear in the early stages of disease. The majority of patients improved with oral steroids ± azathioprine, with resistant cases improving with IVIG [1]. Only one case did not describe improvement in cutaneous mucinosis despite lack of evidence of malignancy; in this case the mucinosis developed after DM had been successfully treated and did not respond to first line treatment [2]. One case was fatal due to respiratory complications of DM and recurrent infection due to long-term high dose steroid use [10]. Of note, in the latter two cases IVIG was not utilized per case documentation.

3.2. Dermatomyositis and Malignancy. DM has a clear temporal link with malignancy. Cancer may present in 15–30% of the adults with DM prior to or at diagnosis or during follow up. DM is most commonly associated with ovarian, breast, lung and colon cancer, melanoma, and non-Hodgkins lymphoma, with adenocarcinomas accounting for 70% of all associated tumors [19]. The pathophysiology relating DM and malignancy is unproven, but the leading proposed hypothesis is that of an autoimmune paraneoplastic mechanism. Myositis specific antigens (MSA), such as antisynthetase and anti-signal recognition particle, have been shown to be expressed at low levels by normal muscles cells and are over expressed during regeneration of muscle fibers during DM [20]. A tumor may overexpress oncoproteins or antigens similar to the myositis antigens, which subsequently stimulate the immune system leading to a lymphocytic reaction causing autoantibody deposition and damage to myofibers [21–23]. Casiola-Rosen showed that solid tumors such as breast and lung may express exact MSA antigens. The damage to muscles causes a release of antigens from the muscle fibers themselves further sensitizing the immune system to the striated muscle. This theory is complemented by the previous theories discussed, correlating serologic antibody titers with DM activity.

As noted previously, malignancy was associated with DM and cutaneous mucinosis in 3 of the 12 cases in the English literature. This proportion of cases with cutaneous mucinosis related to malignancy is proportionate to the number of DM cases relating to malignancy reported in the literature

Table 1: Literature review of all cases of cutaneous mucinosis in the setting of dermatomyositis.

Author, year, diagnosis	Demographics	Clinical description	Pathology (skin biopsy)	Associated condition(s)	Therapy and course
Johnson et al., 1973 [8] DM with lichen myxedematosus	35 African American males	Pruritic papular rash on upper and lower extremities, face, chest, and back. With perifollicular papules on forearms, hands, back, face and lower extremities, dysphagia and proximal muscle weakness of shoulders and pelvic girdle, and nail fold telangiectasia	Fragmented collagen with fibroblast proliferation and mucinous changes extending from the epidermis into the dermis with perivascular lymphocytosis and occasional histiocytes	None	80 mg oral prednisone daily with good response
Igarashi et al., 1985 [9] DM with cutaneous mucinosis	67 Japanese males	Poikilodermatous lesions on face, chest, and extremities	Skin bx: frayed and fragmented collagen bundles with mucinous material in between bundles when stained with alcian blue	Gastric cancer	Unknown
Requena et al., 1990 [3] DM with mucinosis	66 females	Erythematous, indurated plaque on hypogastric region of abdomen with irregular borders, heliotrope rash, violaceous rash on face, and Gottron's papules.	Amorphous mucinous material in epidermis and dermis which stained with alcian blue. The mucinous deposition caused thickening of the dermis and separation of collagen fibers	None	80 mg oral prednisone and 120 mg oral azathioprine daily for 4 weeks with slow taper improved malaise and weakness however only partial improvement of the abdominal mucinous plaque
Kaufmann et al., 1998 [1] Plaque like mucinosis	Case 1: 65 females	Case 1: erythematous plaques on extensor surface of upper extremities and left hip, muscle weakness of shoulder, and pelvic girdle	Case 1: separation of collagen bundles with perivascular lymphoplasmacytic infiltrate with abundant mucin deposition in the papillary and reticular dermis on staining with alcian blue	Case 1: none	Case 1: 80 mg oral prednisone daily, and 100 mg azathioprine daily with clinical response within 3 weeks, full resolution at 1 year
	Case 2: 37 females	Case 2: erythematous plaques over lateral surface of thighs bilaterally, weakness in shoulder and pelvic girdle, and clinical picture developed after fever arthralgia and malaise	Case 2: skin biopsy-separation of collagen vascular bundles with superficial and deep perivascular lymphoplasmacytic infiltrate of dermis with mucin between separated collagen bundles on Alcian blue staining	Case 2: obesity, history of autoimmune thyroiditis, preceded by viral prodrome. No malignancy detected	Case 2: 2 days of IVIG and high dose prednisone and then azathioprine, with excellent response

TABLE 1: Continued.

Author, year, diagnosis	Demographics	Clinical description	Pathology (skin biopsy)	Associated condition(s)	Therapy and course
Del Pozo et al., 2001 [2] DM with cutaneous mucinosis	Case 1: 53 females	Case 1: small violaceous papules on upper extremities and chest; proximal muscle weakness	Case 1: skin biopsy showed hyperkeratosis, colloid bodies, and edema at the dermoepidermal junction with moderate perivascular lymphocytic infiltrate. Collagen bundles separated by mucin deposition	Case 1: ovarian adenocarcinoma	Case 1: recurrence despite prednisone, hydroxychloroquine, methotrexate, and azathioprine. Ovarian carcinoma treated with surgery, paclitaxel and cisplatin, no comment on status of DM or cutaneous findings after treatment
	Case 2: 44 females	Case 2: flesh coloured papules across flexural creases of palms and fingers	Case 2: skin biopsy-epidermal atrophy with perivascular lymphocytic infiltrate and moderate mucin deposition between collagen fibers	Case 2: none	Case 2: mucinosis developed after treatment for DM with 30 mg prednisone po and 250 mg hydroxychloroquine daily, lesions did not improve with this treatment
Tan et al., 2003 [7] DM with cutaneous mucinosis	65 Chinese males	Nontender erythematous plaques on neck, upper back and extensor surfaces of forearms bilaterally. Proximal muscle weakness developed 3 months after initial presentation	Mucin deposition between collagen bundles with surrounding superficial perivascular lymphocytic infiltrate without epidermal changes	Nasopharyngeal carcinoma	Skin lesions resolved after 2 months of radiation therapy
Chen et al., 2005 [10] Dermatomyositis with mucinosis and intestinal vasculopathy	21 Taiwanese females	Erythematous indurated mass on lower abdomen, labia majora and inner thigh with malar rash and periungual telangiectasia, heliotrope rash, Gottron's papules, proximal muscle weakness, and dysphagia	Atrophic epidermis with vacuolar alteration of basal keratinocytes, interstitial mucin deposition, and perivascular lymphocytic infiltrate of dermis and subcutaneous tissue	None	Prednisolone 60 mg/d IV with resolution of CPK however developed dysphagia and pulse steroid therapy initiated. Patient suffered complications and ultimately died after a long hospital course
Edward et al., 2007 [11] Amyopathic DM with mucinosis	31-year-old female	Puritic rash on flexor surface of forearms and chest, violaceous rash of face, Gottron's papules, and nail fold telangiectasia	Dermal accumulation of mucin without inflammatory infiltrate; no evidence of inflammatory myopathy	None	Improved with oral steroids
Wang, 2011 [12] DM with lichen myxedematosus	60-year-old male	Violaceous erythema on face, neck, and chest with flesh coloured papules on arms; muscle weakness of shoulders and dysphagia	Separation of collagen bundles with lymphocytic infiltrate of dermis and mucin deposition between collagen bundles demonstrated with alcian blue stain	None	Oral prednisone 40 mg daily with good response

generally (30%). It is unlikely that the cutaneous mucinosis is independently related to malignancy or that the presence of malignancy increases the chance of cutaneous mucinosis expressed in DM.

4. Conclusion

To date there are 12 cases describing macroscopically evident cutaneous mucin in DM. Our case describes a middle aged man with NSCLC in remission presenting with a puritic, diffuse, and violaceous rash. Histologic evidence showed mucin deposition in the dermis without dermal thickening alongside clinical, immunoserologic, and MRI findings consistent with DM, and even though our patient also had serologies suggestive of systemic lupus erythematosus, the predominant clinical picture was that of DM. The patient's cutaneous findings were highly resistant to first and second line treatments and only improved with the initiation of IVIG. While mucin deposition is a common microscopic finding in connective tissue diseases, it is rarely seen macroscopically. The pathophysiologic mechanism of cutaneous mucin production in these clinical scenarios is unclear. The link between hypoxic states and mucin deposition is a new concept, which has not been explored in the setting of dermatomyositis. Of the cases of cutaneous mucinosis and DM in the literature, the majority of cases improved with first line treatment for DM and in resistant cases positive results were seen using IVIG.

Conflict of Interests

The authors declare that there is no conflict of interests regarding to the publication of this paper.

References

[1] R. Kaufmann, D. Greiner, P. Schmidt, and M. Wolter, "Dermatomyositis presenting as plaque-like mucinosis," *British Journal of Dermatology*, vol. 138, no. 5, pp. 889–892, 1998.

[2] J. Del Pozo, M. Almagro, W. Martínez et al., "Dermatomyositis and mucinosis," *International Journal of Dermatology*, vol. 40, no. 2, pp. 120–124, 2001.

[3] L. Requena, A. Aquilar, and Y. E. Sanchez, "A corrugated plaque on the abdominal wall. Cutaneous mucinosis secondary to dermatomyositis," *Archives of Dermatology*, vol. 126, no. 12, pp. 1639–1640, 1990.

[4] A. M. Shekari, M. Ghiasi, E. Ghasemi, and Z. A. Kani, "Papulonodular mucinosis indicating systemic lupus erythematosus," *Clinical and Experimental Dermatology*, vol. 34, no. 8, pp. e558–e560, 2009.

[5] M. Allam and M. Ghozzi, "Scleromyxedema: a case report and review of the literature," *Case Reports in Dermatology*, vol. 5, no. 2, pp. 168–175, 2013.

[6] M. C. Dalakas, "Pathophysiology of inflammatory and autoimmune myopathies," *Presse Medicale*, vol. 40, no. 4, pp. e237–e247, 2011.

[7] E. Tan, S. H. Tan, and S. K. Ng, "Cutaneous mucinosis in dermatomyositis associated with a malignant tumor," *Journal of the American Academy of Dermatology*, vol. 48, no. 5, pp. S41–S42, 2003.

[8] B. L. Johnson, I. R. Horowitz, C. R. Charles, and D. L. Cooper, "Dermatomyositis and lichen myxedematosus: a clinical, histopathological and electron microscopic study," *Dermatologica*, vol. 147, no. 2, pp. 109–122, 1973.

[9] M. Igarashi, H. Aizawa, Y. Tokudome, and H. Tagami, "Dermatomyositis with prominent mucinous skin change. Histochemical and biochemical aspects of glycosaminoglycans," *Dermatologica*, vol. 170, no. 1, pp. 6–11, 1985.

[10] G.-Y. Chen, M.-F. Liu, J. Y.-Y. Lee, and W. Chen, "Combination of massive mucinosis, dermatomyositis, pyoderma gangrenosum-like ulcer, bullae and fatal intestinal vasculopathy in a young female," *European Journal of Dermatology*, vol. 15, no. 5, pp. 396–400, 2005.

[11] M. Edward, L. Fitzgerald, C. Thind, J. Leman, and A. D. Burden, "Cutaneous mucinosis associated with dermatomyositis and nephrogenic fibrosing dermopathy: fibroblast hyaluronan synthesis and the effect of patient serum," *British Journal of Dermatology*, vol. 156, no. 3, pp. 473–479, 2007.

[12] S. Wang, "Annular lichen myxedematosus in a patient with dermatomyositis," *International Journal of Dermatology*, vol. 50, no. 3, pp. 370–372, 2011.

[13] J. T. Kissel, J. R. Mendell, and K. W. Rammohan, "Microvascular deposition of complement membrane attack complex in dermatomyositis," *The New England Journal of Medicine*, vol. 314, no. 6, pp. 329–334, 1986.

[14] F. Rongioletti and A. Rebora, "Cutaneous mucinoses: microscopic criteria for diagnosis," *The American Journal of Dermatopathology*, vol. 23, no. 3, pp. 257–267, 2001.

[15] A. G. Pandya, R. D. Sontheimer, C. J. Cockerell, A. Takashima, and M. Piepkorn, "Papulonodular mucinosis associated with systemic lupus erythematosus: possible mechanisms of increased glycosaminoglycan accumulation," *Journal of the American Academy of Dermatology*, vol. 32, no. 2, pp. 199–205, 1995.

[16] R. Pugashetti, D. C. Zedek, E. V. Seiverling, P. Rajendran, and T. Berger, "Dermal mucinosis as a sign of venous insufficiency," *Journal of Cutaneous Pathology*, vol. 37, no. 2, pp. 292–296, 2010.

[17] K. Hashimoto, K. Fukuda, K. Yamazaki et al., "Hypoxia-induced hyaluronan synthesis by articular chondrocytes: the role of nitric oxide," *Inflammation Research*, vol. 55, no. 2, pp. 72–77, 2006.

[18] M. C. Dalakas, "Inflammatory myopathies: management of steroid resistance," *Current Opinion in Neurology*, vol. 24, no. 5, pp. 457–462, 2011.

[19] S. M. Levine, "Cancer and myositis: new insights into an old association," *Current Opinion in Rheumatology*, vol. 18, no. 6, pp. 620–624, 2006.

[20] L. Casciola-Rosen, K. Nagaraju, P. Plotz et al., "Enhanced autoantigen expression in regenerating muscle cells in idiopathic inflammatory myopathy," *Journal of Experimental Medicine*, vol. 201, no. 4, pp. 591–601, 2005.

[21] S. Zampieri, M. Valente, N. Adami et al., "Polymyositis, dermatomyositis and malignancy: a further intriguing link," *Autoimmunity Reviews*, vol. 9, no. 6, pp. 449–453, 2010.

[22] A. Chakroun, J. Guigay, A. Lusinchi, P. Marandas, F. Janot, and D. M. Hartl, "Paraneoplastic dermatomyositis and nasopharyngeal carcinoma: diagnosis, treatment and prognosis," *Annales Francaises d'Oto-Rhino-Laryngologie et de Pathologie Cervico-Faciale*, vol. 128, no. 3, pp. 148–152, 2011.

[23] P. Ungprasert, N. K. Bethina, and C. H. Jones, "Malignancy and idiopathic inflammatory myopathies," *North American Journal of Medical Sciences*, vol. 5, no. 10, pp. 569–572, 2013.

51

Acute Methotrexate Toxicity: A Fatal Condition in Two Cases of Psoriasis

Pankti Jariwala,[1] Vinay Kumar,[1] Khyati Kothari,[1] Sejal Thakkar,[2] and Dipak Dayabhai Umrigar[1]

[1] Department of Skin & VD, Government Medical College & New Civil Hospital, Surat, Gujarat 395001, India
[2] Department of Skin & VD, GMERS Medical College & General Hospital, Gotri 202, Wings Ville 41, Arunoday Society, Alkapuri, Vadodara, Gujarat 390001, India

Correspondence should be addressed to Sejal Thakkar; drsejal98@gmail.com

Academic Editor: Jeung-Hoon Lee

We describe two fatal cases of low dose methotrexate (MTX) toxicity in patients with psoriasis, emphasizing the factors that exacerbate MTX toxicity. The first patient was a 50-year-old male of psoriasis on intermittent treatment with MTX. After a treatment-free period of six months, he had self-medication of MTX along with analgesic for joint pain for one week which followed ulceration of the lesions, bone marrow suppression, and eventually death. The second patient was a 37-year-old male of psoriasis, who has taken MTX one week earlier without prior investigations. He had painful ulcerated skin lesions and bone marrow suppression. On investigations, he showed high creatinine level and atrophied, nonfunctioning right kidney on ultrasonography. In spite of dialysis, he succumbed to death. MTX is safe and effective if monitored properly, but inadvertent use may lead to even death also. Prior workup and proper counseling regarding the drug interactions as well as self-medication should be enforced.

1. Introduction

Methotrexate (MTX), when used in low doses, has anti-inflammatory and immunosuppressive action. Low dose MTX is an effective and safe treatment for psoriasis being used for more than 50 years [1]. Renal excretion is the primary route of elimination and is dependent upon dosage and route of administration [2]. It is also affected by concomitant ingestion of certain drugs which are protein bound like non-steroidal anti-inflammatory drugs (NSAIDs), sulfonamides, and barbiturates. This demands careful monitoring of renal function tests and blood counts, along with carefully looking for mucosal lesions or ulcerations in skin to identify acute MTX toxicity. Failure to adhere to guidelines may lead to severe toxicity, even death. There are few publications mentioning adverse reactions of MTX, but very few are there mentioning fatality because of such a safe drug. Here, we report two cases that died of MTX toxicity because of just not abiding by the standard protocol.

2. Case Reports

2.1. Case 1. A 50-year-old male presented with generalized skin lesions with ulcerations along with erosions over lips and oral cavity and difficulty in swallowing for 2 days. He also had fever with chills.

He was a known case of psoriasis for 5 years, on MTX (7.5 mg) once weekly for two years. He was under remission and stopped MTX six months earlier. He had aggravation of lesions along with knee joint pains for two weeks. He took oral MTX (7.5 mg/day) daily for one week along with some pain killers by himself. After two days he developed ulcerations over existing lesions along with erosions on lips and oral cavity (Figure 1).

The patient was conscious with body temperature 103°F, pulse rate 120/minute, and normal respiration and blood pressure. Cutaneous examination revealed generalized multiple annular ulcerated plaques with mucosal erosions. On admission, investigations showed myelosuppression (Hb 6.7

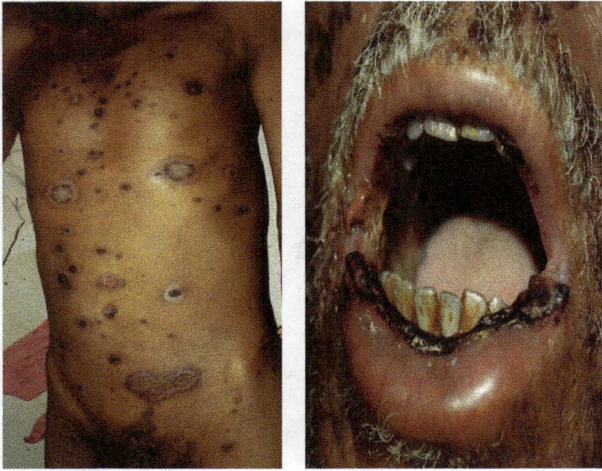

FIGURE 1: Ulceration over psoriatic lesions with crusting on lips (Case 1).

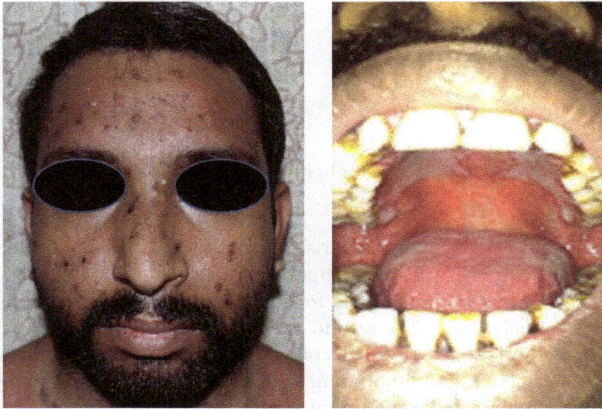

FIGURE 2: Pustules on face with mucositis in oral cavity (Case 2).

gms, WBC 1200, and 69,000 platelet count) with normal renal and liver profile.

Patient was diagnosed as a case of acute MTX toxicity and treated with intravenous antibiotics and leucovorin and neukine (GM-CSF) injection subcutaneously. He was investigated periodically which showed persistent myelosuppression which was worsening day by day. He was supported with packed cell volume and platelet transfusions. On the fifth day, he was transferred to the intensive care unit for better monitoring. His platelet count increased to 45000/mm^3 and WBCs to 1300/mm^3 on the 10th day. His liver function deteriorated with bilirubin 8.1 grams on the 10th day. Unfortunately, he expired due to acute respiratory failure after six hours of onset on the 10th day.

2.2. Case 2. A 37-year-old male, a known case of psoriasis, presented with complaint of reduced oral intake due to painful lesions in the oral cavity, along with fever and chills for three days. He also complained of pain with ulceration in the existing lesions. On careful history taking, it was revealed

that he took an unknown amount of oral MTX one week back without prior investigations.

On examination, he was conscious but febrile with 102°F temperature with normal vitals. Cutaneous examination showed ulcerated and necrotic psoriatic plaques with erythema and tenderness. There were few new pustules on chest and face (Figure 2). He also had crusting and fissuring of the lips along with erosions in oral cavity. On admission, investigations suggested bone marrow suppression (hemoglobin 8.2 grams, WBC 1600 cells/mm^3, and platelet count 1,06,000 cells/mm^3) and altered renal functions (blood urea 72 and creatinine level 4.8).

Based on the clinical and laboratory findings, he was diagnosed having MTX toxicity and was covered with broad spectrum empirical antibiotics and injectable leucovorin. Sodium bicarbonate was added to aid in the excretion of drug by alkalinization of the urine and was hydrated aggressively. Despite aggressive therapy, there was gradual worsening with odynophagia/dysphagia and the blood counts still falling with no improvement in the renal functions. The patient was transferred to medicine ward. He was given platelet transfusions and taken for dialysis for two days, during which he succumbed to death.

3. Discussion

Low dose MTX in psoriasis rarely produces toxicity, and most of such cases occur due to failure to adhere to the recommended guidelines [1]. The risk of toxicity is greater if additional methotrexate is administered sooner than the usual scheduled weekly dose [3]. In the first case, it was a self-administration of the higher, consecutive dose which acted as a precipitating factor.

MTX toxicity has its impact on skin, gastrointestinal mucosa, liver, kidneys, and bone marrow. Ulcerations in skin due to MTX toxicity are restricted to the psoriatic plaques probably because of higher uptake of methotrexate by the hyperproliferative psoriatic plaques than normal skin [4]. Both of the cases presented with ulceration on existing plaques of psoriasis.

Pancytopenia due to MTX is attributed to the patients with renal dysfunction, presence of infection, folic acid deficiency, hypoalbuminemia, concomitant use of drugs such as trimethoprim, and advanced age [5]. Both of our patients had mucositis along with myelosuppression as a presenting feature of MTX toxicity. The probable cause of myelosuppression in the first patient could be advanced age, concomitant use of NSAID, and inadvertent use of MTX dose, while, in the second patient, it was renal dysfunction which was not picked up before initiation of the treatment.

Drugs can increase the risk of methotrexate toxicity either by decreasing renal elimination of methotrexate (aminoglycosides, cyclosporine, nonsteroidal anti-inflammatory agents, sulfonamides, probenecid, salicylates, penicillins, colchicines, cisplatin, and other renotoxic drugs) or by displacing methotrexate from protein binding sites in the plasma (salicylates, probenecid, sulfonamides, barbiturates, phenytoin, retinoids, sulfonylureas, and tetracyclines). NSAID taken for joint pain had contributed to the MTX toxicity in the first case.

Unfortunately, we could not measure the drug level of MTX because of lack of facility. But the common feature in both of them was inadvertent dosage of MTX which is the major contributory factor for the toxicity.

It is a must to avoid self-administration of such drugs. There should be proper counseling of the patient for not taking the drugs on their own without consulting a dermatologist as well as not to combine with any other drug without taking doctors' consent. Selling such drugs without prescription should be banned.

The second case had consumed MTX without following the standard investigative as well as therapeutic protocol. Already compromised renal functions were missed out and impairment in renal clearance could have played a role in MTX toxicity. Prior workup is mandatory for MTX which is otherwise really safe and effective in cases of psoriasis.

Key Messages

Pretreatment investigations are a must if MTX is to be prescribed. Proper monitoring and strict avoidance of self-administration of MTX are mandatory. Coadministration of the drugs like NSAIDs should be judicious.

Conflict of Interests

The authors declare that there is no conflict of interests regarding the publication of this paper.

References

[1] H. H. Roenigk Jr., H. I. Maibach, and G. D. Weinstein, "Use of methotrexate in psoriasis," *Archives of Dermatology*, vol. 105, no. 3, pp. 363–365, 1972.

[2] E. A. Olsen, "The pharmacology of methotrexate," *Journal of the American Academy of Dermatology*, vol. 25, pp. 300–318, 1993.

[3] W. A. Bleyer, "Methotrexate: clinical pharmacology, current status and therapeutic guidelines," *Cancer Treatment Reviews*, vol. 4, no. 2, pp. 87–101, 1977.

[4] D. L. Kaplan and E. A. Olsen, "Erosion of psoriatic plaques after chronic methotrexate administration," *International Journal of Dermatology*, vol. 27, no. 1, pp. 59–62, 1988.

[5] S. Gutierrez-Ureña, J. F. Molina, C. O. Garcia, M. L. Cuellar, and L. R. Espinoza, "Pancytopenia secondary to methotrexate therapy in rheumatoid arthritis," *Arthritis and Rheumatism*, vol. 39, pp. 272–276, 1996.

52

Peripheral Ulcerative Keratitis with Pyoderma Gangrenosum

Adrián Imbernón-Moya,[1] **Elena Vargas-Laguna,**[1] **Antonio Aguilar,**[1]
Miguel Ángel Gallego,[1] **Claudia Vergara,**[2] **and María Fernanda Nistal**[2]

[1]*Department of Dermatology, Hospital Universitario Severo Ochoa, Avenida de Orellana, Leganés, 28911 Madrid, Spain*
[2]*Department of Ophthalmology, Hospital Universitario Severo Ochoa, Avenida de Orellana, Leganés, 28911 Madrid, Spain*

Correspondence should be addressed to Adrián Imbernón-Moya; adrian_imber88@hotmail.com

Academic Editor: Akimichi Morita

Pyoderma gangrenosum is an unusual necrotizing noninfective and ulcerative skin disease whose cause is unknown. Ophthalmic involvement in pyoderma gangrenosum is an unusual event. Only a few cases have been reported, from which we can highlight scleral, corneal, and orbital cases. Peripheral ulcerative keratitis is a process which destroys the peripheral cornea. Its cause is still unknown although it is often associated with autoimmune conditions. Pyoderma gangrenosum should be included in the differential diagnosis of peripheral ulcerative keratitis. Early recognition of these manifestations can vary the prognosis by applying the appropriate treatment. We introduce a 70-year-old woman who suffered pyoderma gangrenosum associated with peripheral ulcerative keratitis in her left eye. The patient's skin lesions and peripheral keratitis responded successfully to systemic steroids and cyclosporine A.

1. Introduction

Pyoderma gangrenosum (PG) is an unusual necrotizing noninfective and ulcerative skin disease of unknown cause that has been included among the so-called neutrophilic dermatoses. The condition is clinically characterized by necrotic and deep ulcers that are previously preceded by inflammatory pustules [1, 2].

Under the term peripheral ulcerative keratitis (PUK), a group of inflammatory corneal diseases clinically characterized by peripherical corneal thinning, cellular infiltration, ulceration, and variable degree vasoocclusion and injection of the adjacent vascular network are included [3, 4].

Ophthalmic involvement in pyoderma gangrenosum is not a usual event. Only a few cases have been reported, from which we can highlight scleral, corneal, and orbital cases [5–10]. We report a case of PG associated with PUK in a 70-year-old woman. The patient's skin lesions and peripheral keratitis responded successfully to systemic steroids and cyclosporine A.

2. Case Presentation

A 70-year-old woman with a personal history of non-insulin-dependent diabetes mellitus was seen on consultation because of rapid development of an eruption consisting in several ulcerative and painful lesions located on her left leg. Initial lesions were boggy violaceous plaques with pustules that rapidly enlarged for two weeks prior to presentation. The patient was treated with oral and topical antibiotics without results. At the same time, the patient had fever and discomfort and complained of redness and pain and visual acuity decreased in her left eye.

Cutaneous examination revealed scattered shallow ulcers with a necrotic base which were confined to the left leg. The ulcer border was raised, serpiginous, and irregular and it was surrounded by an inflammatory area of erythema (Figure 1). There were no other cutaneous findings.

A wedge-shaped cutaneous biopsy showed neutrophilic abscess formation under areas of ulceration, as well as a dense inflammatory dermal infiltrate composed primarily

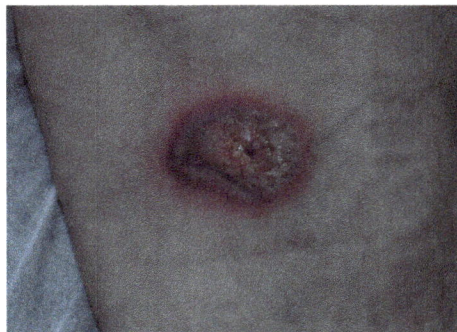

FIGURE 1: Ulcer with a necrotic base, raised border, and halo erythema on the left leg.

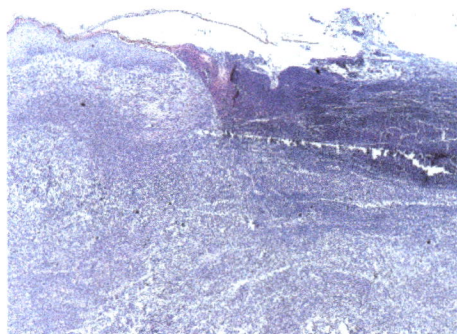

FIGURE 3: Ulceration and peripheral stromal infiltrates in the upper and lower limb (slit lamp).

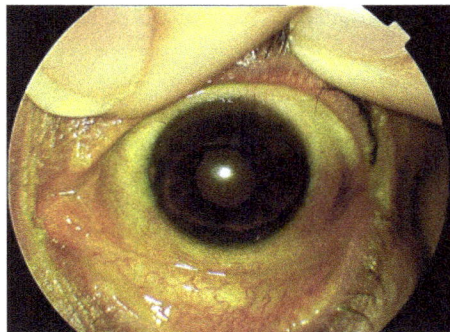

FIGURE 2: Neutrophilic abscess formation under areas of ulceration, as well as a dense inflammatory dermal infiltrate composed primarily of polymorphonuclear leukocytes (H-E ×10).

of polymorphonuclear leukocytes but including occasional mature lymphocytes. No vascular involvement was observed (Figure 2). Cultures from the skin lesions were negative for fungi, mycobacteria, and bacteria.

Ocular examination with slit lamp revealed ulceration and peripheral stromal infiltrates in the upper and lower limb on her left eye (Figure 3).

All the following laboratory evaluations were in the normal range: biochemical parameters, complete blood cell count, white blood cell count, differential count, erythrocyte sedimentation rates, serum protein electrophoresis, quantitative serum immunoglobulins, C3 and C4 levels, antinuclear antibodies, anti-double stranded DNA antibodies, rheumatoid factor, and Venereal Disease Research Laboratory (VDRL) test. Chest X-ray examination, ultrasound examination, and thoracic-abdominal-pelvic computed tomography were all carried out although no systematic involvement was found.

The patient was diagnosed with pyoderma gangrenosum and unilateral peripheral ulcerative keratitis. Therapy was started with a course of systemic corticosteroid (prednisone 1 mg/Kg daily) obtaining a favourable response with improvement of the skin ulcers and the ocular damage after four weeks of treatment. When the dose of prednisone was reduced to 0,5 mg/Kg daily, mild relapse of the cutaneous and ocular lesions occurred, so the patient was treated with

cyclosporine A 3 mg/Kg daily and prednisone 20 mg daily. After three months, the disease was totally resolved with no ocular residual damage and no new active skin lesions were detected.

3. Discussion

PG may appear in healthy patients or in those associated with a variety of systemic diseases. These diseases are present in more than 50% of patients. The most common is the comorbidity inflammatory bowel disease followed by rheumatoid arthritis. Others include immunologic abnormalities, hematologic disorders like monoclonal gammopathy and polycythemia vera, and hematologic malignancies like myeloma, leukemia, lymphoma, and myelodysplasia [1, 2, 5, 7–10]. This relationship supports the hypothesis that the disease may be caused due to underlying defects in the immune system such as abnormalities of cellular or humoral immunity, reduced production of macrophage inhibitory factor, disorder of chemotaxis, and phagocytosis by neutrophils and monocytes. However, a specific immune defect has not been demonstrated [1, 2, 5, 8, 10].

The skin lesions have classic appearance and evolution, starting as a papule or pustules that rapidly progress to a well defined and very painful ulcer with necrotic or mucopurulent debris at the base. The ulcer is surrounded by violaceous undermined borders and an inflammatory halo of erythema. Cutaneous lesions may be present at any site of the skin surface but mucosal membranes are usually spread. It has a propensity to appear on the lower limbs or the trunk and sometimes occurs at areas of the skin previously damaged by trauma or surgical wounds (pathergic phenomenon). The diagnosis of PG is essentially clinical and PG is considered a diagnosis of exclusion. The histopathologic findings are not specific and there are no diagnostic laboratory test markers of the disease [1, 2, 10].

PUK is a destructive process of the peripheral cornea that is often associated with autoimmune conditions including rheumatoid arthritis, Sweet syndrome, systemic lupus erythematosus, Wegener's granulomatosis, and polyarteritis nodosa. Patients may present decreased visual acuity,

TABLE 1: Description of cases reported of pyoderma gangrenosum with peripheral ulcerative keratitis (PUK). Literature review.

Authors	Gender	Age	PUK	Association	Therapy	Response to therapy
Bouchard et al. [5]	Male	37	Bilateral	Chronic myelogenous leukaemia	Systemic corticosteroids	Complete response
Bishop and Tullo [6]	Female	59	Left eye	Monoarticular arthritis	Cyclophosphamide and systemic corticosteroids	Improved but with intermittent flares of ocular diseases
Bishop and Tullo [6]	Male	56	Right eye	Leukocytoclastic vasculitis	Systemic corticosteroids	Improved but with recurrence of ocular disease
Wilson et al. [7]	Female	60	Left eye	Rheumatoid arthritis and leukocytoclastic vasculitis	Cyclosporine A and systemic corticosteroids	Improved but with intermittent flares of ocular and skin diseases
Brown et al. [8]	Male	54	Right eye	Chronic obstructive pulmonary disease and diabetes mellitus	Systemic corticosteroids and azathioprine	Complete response
Teasley et al. [9]	Female	30	Left eye	Graves' disease	Dapsone	Complete response
Fournié et al. [10]	Male	78	Left eye	Multiple myeloma	Cyclophosphamide, systemic corticosteroids, and human intravenous immunoglobulins	Complete response

blindness, eye pain, redness, or irritation. The diagnosis is confirmed by slit lamp examination [3, 4, 7–10].

As with PG the aetiology of PUK is poorly understood, the postulated reasons include autoimmune reactions to corneal antigens, circulating immunocomplex deposition, vasculitis, and hypersensitivity reactions to exogenous antigens. PUK may result from humoral or cell-mediated immune mechanisms or both, causing obliterative microangiitis at the level of the limbal vascular arcades. Subsequent leakage of inflammatory cells with destructive collagenases and proteases leads to scleral inflammation and destruction [3–5, 8, 10].

There have been only seven reported cases of PUK associated with PG [5–10] (Table 1). There have been four reported cases in males and three cases in females. The age of clinical appearance varies between 30 and 78 years. PUK is usually unilateral and the left eye is the most frequently affected. There is only one case of bilateral ocular involvement [5]. Other autoimmune disorders were associated like monoarticular arthritis [6], rheumatoid arthritis [7], leukocytoclastic vasculitis [6, 7], and Graves' disease [9], as well as diseases producing immunosuppression like chronic obstructive pulmonary disease [8], diabetes mellitus [8], multiple myeloma [10], and chronic myelogenous leukemia [5]. All the patients were prescribed systemic corticosteroids. All but 1 were treated with immunosuppressive agents. These include cyclophosphamide, cyclosporine A, azathioprine, dapsone, and human intravenous immunoglobulins. All the patients had an initial adequate response but the course of the disease varied between cases with some relapsing cases. PG and PUK do not follow a parallel course.

Our patient had no other autoimmune disease associated and she had a complete response of PG and PUK with cyclosporine A and systemic corticosteroids. PG and other autoimmune disorders or diseases producing immunosuppression should be considered in the differential diagnosis of PUK. Early recognition of these manifestations can lead to the application of appropriate treatment improving the prognosis [3–10].

Acronyms

PG: Pyoderma gangrenosum
PUK: Peripheral ulcerative keratitis.

Conflict of Interests

The authors declare no conflict of interests.

References

[1] E. Cozzani, G. Gasparini, and A. Parodi, "Pyoderma gangrenosum: a systematic review," *Giornale Italiano di Dermatologia e Venereologia*, vol. 149, no. 5, pp. 587–600, 2014.

[2] A. Alavi, D. Sajic, F. B. Cerci, D. Ghazarian, M. Rosenbach, and J. Jorizzo, "Neutrophilic dermatoses: an update," *American Journal of Clinical Dermatology*, vol. 15, no. 5, pp. 413–423, 2014.

[3] N. E. Knox Cartwright, D. M. Tole, P. Georgoudis, and S. D. Cook, "Peripheral ulcerative keratitis and corneal melt: a 10-year single center review with historical comparison," *Cornea*, vol. 33, no. 1, pp. 27–31, 2014.

[4] A. Galor and J. E. Thorne, "Scleritis and peripheral ulcerative keratitis," *Rheumatic Disease Clinics of North America*, vol. 33, no. 4, pp. 835–854, 2007.

[5] C. S. Bouchard, M. A. Meyer, and J. F. McDonnell, "Bilateral peripheral ulcerative keratitis associated with pyoderma gangrenosum," *Cornea*, vol. 16, no. 4, pp. 480–482, 1997.

[6] P. Bishop and A. Tullo, "Pyoderma gangrenosum and necrotising sclerokeratitis," *Cornea*, vol. 17, no. 3, pp. 346–347, 1998.

[7] D. M. Wilson, G. R. John, and J. P. Callen, "Peripheral ulcerative keratitis—an extracutaneous neutrophilic disorder: report of a patient with rheumatoid arthritis, pustular vasculitis, pyoderma gangrenosum, and Sweet's syndrome with an excellent response to cyclosporine therapy," *Journal of the American Academy of Dermatology*, vol. 40, no. 2, pp. 331–334, 1999.

[8] B. A. Brown, C. T. Parker, and K. S. Bower, "Effective steroid-sparing treatment for peripheral ulcerative keratitis and pyoderma gangrenosum," *Cornea*, vol. 20, no. 1, pp. 117–118, 2001.

[9] L. A. Teasley, C. S. Foster, and S. Baltatzis, "Sclerokeratitis and facial skin lesions: a case report of pyoderma gangrenosum and its response to dapsone therapy," *Cornea*, vol. 26, no. 2, pp. 215–219, 2007.

[10] P. Fournié, F. Malecaze, J. Coullet, and J.-L. Arné, "Pyoderma gangrenosum with necrotizing sclerokeratitis after cataract surgery," *Journal of Cataract and Refractive Surgery*, vol. 33, no. 11, pp. 1987–1990, 2007.

53

Subcutaneous Histiocytoid Sweet Syndrome Associated with Crohn Disease in an Adolescent

Rosa María Fernández-Torres,[1] **Susana Castro,**[2] **Ana Moreno,**[2]
Roberto Álvarez,[3] **and Eduardo Fonseca**[1]

[1] Department of Dermatology, University Hospital of La Coruña, Xubias de Arriba 84,
   15006 La Coruña, Spain
[2] Department of Pediatrics, University Hospital of La Coruña, Xubias de Arriba 84,
   15006 La Coruña, Spain
[3] Department of Pathology, University Hospital of La Coruña, Xubias de Arriba 84,
   15006 La Coruña, Spain

Correspondence should be addressed to Rosa María Fernández-Torres; rosaftorres@gmail.com

Academic Editors: K. Jimbow and H. Nakano

We report a case of subcutaneous histiocytoid Sweet syndrome in an adolescent with Crohn disease. A 14-year-old boy with a 1-year history of ileocolonic and perianal Crohn disease, treated with infliximab and azathioprine, was admitted to the Pediatrics Department with malaise, abdominal pain, bloody diarrhea, and fever (39°C) from 15 days ago. Two days later, he developed cutaneous lesions consisting of tender, erythematous, and violaceous papules and nodules scattered over his legs, soles, and upper extremities. Laboratory studies revealed neutrophilia, microcytic anemia, and elevation of both erythrocyte sedimentation rate and C-reactive protein rate. A skin biopsy specimen showed deep dermal and predominantly septal inflammatory infiltrate in the subcutaneous tissue composed of polymorphonuclears, eosinophils, and mononuclear cells of histiocytic appearance. These histiocytoid cells stained positive for myeloperoxidase. Subcutaneous Sweet syndrome is a rare subtype of acute neutrophilic dermatosis, in which the infiltrate is exclusively or predominantly located in the subcutaneous tissue, causing lobular or septal panniculitis. It is often described in patients with an underlying haematological disorder or caused by drugs, but very rare in patients with inflammatory bowel disease, especially in childhood or adolescence. To our knowledge, this is the first case of subcutaneous histiocytoid type in a paediatric patient.

1. Introduction

Sweet syndrome, also referred to as acute febrile neutrophilic dermatosis, is a reactive condition of unknown etiology characterized by an abrupt onset of cutaneous lesions consisting of painful, erythematous plaques, papules, and nodules accompanied by fever and neutrophilia. It has been reported in association with several drugs and inflammatory, neoplastic, and infectious diseases [1].

Cases of Sweet syndrome in patients with Crohn disease have been sporadically reported. Herein, we report a case of this association with the peculiarities being the subcutaneous histiocytoid variant of Sweet syndrome and occurring in an adolescent.

2. Case Presentation

A 14-year-old boy with a 1-year history of recurrent ileocolonic and perianal Crohn disease, treated with infliximab and azathioprine, was admitted to the Pediatrics Department with malaise, abdominal pain, bloody diarrhea, and fever (39°C) from 15 days ago. Due to suspicion of concurrent intra-abdominal infection, treatment with teicoplanin, meropenem, and metronidazole was started. Two days after hospital admission, he developed cutaneous lesions consisting of tender, erythematous, and violaceous papules and nodules scattered over his legs, soles, and upper extremities (Figure 1). Laboratory studies revealed a total white cell count of 18.85×10^9 g/L with 76.4% neutrophils,

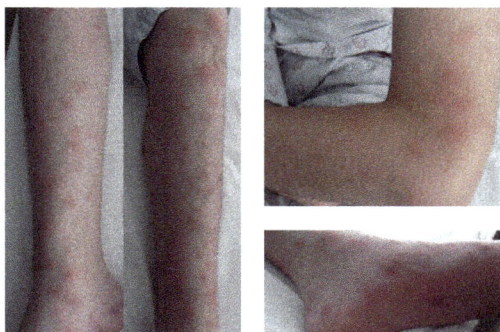

FIGURE 1: Erythematous nodules and plaques on the legs, arms, and soles.

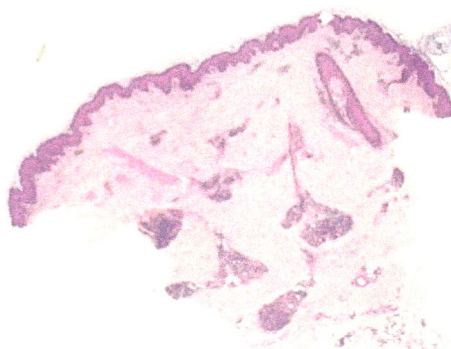

(a)

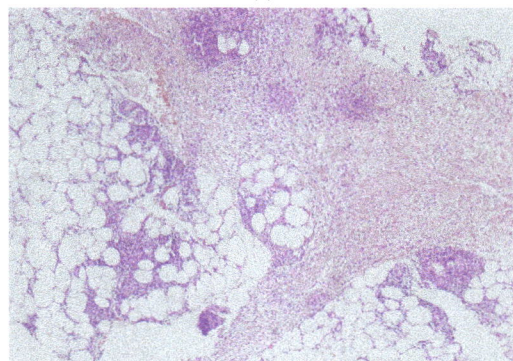

(b)

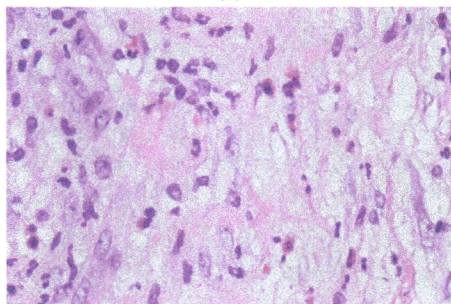

(c)

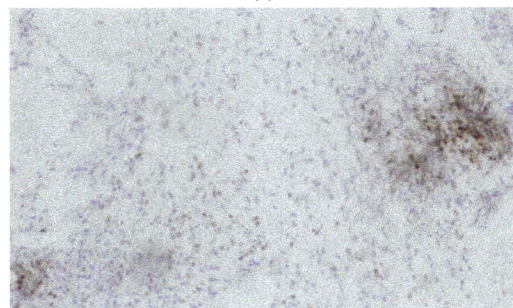

(d)

FIGURE 2: (a) Normal epidermis and dermis. Inflammatory infiltrate affecting exclusively the adipose tissue (hematoxylin-eosin, original magnification ×2). (b) Inflammatory infiltrate in the subcutaneous tissue, predominating in the septa, but also in the fat lobules (hematoxylin-eosin, original magnification ×10). (c) Infiltrate of polymorphonuclear cells, eosinophils, and large, mononuclear cells with histiocytoid appearance (hematoxylin-eosin, original magnification ×20). (d) Immunoreactivity for myeloperoxidase in most of the cells of the inflammatory infiltrate.

microcytic anemia (serum hemoglobin: 11.20 g/dL), and elevation of both erythrocyte sedimentation rate (101 mm/hour; normal value <20 mm/hour) and C-reactive protein rate (15.30 mg/dL; normal value <1 mg/L). All other laboratory parameters were within the normal range. Blood, urine, and stool cultures were all negative as well as serology for HIV, hepatitis B, hepatitis C, and autoimmunity studies.

A skin biopsy specimen showed deep dermal and predominantly septal inflammatory infiltrate in the subcutaneous tissue composed of polymorphonuclear cells, eosinophils, and mononuclear cells of histiocytic appearance. These histiocytoid cells stained positive for myeloperoxidase (Figure 2).

Based on these findings, the diagnosis of subcutaneous histiocytoid Sweet syndrome associated with Crohn disease was established.

Methylprednisolone therapy was started at dose of 1 mg/kg daily with tapering over the next four weeks. Significant improvement was observed since the start of treatment with disappearance of fever within 24 hours and gradual involution of skin lesions.

3. Discussion

Sweet syndrome is a type of neutrophilic dermatosis characterized by pyrexia, elevated neutrophil counts, tender erythematous papules, nodules or plaques, and a predominantly mature neutrophilic dermal infiltrate. Subcutaneous Sweet syndrome is a rare subtype, in which the neutrophilic infiltrate is exclusively or predominantly located in the subcutaneous tissue, causing lobular or septal panniculitis [1].

In recent years, there have been several reports of a distinct variant of Sweet syndrome, the so-called histiocytoid Sweet syndrome, characterized by an infiltrate composed of histiocytoid mononuclear cells, often with elongated vesicular nuclei and ample cytoplasm, which can lead to consider histiocytic, lymphocytic, or myeloid lineages as possibilities. The most striking immunohistochemical finding is the reactivity for myeloperoxidase in most of these cells, suggesting that they are immature myeloid cells, specifically neutrophil precursors [2]. Clinically, the lesions often present as dermal nodules which may mimic erythema nodosum, especially when they are located on the legs, but can be distinguished by different histological findings.

Sweet syndrome may represent a hypersensitivity or immunological phenomenon and is known to occur in association with many drugs, paraneoplastic and inflammatory conditions as inflammatory bowel disease, haematopoietic malignancies, or solid tumours [3]. Sweet syndrome is an unusual extraintestinal manifestation of Crohn's disease. In the few cases reported, there is predilection for adult women (87%), patients with colonic disease (100%), and those with other extraintestinal manifestations (77%) [4]. Although the relationship between skin and intestinal disease is variable, cutaneous manifestations were associated with active intestinal disease in 67–80% of cases but may precede the onset of intestinal symptoms in 21% [4].

We report a case of subcutaneous histiocytoid Sweet syndrome, a rare histopathological variant often described in patients with an underlying haematological disorder or caused by several drugs, but very rare in patients with inflammatory bowel disease [5, 6].

Our patient was an adolescent with Crohn's disease receiving pharmacological treatment. Although Sweet syndrome has been associated with certain drugs as azathioprine [7], in this case, skin lesions completely cleared despite continuing with all of the drugs.

Treatment is the same as in classic Sweet syndrome, with an excellent response to oral corticosteroids, alone or in combination with metronidazole, acting synergistically.

4. Conclusion

We report a case of histiocytoid Sweet syndrome with the distinct features of being the subcutaneous variant occurring in an adolescent with Crohn's disease. To our knowledge, this is the first case of subcutaneous histiocytoid Sweet syndrome in a paediatric patient.

Conflict of Interests

The authors declare that there is no conflict of interests regarding the publication of this paper.

References

[1] G. Guhl and A. García-Díez, "Subcutaneous Sweet síndrome," *Dermatologic Clinics*, vol. 26, pp. 541–551, 2008.

[2] L. Requena, H. Kutzner, G. Palmedo et al., "Histiocytoid Sweet syndrome: a dermal infiltration of immature neutrophilic granulocytes," *Archives of Dermatology*, vol. 141, no. 7, pp. 834–842, 2005.

[3] C. Y. Neoh, A. W. H. Tan, and S. K. Ng, "Sweet's syndrome: a spectrum of unusual clinical presentations and associations," *British Journal of Dermatology*, vol. 156, no. 3, pp. 480–485, 2007.

[4] S. Travis, N. Innes, M. G. Davies, T. Daneshmend, and S. Hughes, "Sweet's syndrome: an unusual cutaneous feature of Crohn's disease or ulcerative colitis. The South West Gastroenterology Group," *European Journal of Gastroenterology and Hepatology*, vol. 9, no. 7, pp. 715–720, 1997.

[5] S. Chow, S. Pasternak, P. Green et al., "Histiocytoid neutrophilic dermatoses and panniculitides: variations on a theme," *The American Journal of Dermatopathology*, vol. 29, no. 4, pp. 334–341, 2007.

[6] A. J. Wu, T. Rodgers, and D. R. Fullen, "Drug-associated histiocytoid Sweet's syndrome: a true neutrophilic maturation arrest variant," *Journal of Cutaneous Pathology*, vol. 35, no. 2, pp. 220–224, 2008.

[7] X. Treton, F. Joly, A. Alves, Y. Panis, and Y. Bouhnik, "Azathioprine-induced Sweet's syndrome in Crohn's disease," *Inflammatory Bowel Diseases*, vol. 14, no. 12, pp. 1757–1758, 2008.

54

Topical Pimecrolimus as a New Optional Treatment in Cutaneous Sarcoidosis of Lichenoid Type

Antonella Tammaro,[1] **Claudia Abruzzese,**[1] **Alessandra Narcisi,**[1]
Giorgia Cortesi,[1] **Francesca Romana Parisella,**[2] **Pier Paolo Di Russo,**[1]
Gabriella De Marco,[1] **and Severino Persechino**[1]

[1] *NESMOS Department, UOC Dermatology, Faculty of Medicine and Psychology, University of Rome "Sapienza", 00189 Rome, Italy*
[2] *Faculty of Medicine, University of Towson, Towson, MD 21204, USA*

Correspondence should be addressed to Claudia Abruzzese; abruzzeseclaudia@gmail.com

Academic Editors: L. Bianchi, X.-H. Gao, T. Hoashi, G. E. Piérard, H. Wong, and T. Yamamoto

We report the case of cutaneous sarcoidosis of lichenoid type successfully treated with pimecrolimus. For the first time in the literature, we propose the use of this topical calcineurin inhibitor for the treatment of the cases refractory to common therapy regimens.

1. Introduction

Lichenoid sarcoidosis is an extremely rare cutaneous manifestation of sarcoidosis, occurring in 1%-2% of all cases and presenting with multiple erythematous or violaceous, slightly scaling maculopapules localized on the trunk, limbs, and face, without systemic involvement. Different therapeutic approaches have been described for the treatment of cutaneous sarcoidosis, but the lesions are often refractory to the common treatments. We described the case of a female patient affected by cutaneous sarcoidosis of lichenoid type successfully treated with topical calcineurin inhibitor Pimecrolimus, never been reported in the literature until now.

2. A Case Report

A 66-year-old woman was referred to our department with a 6-month history of 1-2 mm diameter, violaceous, nonfollicular, infiltrated lichenoid papules with a tendency to group, located on the right knee (Figure 1(a)). The onset had been abrupt and no antecedent of trauma was found. She had been using a clobetasol ointment once daily for 2 months with no improvement of the lesions.

She did not complain of any systemic symptoms or take any kind of drugs. In the past medical history, no relevant diseases were referred, except for a papillary thyroid carcinoma excised 4 years before. General physical examination did not reveal any abnormality or lymphadenopathy. Cutaneous biopsy of one of the lesions revealed mild thinning of the epidermis, and a nonnecrotizing lymphohstiociytic granulomatous infiltrate in the superficial and deep dermis (Figures 2 and 3). Neither eosinophils nor mucin were seen. Gram stain, stain for fungi, and special stains for mycobacteria were negative. We also performed a videodermoscopy evaluation of the lesions, showing a round to oval yellow-brown lesion with absence of white Wickham striae (Figure 4).

Chest X-ray, eye examination, and blood tests, including complete blood count, hepatic and renal functions, serum angiotensin-converting enzyme, blood and urinary calcium, and beta-2-microglobulin, were all normal. A tuberculin reaction was also negative. Clinical and histological findings led to a diagnosis of cutaneous lichenoid sarcoidosis without systemic involvement. As treatment with topical corticosteroids had been ineffective, topical 1% pimecrolimus cream twice daily was prescribed. The patient was followed up monthly and after 6 months of treatment, we noted a

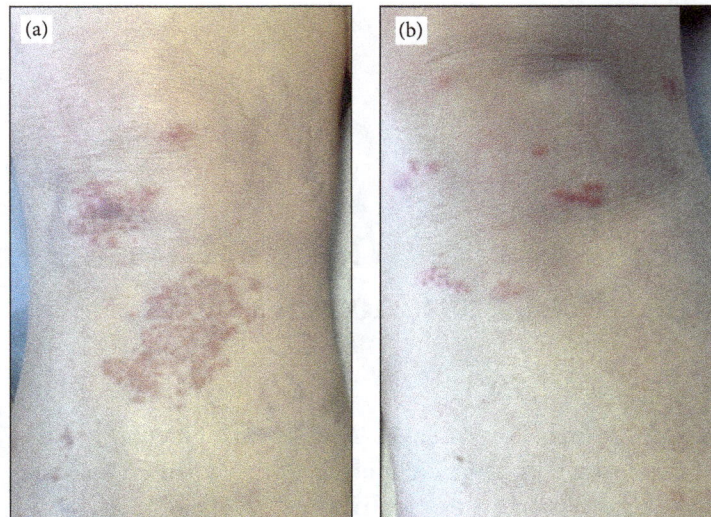

FIGURE 1: (a) Infiltrated, nonfollicular, lichenoid papules with a tendency to group, located on both knees; (b) a nearly complete remission of the lesions after 6-months therapy with topical 1% pimecrolimus.

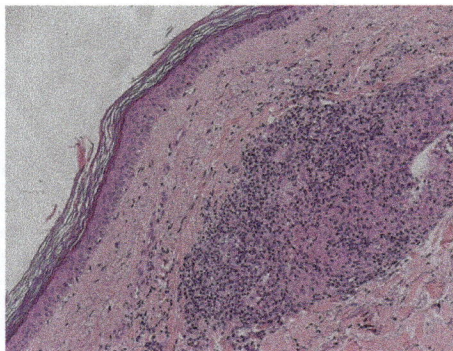

FIGURE 2: H&E staining, 100x magnification. Epidermis presents rete ridges flattening and orthotopic hyperkeratosis. In the deep dermal layer a sarcoidosis-like granulomatous reaction is visible.

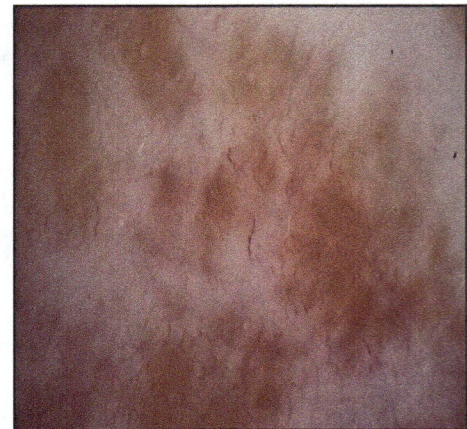

FIGURE 4: Videodermoscopic features: round to oval yellow-brown lesion with absence of white Wickham striae.

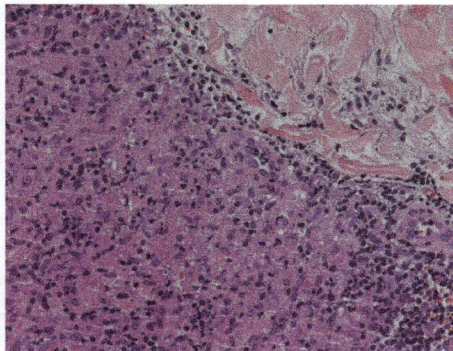

FIGURE 3: H&E staining, 200x magnification. Sarcoidosis-like granulomas are composed by epithelioid macrophages aggregates, surrounded by a scarce rime of small lymphocytes. Neither asteroid bodies nor Schaumann bodies were observed.

nearly complete remission of the lesions on the knee, with no topical and systemic adverse effects referred to by the patient (Figure 1(b)) and no relapses of the lesions at 12-month follow up.

3. Discussion

Sarcoidosis is a chronic multisystemic granulomatous disease of unknown etiology, characterized by the formation of noncaseating granulomas in the involved organs. Cutaneous involvement is about 25% and the most common clinical manifestations are maculopapular lesions, whereas lupus pernio is the most characteristic skin lesion.

The lichenoid-type lesion is an extremely rare cutaneous manifestation of sarcoidosis and is estimated in 1%-2% of all cases of skin sarcoidosis [1]. Clinically, the lichenoid type presents with multiple 1 to 3 mm, erythematous or violaceous, slightly scaling maculopapules involving an extensive area of the skin. They occur singly or in groups, especially localized on the trunk, limbs, and face. Dermoscopy usually shows round to oval yellow-brown lesion with absence of white Wickham striae; even if this pattern is not specific for sarcoidosis, these homogeneus patches are indicative of a granulomatous skin disease [2].

Lichenoid lesions have been particularly reported in young children, frequently presenting together with eye and joint complications, but respiratory involvement is usually absent [3, 4].

Diverse therapeutic approaches, including topical, intralesional, and systemic corticosteroids, antimalarials, methotrexate, tetracycline, infliximab, thalidomide, allopurinol, and isotretinoin, have been described in the management of cutaneous sarcoidosis; however, their efficacy varies and adverse effects, like the skin atrophy, sometimes limit their use. In the last decade an increasing interest derived from the use of topical calcineurin inhibitors (TCIs) in the treatment of cutaneous sarcoidosis [3, 5, 6].

Tacrolimus is a macrolide immunosuppressive agent isolated from *Streptomyces tsukubaensis* and modulates T-cell-mediated responses by inhibiting calcineurin-dependent dephosphorylation activation of the transcription factor NF-AT [7].

Pimecrolimus is a lipophilic macrolactamic agent isolated from ascomycin; it selectively modulates T-cell-mediated response binding with high affinity to macrophilin-12 and inhibiting calcineurin calcium-dependent phosphatase. These drugs, blocking the production and release of proinflammatory T helper1 cytokines and activation of T lymphocytes, have been successfully used in atopic dermatitis for many years [8].

It is supposed that, in sarcoidosis, granulomas may be caused by a series of factors, including Th1 cell activation by antigen-presenting cells (APC) and their cytokine release (IL2 and interferon-gamma) with a subsequent inflammatory cell recruitment and tissue infiltration; in addition, T lymphocytes and macrophages are responsible for an overproduction of TNF-alpha, amplifying the granulomatous reaction [6].

The ability of tacrolimus to inhibit both hapten-induced production of Th1 cytokines and the production of TNF-alpha by T cells and macrophages constitutes an effective rational for its use in the treatment of sarcoidosis [9]. In the literature are described few cases of cutaneous sarcoidosis treated with tacrolimus and only one case of lichenoid-type sarcoidosis treated with tacrolimus is reported [9–13].

Pimecrolimus has the same actions of tacrolimus but is more selective than tacrolimus in the modulation of immune cells: in fact it acts specifically on T lymphocytes and mast cells with a more antiinflammatory than immunosuppressive action, whereas tacrolimus also downregulates Langerhans cells and basophilic cells [14].

Moreover, pimecrolimus is more lipophilic and binds with higher affinity to structural skin proteins than tacrolimus, having a lower penetration rate in the dermis and a minor systemic biodisponibility [15].

These features allow a better efficacy and tolerability profile than tacrolimus, reducing the possibility of adverse systemic effects [16].

Based on the data in the literature about the use of topical tacrolimus in cutaneous sarcoidosis, we experienced the possibility to use also topical pimecrolimus in the treatment of lichenoid type of cutaneous sarcoidosis, deciding for a long-term treatment of six months for the appearance of relapses with a shorter therapy period, as described in previous cases reported in the literature [3].

The promising results we obtained let us define pimecrolimus as a useful therapeutic option for refractory forms of cutaneous sarcoidosis, besides representing a valuable alternative to tacrolimus for its better efficacy and tolerability profile.

Conflict of Interests

The authors declare that there is no conflict of interests regarding the publication of this paper.

References

[1] K. Fujii, H. Okamoto, M. Onuki, and T. Horio, "Recurrent follicular and lichenoid papules of sarcoidosis," *European Journal of Dermatology*, vol. 10, no. 4, pp. 303–305, 2000.

[2] F. Vazquez-Lopez, L. Palacios-Garcia, S. Gomez-Diez, and G. Argenziano, "Dermoscopy for discriminating between lichenoid sarcoidosis and lichen planus," *Archives of Dermatology*, vol. 147, no. 9, p. 1130, 2011.

[3] H. Tsuboi, K. Yonemoto, and K. Katsuoka, "A 14-year-old girl with lichenoid sarcoidosis successfully treated with tacrolimus," *Journal of Dermatology*, vol. 33, no. 5, pp. 344–348, 2006.

[4] S. K. Seo, J. S. Yeum, J. C. Suh, and G. Y. Na, "Lichenoid sarcoidosis in a 3-year-old girl," *Pediatric Dermatology*, vol. 18, no. 5, pp. 384–387, 2001.

[5] C. Badgwell and T. Rosen, "Cutaneous sarcoidosis therapy updated," *Journal of the American Academy of Dermatology*, vol. 56, no. 1, pp. 69–83, 2007.

[6] R. J. Young III, R. T. Gilson, D. Yanase, and D. M. Elston, "Cutaneous sarcoidosis," *International Journal of Dermatology*, vol. 40, no. 4, pp. 249–253, 2001.

[7] S. Sawada, G. Suzuki, Y. Kawase, and F. Takaku, "Novel immunosuppressive agent, FK506: in vitro effects of the cloned T cell activation," *Journal of Immunology*, vol. 139, no. 6, pp. 1797–1803, 1987.

[8] E. J. M. Van Leent, M. Gräber, M. Thurston, A. Wagenaar, P. I. Spuls, and J. D. Bos, "Effectiveness of the ascomycin macrolactam SDZ ASM 981 in the topical treatment of atopic dermatitis," *Archives of Dermatology*, vol. 134, no. 7, pp. 805–809, 1998.

[9] S. Vano-Galvan, M. Fernandez-Guarino, L. P. Carmona, A. Harto, R. Carrillo, and P. Jaén, "Lichenoid type of cutaneous sarcoidosis: great response to topical tacrolimus," *European Journal of Dermatology*, vol. 18, no. 1, pp. 89–90, 2008.

[10] V. de Francesco, A. S. Cathryn, and F. Piccirillo, "Successful topical treatment of cutaneous sarcoidosis with macrolide immunomodulators," *European Journal of Dermatology*, vol. 17, no. 5, pp. 454–455, 2007.

[11] R. Gutzmer, B. Völker, A. Kapp, and T. Werfel, "Successful topical treatment of cutaneous sarcoidosis with tacrolimus ointment," *Hautarzt*, vol. 54, no. 12, pp. 1193–1197, 2003.

[12] C. M. Green, "Topical tacrolimus for the treatment of cutaneous sarcoidosis," *Clinical and Experimental Dermatology*, vol. 32, no. 4, pp. 457–458, 2007.

[13] N. Katoh, H. Mihara, and H. Yasuno, "Cutaneous sarcoidosis successfully treated with topical tacrolimus," *British Journal of Dermatology*, vol. 147, no. 1, pp. 154–156, 2002.

[14] T. Zuberbier, S. U. Chong, K. Grunow et al., "The ascomycin macrolactam pimecrolimus (Elidel, SDZ ASM 981) is a potent inhibitor of mediator release from human dermal mast cells and peripheral blood basophils," *Journal of Allergy and Clinical Immunology*, vol. 108, no. 2, pp. 275–280, 2001.

[15] H. P. Gschwind, F. Waldmeier, M. Zollinger, A. Schweitzer, and M. Grassberger, "Pimecrolimus: skin disposition after topical administration in minipigs in vivo and in human skin in vitro," *European Journal of Pharmaceutical Sciences*, vol. 33, no. 1, pp. 9–19, 2008.

[16] H. M. Weiss, M. Fresneau, T. Moenius, A. Stuetz, and A. Billich, "Binding of pimecrolimus and tacrolimus to skin and plasma proteins: implications for systemic exposure after topical application," *Drug Metabolism and Disposition*, vol. 36, no. 9, pp. 1812–1818, 2008.

55

Treatment of a Refractory Skin Ulcer Using Punch Graft and Autologous Platelet-Rich Plasma

Mauro Carducci,[1] **Marcella Bozzetti,**[1] **Marco Spezia,**[2]
Giorgio Ripamonti,[3] **and Giuseppe Saglietti**[4]

[1]*Department of Dermatologic Surgery, Centro Ortopedico di Quadrante Hospital, 28882 Omegna, Italy*
[2]*Department of Orthopedics, Centro Ortopedico di Quadrante Hospital, 28882 Omegna, Italy*
[3]*Department of Medicine, Centro Ortopedico di Quadrante Hospital, 28882 Omegna, Italy*
[4]*Department of Metabolic Disease and Diabetology, ASL VCO, 28925 Verbania, Italy*

Correspondence should be addressed to Mauro Carducci; mauro.carducci@ospedalecoq.it

Academic Editor: Elizabeth Helen Kemp

Background. Chronic ulceration of the lower legs is a relatively common condition amongst adults: one that causes pain and social distress and results in considerable healthcare and personal costs. The technique of punch grafting offers an alternative approach to the treatment of ulcers of the lower limbs. *Objective.* Combining platelet-rich plasma and skin graft enhances the efficacy of treating chronic diabetic wounds by enhancing healing rate and decreasing recurrence rate. Platelet-rich plasma could, by stimulating dermal regeneration, increase the take rate after skin grafting or speed up reepithelialization. *Methods and Materials.* The ulcer was prepared by removing fibrin with a curette and the edges of the ulcer were freshened. The platelet-rich plasma has been infiltrated on the bottom and edges of the ulcer. The punch grafts were placed in 5 mm holes arranged. The ulcer was medicated with hydrogel and a pressure dressing was removed after 8 days. *Results.* After a few days the patient did not report more pain. Granulation tissue appeared quickly between implants. Most of the grafts were viable in 2-3 weeks. The grafts gradually came together to close the ulcer and were completed in four months.

1. Introduction

Chronic ulceration of the lower legs is a relatively common condition amongst adults: one that causes pain and social distress and results in considerable healthcare and personal costs [1, 2].

The 3 main types of lower extremity ulcers are venous, arterial, and neuropathic. Venous ulcers constitute the majority of all leg ulcers, whereas foot ulcers are more likely to be due to arterial insufficiency or neuropathy. Up to 80% of leg ulcers are caused by venous disease.

Treatment goals for patients with chronic venous insufficiency include reduction of edema, alleviation of pain, improvement of lipodermatosclerosis, healing of ulcers, and prevention of recurrence. Better understanding of the pathophysiology of venous disease and leg ulceration has in turn suggested new approaches to the management of ulcer disease with new types of wound dressings, compression bandages, topical and systemic therapeutic agents, and surgical modalities [3].

Surgical treatment of venous ulcers may be directed toward modifying the cause of venous hypertension or treating the ulcer itself by a graft. There are no specific indications for when skin grafting for lower extremity ulcers should be used. Larger or refractory ulcers are two instances when grafting should be considered. Even if grafts do not take, they likely stimulate wound that may rapidly and markedly relieve pain [4].

Wound healing is a complex process mediated by interacting molecular signals involving mediators and cellular events. Platelets play two important roles in wound healing: hemostasis and initiation of wound healing. After platelet activation and clot formation, growth factors are released from granules located in the thrombocyte cell membrane.

Growth factors work as biologic mediators to promote cellular activity by binding to specific cell surface receptors [5, 6].

Recent studies have found that autologous platelet concentrate with growth factors (APGF) or platelet-rich plasma (PRP) may accelerate wound healing [7].

There is also indication that platelet-rich plasma has infection-fighting properties and it has been proposed as an adjunct for the treatment of diabetic foot ulcers [8, 9]. Platelet-rich plasma is most often mixed with thrombin before application in order to generate a fibrin gel, often called platelet gel, and platelet-growth-factors-rich exudates [10].

The technique of punch grafting offers an alternative approach to the treatment of ulcers of the lower limbs. The method was first described by Reverdin [11] and later developed by Davis [12]; it is a relatively simple technique without immobilization of the patient, suited to the treatment of outpatients [13].

Good results were obtained regarding the reduction of pain and improvement in quality of life [14]. Similar results were obtained more recently by Swedish authors [15].

The method is also taken into consideration in the past American guidelines for the management of ulcers [16].

Combining platelet-rich plasma and skin graft enhances the efficacy of treating chronic diabetic wounds by enhancing healing rate and decreasing recurrence rate [17].

Autologous platelet gel could help to create a vascularised matrix, aiding the success of skin grafting in patients. Platelet-rich plasma could, by stimulating dermal regeneration, increase the take rate after skin grafting or speed up reepithelialization [18].

2. Case Presentation

Patient is a male, 77 years old, diabetic, and treated with oral hypoglycemic drugs and antihypertensive therapy, with good overall clinical condition. A mixed arterial and venous wide ulcer was localized in left ankle from three years. The patient has been followed up by an outpatient service of diabetes with topical treatments and advanced dressing with mixed results. The ulcer was extended over 50% of the circumference of the left ankle. The Achilles tendon was partially exposed. The patient was subjected to periodic Doppler ultrasound to check the venous and arterial circulation. The foot pulses were retained. The lesion was painful, in particular in the night hours. The ulcer was prepared by removing fibrin with a curette and the edges of the ulcer were freshened (Figure 1). Local anesthesia has been practiced around the ulcer and in the donor site graft. Platelet rich plasma was prepared using gravitational platelet heparinazed system. Briefly, the patient's phlebotomization consisted of 27 mL of whole blood and was drawn from the median cubital vein with a 21-gauge needle. One 30 mL syringe with 3 mL of anticoagulant citrate dextrose (ACD) solution formula 3 cc of platelet-rich plasma was extracted. Holes were drilled in the ulcer using a punch 5 mm while maintaining a distance of one centimeter between the holes (Figure 2).

The platelet-rich plasma has been infiltrated on the bottom and edges of the ulcer (Figure 3).

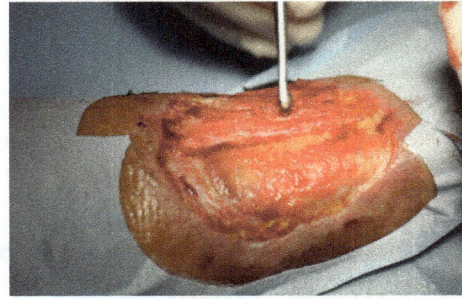

FIGURE 1: Right ankle: the ulcer was prepared by removing fibrin with a curette and the edges of the ulcer were freshened.

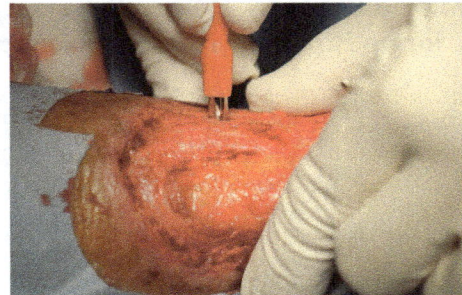

FIGURE 2: Holes were drilled in the ulcer using a punch 5 mm while maintaining a distance of one centimeter between the holes.

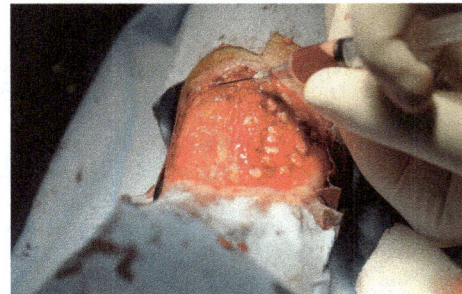

FIGURE 3: The platelet-rich plasma has been infiltrated on the bottom of the punch graft and edges of the ulcer.

From the donor sites, skin was harvested with a 6 mm biopsy punch. The grafts were removed with scissors and tweezers and placed on sterile, saline-moistened cotton dressings; the punch grafts were taken from the arm. The grafts were placed in 5 mm holes arranged. Local anesthesia has been practiced in the ulcer compared to the donor site graft. The ulcer was medicated with hydrogel and a pressure dressing was removed after 8 days, in successive weeks the wound was medicated with paraffin gauze.

If the ulcers are very extensive, you can perform surgery in 2 or 3 steps (Figure 5).

After a few days the patient no longer reported pain. Granulation tissue appeared quickly between the grafts. Most of the grafts took root after 2-3 weeks and started the development of the islands of epithelial tissue that gradually

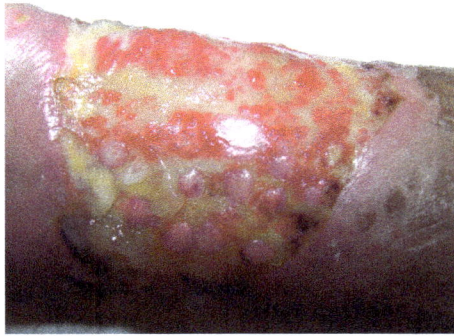

FIGURE 4: Epithelialization of the edge and epithelial islands inside the ulcer, one month later surgery treatment with punch grafting and platelet-rich plasma.

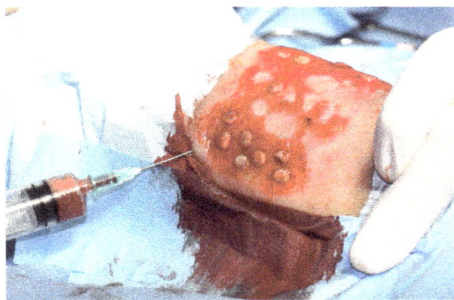

FIGURE 5: After 2 months we repeat intervention in areas not treated the first time. You can see the islands of reepithelialization of the previous treatment.

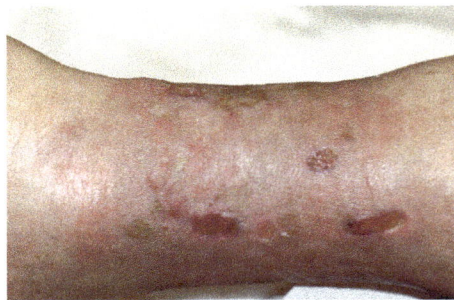

FIGURE 6: Complete reepithelialization after four months confirmed in follow-up, one year later.

came together to close the ulcer (Figure 4). The process of reepithelialization was completed in four months (Figure 6). The conditions of life of the patient are significantly improved by the absence of pain and the limited number of dressings.

3. Conclusion

The repair of leg ulcers causes discomfort to the patient with a high social cost.

The rapid healing of ulcers improves the patient's life by reducing the inconvenience of constant medication. The use of punch graft is a simple technique manageable even on

an outpatient that quickly reduces the pain and eases the reepithelialization ulcer. The use of punch graft increases the possibility that epithelial cells are developed and the fragmentation of the islands reduces the risk of failures (Figure 2).

We believe that the combined technique can benefit from the advantages of both methods.

Autologous platelet gel could help to create a vascularised matrix, aiding the success of skin grafting in patients. Platelet-rich plasma could, by stimulating dermal regeneration, increase the take rate after skin grafting or speed up reepithelialization. The repair process is accelerated by the use of platelet-rich plasma. The technique has been applied to a limited number of patients, but they all had an important reduction in pain and all ulcers treated were completely closed in a time ranging between 3 and 6 months. The follow-up at one year confirms the result (Figure 6).

We treated 9 patients with 11 ulcers resistant to conventional topical therapies. Three patients with 5 ulcers are still in follow-up.

Conflict of Interests

The authors declare that there is no conflict of interests regarding the publication of this paper.

References

[1] E. Lindsay, "The social dimension in leg ulcer management," *Primary Intention: The Australian Journal of Wound Management*, vol. 9, no. 1, pp. 31–33, 2001.

[2] O. R. Herber, W. Schnepp, and M. A. Rieger, "A systematic review on the impact of leg ulceration on patients' quality of life," *Health and Quality of Life Outcomes*, vol. 5, article 44, 2007.

[3] M. P. Goldman and A. Fronek, "Consensus paper on venous leg ulcer," *The Journal of Dermatologic Surgery and Oncology*, vol. 18, no. 7, pp. 592–602, 1992.

[4] R. S. Kirsner and V. Falanga, "Techniques of split-thickness skin grafting for lower extremity ulcerations," *Journal of Dermatologic Surgery and Oncology*, vol. 19, no. 8, pp. 779–783, 1993.

[5] E. Canalis, "Clinical review 35: growth factors and their potential clinical value," *Journal of Clinical Endocrinology and Metabolism*, vol. 75, no. 1, pp. 1–4, 1992.

[6] M. Rothe and V. Falanga, "Growth factors. Their biology and promise in dermatologic diseases and tissue repair," *Archives of Dermatology*, vol. 125, no. 10, pp. 1390–1398, 1989.

[7] R. L. Knox, A. R. Hunt, J. C. Collins, M. DeSmet, and S. Barnes, "Platelet-rich plasma combined with skin substitute for chronic wound healing: a case report," *Journal of Extra-Corporeal Technology*, vol. 38, no. 3, pp. 260–264, 2006.

[8] D. J. Margolis, J. Kantor, J. Santanna, B. L. Strom, and J. A. Berlin, "Effectiveness of platelet releasate for the treatment of diabetic neuropathic foot ulcers," *Diabetes Care*, vol. 24, no. 3, pp. 483–488, 2001.

[9] V. R. Driver, J. Hanft, C. P. Fylling, and J. M. Beriou, "A prospective, randomized, controlled trial of autologous platelet-rich plasma gel for the treatment of diabetic foot ulcers," *Ostomy Wound Management*, vol. 52, no. 6, pp. 68–74, 2006.

[10] P. Borzini and L. Mazzucco, "Platelet gels and releasates," *Current Opinion in Hematology*, vol. 12, no. 6, pp. 473–479, 2005.

[11] J. L. Reverdin, "Greffe épidermique—expérience faite dans le service de M. le docteurGuyon, à l'hôpital Necker," *Bulletin de la Société Impériale de Chirurgie de Paris*, vol. 10, pp. 511–515, 1869.

[12] J. Davis, "The use of small deep skin grafts," *The Journal of the American Medical Association*, vol. 63, no. 12, pp. 985–989, 1914.

[13] K. Steele, "Pinch grafting for chronic venous leg ulcers in general practice," *The Journal of the Royal College of General Practitioners*, vol. 35, no. 281, pp. 574–575, 1985.

[14] R. F. Öien, A. Håkansson, B. U. Hansen, and M. Bjellerup, "Pinch grafting of chronic leg ulcers in primary care: fourteen years' experience," *Acta Dermato-Venereologica*, vol. 82, no. 4, pp. 275–278, 2002.

[15] A. Nordström and C. Hansson, "Punch-grafting to enhance healing and to reduce pain in complicated leg and foot ulcers," *Acta Dermato-Venereologica*, vol. 88, no. 4, pp. 381–391, 2008.

[16] *Association for the Advancement of Wound Care (AAWC) Venous Ulcer Guideline*, Revised 2010, 2005.

[17] Y.-S. Tzeng, S.-C. Deng, C.-H. Wang, J.-C. Tsai, T.-M. Chen, and T. Burnouf, "Treatment of nonhealing diabetic lower extremity ulcers with skin graft and autologous platelet gel: a case series," *BioMed Research International*, vol. 2013, Article ID 837620, 9 pages, 2013.

[18] N. Pallua, T. Wolter, and M. Markowicz, "Platelet-rich plasma in burns," *Burns*, vol. 36, no. 1, pp. 4–8, 2010.

56

A 27-Year-Old Severely Immunosuppressed Female with Misleading Clinical Features of Disseminated Cutaneous Sporotrichosis

Atiyah Patel,[1] Victor Mudenda,[2] Shabir Lakhi,[1] and Owen Ngalamika[3]

[1]*Department of Medicine, University of Zambia School of Medicine, University Teaching Hospital, Lusaka, Zambia*
[2]*Pathology Department, University Teaching Hospital, Lusaka, Zambia*
[3]*Dermatovenereology Section, Department of Medicine, University of Zambia School of Medicine, University Teaching Hospital, Lusaka, Zambia*

Correspondence should be addressed to Owen Ngalamika; owen_ngalamika@yahoo.com

Academic Editor: Ravi Krishnan

Sporotrichosis is a subacute or chronic granulomatous mycosis caused by fungus of the *Sporothrix schenckii* complex. It is considered to be a rare condition in most parts of the world. It mostly causes cutaneous infection but can also cause multisystemic disease. Unlike most deep cutaneous mycoses which have a primary pulmonary focus, it is usually caused by direct inoculation of the fungus into the skin causing a classical linear, lymphocutaneous nodular eruption. However, atypical presentations of the condition can occur especially in immunosuppressed individuals. We report the case of a severely immunosuppressed female who presented with disseminated cutaneous sporotrichosis which was initially diagnosed and treated as disseminated cutaneous Kaposi's sarcoma.

1. Introduction

Sporotrichosis is a subacute or chronic granulomatous mycosis caused by fungus of the *Sporothrix schenckii* complex (including *S. albicans, S. brasiliensis, S. globosa, S. luriei, S. mexicana,* and *S. schenckii*) [1]. It occurs worldwide particularly in tropical/subtropical areas and temperate zones with warm and humid climates favoring the growth of saprophytic fungus. Cutaneous infection falls in the category of deep cutaneous mycoses. Unlike most deep cutaneous mycoses, infection is primarily through direct inoculation in the skin rather than dissemination from a primary pulmonary focus.

Since infection occurs following traumatic implantation of the causative fungus (naturally found in soil, plants, hay, and sphagnum moss), the most common clinical presentations include lymphocutaneous and fixed-cutaneous sporotrichosis occurring in persons handling soil or decaying plant material (miners, farmers, gardeners, florists, foresters, etc.) [2, 3]. Occasionally, inhalation of conidia may occur and cause pulmonary and disseminated infection [4]. However,

zoonotic transmission of the mycosis from infected animals like cats may also occur.

Disseminated cutaneous sporotrichosis or involvement of multiple visceral organs occurs most commonly in persons with immunosuppression [4]. However, there have been no documented cases of sporotrichosis in Zambia despite having a large burden of HIV disease. In this paper, we report the case of a 27-year-old HIV-positive female with severe immunosuppression who presented with atypical skin lesions of disseminated cutaneous sporotrichosis initially diagnosed and treated as disseminated cutaneous Kaposi's sarcoma (KS).

2. Case Report

A 27-year-old female was referred from a primary health care centre to the University Teaching Hospital (UTH) with a 3-week history of ill health. She complained of general body malaise, fever, night sweats, and a skin rash. She described the skin rash as having begun on the nose and subsequently spread to involve the upper limbs and trunk.

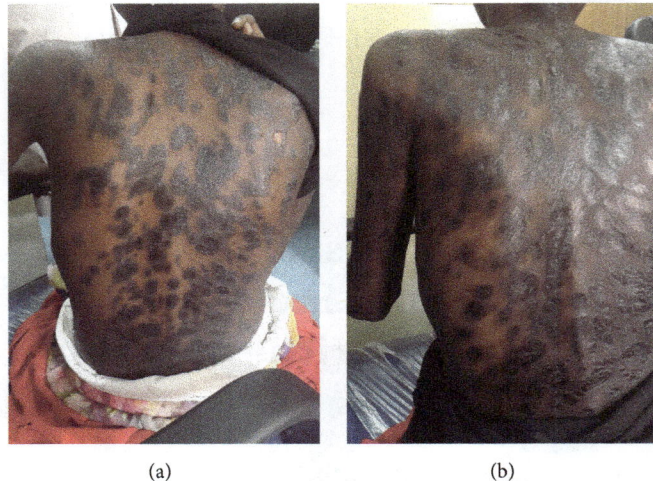

(a)   (b)

FIGURE 1: (a) Hyperpigmented plaques (elevated lesions) seen before commencement of treatment; (b) shiny hyperpigmented patches (flat lesions) of postinflammatory hyperpigmentation seen after 3 months of antifungal treatment.

TABLE 1: Initial investigations done at presentation.

Test	Result	Reference range
White cell count	1.56×10^9/L	4.00–10.00
Red cell count	2.73×10^{12}/L	4.13–5.67
Haemoglobin	6.4 g/dL	12.1–16.3
HCT	24.5%	35.0–47.0
MCV	89.7 fL	79.1–98.9
MCH	23.4 pg	27.0–32.0
MCHC	26.1 g/dL	32.0–36.0
Platelets	88×10^9/L	178–400
Kidney function tests	Normal	—
Liver function tests	Normal	—
CD4 absolute count	43 cells/μL	410–1590
Chest X-ray	Normal	—

HCT: haemotocrit, MCV: mean corpuscular volume, MCH: mean corpuscular haemoglobin, MCHC: mean corpuscular haemoglobin concentration.

She was also HIV-positive and had been commenced on antiretroviral therapy at the primary health care centre prior to presentation. Her baseline CD4 count was unknown. She had previously worked as a gardener for several years.

On physical examination, she was pale, chronically ill looking, and wasted. She had multiple, annular, hyperpigmented (purplish-black), slightly raised papules and plaques. A few lesions were ulcerated. The lesions were widespread but mostly involving the face, upper limbs, and trunk (Figure 1(a)). The rest of the examination was unremarkable.

Baseline investigations were done. Chest X-ray was normal. The full blood count revealed severe anemia with a pancytopenia for which she was given a blood transfusion. Upon further questioning, she admitted to receiving a cycle of anticancer chemotherapy. Her renal function tests as well as liver function tests were all normal (Table 1). Her CD4 count was 43 cells/μL. A presumptive clinical diagnosis of disseminated cutaneous KS was made based on the skin

lesions and HIV-induced immunosuppression, and a skin biopsy was done. During the course of the admission, the skin lesions were noted to be increasing in number and size. The patient was empirically given triple-agent anticancer chemotherapy for KS whilst awaiting histopathology results. No improvement was noted on anticancer chemotherapy and the patient once again developed severe anemia which was treated with blood transfusion and hematinics.

The histology showed a dermal nonspecific mixed inflammatory infiltrate which was predominantly chronic (lymphocytes and plasma cells). In and amongst the aggregates of inflammatory cells were round-shaped yeast organisms consistent with sporotrichosis. The overlying epidermis showed a mild degree of hyperplasia (Figure 2).

It was not possible to do the fungal culture immediately due to unavailability of culture media. The patient had a normal chest X-ray, no central nervous system manifestations, no joint pains, no bony lesions, and no pulmonary symptoms and signs. In the absence of symptoms and signs of other organ systems (despite anemia and pancytopenia attributed to anticancer chemotherapy) the condition was thought to only affect the skin, and no thorough systemic evaluations were indicated.

Our final diagnosis was disseminated cutaneous sporotrichosis. The patient was commenced on Itraconazole 200 mg once daily in addition to her antiretroviral therapy. Improvement in the skin lesions and general condition was noted after three months of therapy. The lesions became flat, and the nodules disappeared, leaving postinflammatory hyperpigmented patches (Figure 1(b)).

3. Discussion

Although HIV-infected patients are at increased risk of developing potentially life-threatening disseminated deep fungal infections, sporotrichosis is encountered relatively infrequently [5]. There is limited data on HIV/AIDS and

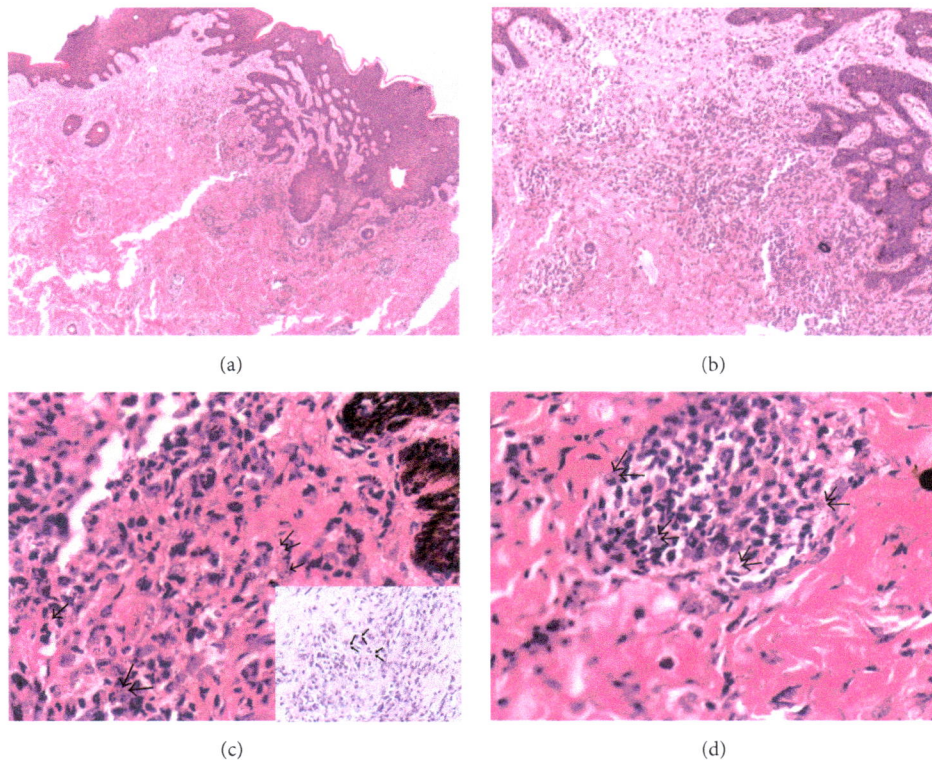

FIGURE 2: (a) Diffuse inflammatory infiltrate composed of chronic inflammatory cells and macrophages (H&E, ×40); (b) yeast-like forms widely dispersed in the dermis (H&E, ×100); (c) yeast-like forms widely dispersed in the dermis, black arrows pointing out the spores (H&E, ×400). Insert shows a period acid-Schiff stain with arrows pointing out the fungal spores; (d) a granuloma composed of macrophages containing *S. schenckii* organisms (H&E, ×400).

sporotrichosis coinfection. When it does occur, it is mostly disseminated and the CD4 count is usually very low [6].

Our patient presented with clinical and histopathological features highly suggestive of disseminated cutaneous sporotrichosis with no evidence of extracutaneous involvement. Considering that the patient was a gardener, it is possible that she was infected by accidental inoculation of the fungus at the primary site of disease.

Our patient was initially misdiagnosed as a case of KS. This is not surprising considering the purplish-black skin lesions that can easily give an impression of KS and the high prevalence of KS in our setting. Furthermore, the subtype of sporotrichosis that she had, the HIV-induced immunosuppression, and the effect of the anticancer chemotherapy may also have led to the misleading atypical clinical features. In immunocompetent individuals and those with the common classical lymphocutaneous sporotrichosis, clinical diagnosis is usually easy.

Culture is the gold standard in diagnosis and is also the most sensitive [7]. However, when culture is not feasible, histopathology can also be very useful, like in our patient, where characteristic histopathology features can guide the diagnosis [8]. Other fungal organisms that may show a similar histopathological picture include *Histoplasma capsulatum*, *Cryptococcus* species, and *Blastomyces dermatitidis*. Unlike sporotrichosis, histoplasmosis is mainly airborne, and

the disseminated form may also affect the mucous membranes. Yeasts of cryptococcosis have variable sizes and appear to have a clear halo on histology, with skin lesions mainly presenting as umbilicated papules with a central hemorrhagic crust. *Blastomyces dermatitidis* infection shows larger, broad-based yeasts on histology, with skin lesions presenting as painless verrucous ulcers. In addition, purely skin involvement without pulmonary involvement is highly unusual in histoplasmosis, cryptococcosis, and blastomycosis.

Treatment for sporotrichosis in immunocompetent hosts is well established. Itraconazole is the drug of choice for cutaneous, lymphocutaneous, and osteoarticular sporotrichosis. Fluconazole can also be used but is less effective than Itraconazole. Amphotericin B is required for severe pulmonary infection and disseminated systemic sporotrichosis [9]. Our patient was commenced on daily Itraconazole with significant clinical improvement noted after about six to eight weeks of treatment. In addition, initiation of highly active antiretroviral therapy was also an integral part in improving clinical response and promoting an adequate immune reconstitution.

Sporotrichosis is regarded to be a very rare disease in Zambia. Nonclassical forms occurring in HIV patients pose a great diagnostic challenge. Clinicians should have a high index of suspicion especially in immunosuppressed individuals who present with atypical skin lesions such as those seen in our patient. When sporotrichosis is suspected, ideally a culture should be obtained. In cases such as ours, where obtaining a culture is not possible, a presumptive diagnosis can be made based on highly suggestive clinical and histopathologic findings and treatment should be initiated. Should the patient not respond to treatment, alternative diagnoses should be strongly considered.

Conflict of Interests

The authors declare that there is no conflict of interests regarding the publication of this paper.

References

[1] E. López-Romero, M. D. R. Reyes-Montes, A. Pérez-Torres et al., "Sporothrix schenckii complex and sporotrichosis, an emerging health problem," *Future Microbiology*, vol. 6, no. 1, pp. 85–102, 2011.

[2] A. Bonifaz, A. Peniche, P. Mercadillo, and A. Saúl, "Successful treatment of AIDS-related disseminated cutaneous sporotrichosis with itraconazole," *AIDS Patient Care and STDS*, vol. 15, no. 12, pp. 603–606, 2001.

[3] V. K. Mahajan, "Sporotrichosis: an overview and therapeutic options," *Dermatology Research and Practice*, vol. 2014, Article ID 272376, 13 pages, 2014.

[4] M. T. M. Carvalho, A. P. de Castro, C. Baby, B. Werner, J. F. Neto, and F. Queiroz-Telles, "Disseminated cutaneous sporotrichosis in a patient with AIDS: report of a case," *Revista da Sociedade Brasileira de Medicina Tropical*, vol. 35, no. 6, pp. 655–659, 2002.

[5] S. A. Marques, A. M. Robles, A. M. Tortorano, M. A. Tuculet, R. Negroni, and R. P. Mendes, "Mycoses associated with AIDS in the third world," *Medical Mycology*, vol. 38, no. 1, pp. 269–279, 2000.

[6] J. A. S. Moreira, D. F. S. Freitas, and C. C. Lamas, "The impact of sporotrichosis in HIV-infected patients: a systematic review," *Infection*, vol. 43, no. 3, pp. 267–276, 2015.

[7] M. B. D. L. Barros, R. de Almeida Paes, and A. O. Schubach, "Sporothrix schenckii and sporotrichosis," *Clinical Microbiology Reviews*, vol. 24, no. 4, pp. 633–654, 2011.

[8] L. P. Quintella, S. R. Lambert Passos, A. C. Francesconi do Vale et al., "Histopathology of cutaneous sporotrichosis in Rio de Janeiro: a series of 119 consecutive cases," *Journal of Cutaneous Pathology*, vol. 38, no. 1, pp. 25–32, 2011.

[9] C. A. Kauffman, R. Hajjeh, and S. W. Chapman, "Practice guidelines for the management of patients with sporotrichosis. For the mycoses study group. Infectious diseases society of America," *Clinical Infectious Diseases*, vol. 30, no. 4, pp. 684–687, 2000.

57

Expansion of Natural Killer Cells in Peripheral Blood in a Japanese Elderly with Human T-Cell Lymphotropic Virus Type 1-Related Skin Lesions

Shinsaku Imashuku,[1] Naoko Kudo,[1] Kagekatsu Kubo,[2] and Kouichi Ohshima[3]

[1] *Division of Hematology, Takasago Seibu Hospital, 1-10-41 Nakasuji, Takasago 676-0812, Japan*
[2] *Division of Internal Medicine, Takasago Seibu Hospital, Takasago 676-0812, Japan*
[3] *Department of Pathology, School of Medicine, Kurume University, Kurume 830-0011, Japan*

Correspondence should be addressed to Shinsaku Imashuku; shinim95@mbox.kyoto-inet.or.jp

Academic Editor: Naoki Oiso

Natural killer (NK) cells were proposed to play an important role in the pathogenesis of human T-cell lymphotropic virus type 1-(HTLV-1-) associated neurologic disease. Our patient was a 77-year-old Japanese man, who had been treated for infective dermatitis associated with HTLV-1 for nearly 10 years. When referred to us, he had facial eczema/edema as well as extensive dermatitis at the neck/upper chest and nuchal area/upper back regions. Dermal lesions had CD3+CD4+ cells, but no NK cells. Flow cytometry of his peripheral blood showed a phenotype of CD2+ (97%), CD3+ (17%), CD4+ (12%), CD7+ (94%), CD8+ (6%), CD11c+ (70%), CD16+ (82%), CD19+ (0%), CD20+ (0%), CD56+ (67%), HLA-DR+ (68%), and NKp46+ (36%). Absolute numbers of CD56+NK cells in the peripheral blood were in a range of 986/μL–1,270/μL. The expanded NK cells in the peripheral blood are considered to be reactive, to maintain the confinement of the HTLV-1-positive CD4+ cells in the skin, and to prevent the progression of the disease.

1. Introduction

Among human T-cell lymphotropic virus type 1 (HTLV-1) infected individuals, adult T-cell leukemia/lymphoma (ATLL), and a chronic neurological disease, the HTLV-1-associated myelopathy/tropical spastic paraparesis (HAM/TSP) are two major symptomatic disorders. In addition, dermatological disorders are noted in 5–10% of the HTLV-1 infected patients [1]. The skin lesions could be either infectious or autoimmune dermatitis [2]. The infective dermatitis associated with HTLV-1 (IDH) is a chronic recurrent form of eczema affecting the scalp and retroauricular regions [1]. IDH may also progress to HAM/TSP or to ATLL [3]. Immunological features of IDH are similar to those of HAM/TSP [2]. However, expansion of natural killer (NK) cells has rarely been described in patients with IDH.

2. Case Report

We report here a 77-year-old Japanese man, who had been a carrier of HTLV-1 infection and treated for IDH with oral prednisolone (maximum dose was 40 mg/day) for nearly 10 years. When he was referred to us, he had fatigue, loss of appetite, and exacerbated facial eczema/edema as well as dermatitis at the neck/upper chest and nuchal area and upper back regions (Figure 1). He did not have any lymphadenopathy, hepatosplenomegaly, and clinical symptoms/signs of HAM/TSP. Laboratory data were as follows: WBC 4,700/μL, Hb 12.3 g/dL, platelet counts 91,000/μL, AST 74 U/L, ALT 45 U/L, LDH 882 U/L, BUN 16.5 mg/dL, creatinine 0.94 mg/dL, CRP 2.39 mg/dL, sIL-2R 1,280 U/mL, beta-2-microglobulin 6.5 mg/L, and ANA x40 positive, but complements were within normal. The patient had 22 copy/10e4

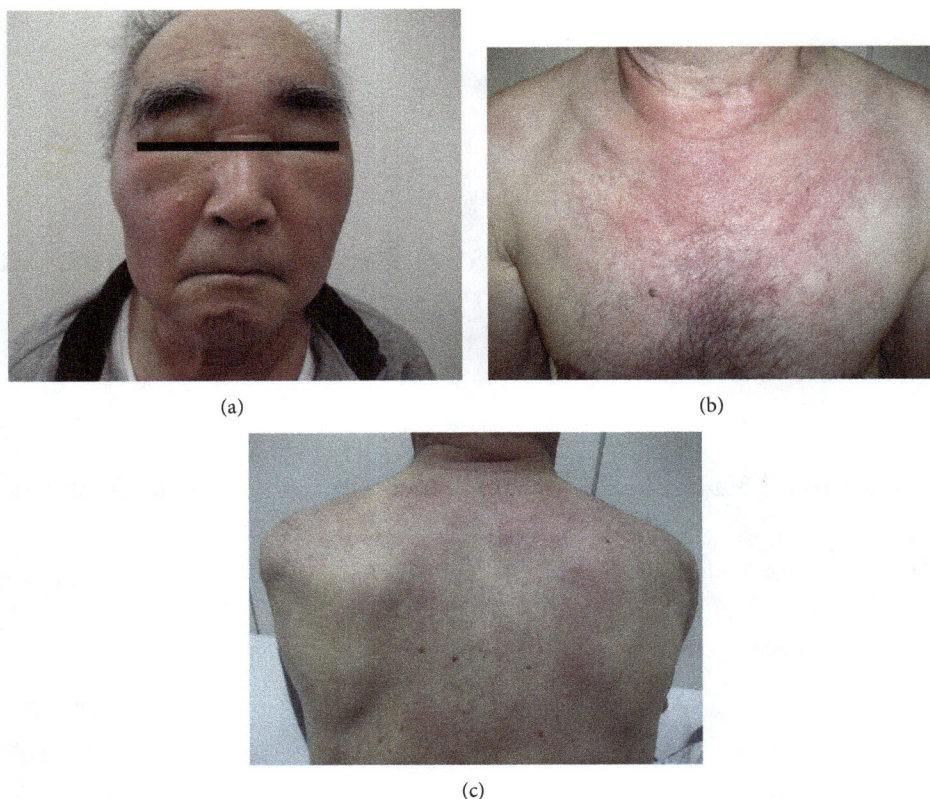

FIGURE 1: Facial edema/rash (a) and skin lesions at the neck/upper chest (b) as well as at the upper back (c).

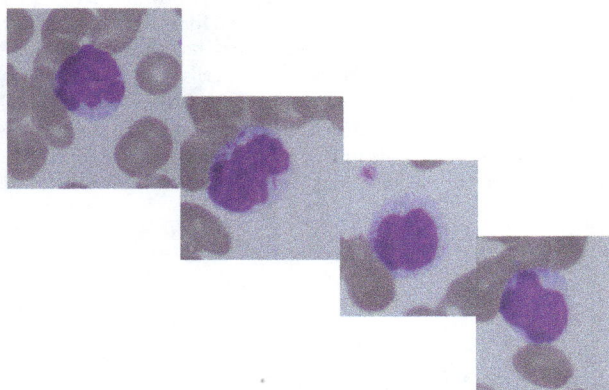

FIGURE 2: NK cells with azurophilic granules in the peripheral blood.

PBMCs of proviral HTLV-1 load (normal <20 copy/10e4), with positive anti-HTLV-1 antibody, consisting of western blot pattern of GP46 (+), p53 (+), p24 (+), and p19 (+). He showed a marked increase of granular lymphocytes with atypical nuclei in this peripheral blood (Figure 2) which were identified to be NK cells, with a phenotype of CD2+ (97%), CD3+ (17%), CD4+ (12%), CD7+ (94%), CD8+ (6%), CD19+ (0%), CD20+ (0%), CD11c+ (70%), CD16+ (82%), CD56+ (67%), HLA-DR+ (68%), and NKp46+ (36%). To rule out if these NK cells were in fact T cells with NK cell phenotype, we tested rearrangement of T-cell receptor (TCR) Cβ1 gene by southern blot analysis in the peripheral blood. Results showed no TCR rearrangement bands (data not shown). Thus, during the pretreatment period, absolute CD56+ NK cell counts in the peripheral blood were in a range of 986/μL–1,270/μL (reference values: 14–634/μL). Bone marrow smear showed hypocellular and hypoplastic marrow, with decreased numbers of megakaryocytes; however no abnormal features were noted. Flow cytometry of bone marrow revealed NK cell dominance as seen in the peripheral blood. Analysis of his peripheral blood as well as bone marrow showed a normal karyotype. On the other hand, infiltrating mononuclear cells in his dermis obtained by the skin biopsy of facial eczema were shown to be CD3+CD4+CD56-EBNA-. Only a few cells in this dermal area were stained with TIA-1 and Granzyme B (Figure 3). These findings were compatible with smoldering and chronic ATLL skin lesions. The patient was given a combination of weekly etoposide (100 mg/body) with dexamethasone (4 mg/body) for a total of 5 courses, when his skin lesions were markedly improved. Thereafter, the treatment was continued up to a total of 12 courses. This treatment resolved skin lesions but did not affect his NK cell-dominant features in the peripheral blood (data not shown).

3. Discussion

The clinical and pathological features of HTLV-1-associated cutaneous disease are diverse [4]. Our patient had chronic dermatitis at the face, neck area, and the upper back over

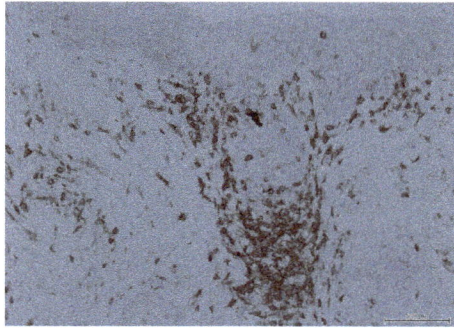

FIGURE 3: Microscopic findings of skin biopsy; CD4+ cells were infiltrated. These cells were CD3+, but no CD56+ cells or EBER+ cells were detectable. Also, only a few cells in this dermal area were stained with TIA-1 and Granzyme B (data not shown).

the period of ten years, in association with HTLV-1 antibody seropositivity but not with HAM/TSP as previously reported [5]. IDH is common in childhood; thus this case may not be a typical IDH, although report on adult-onset IDH was also available [6]. In patients with ATLL, peripheral blood generally shows the phenotype of CD2+CD3+CD4+CD7-CD8-, while in our patient it showed a pattern of CD2+CD3-CD4-CD7+CD8-CD16+CD56+, strongly suggesting NK cells. Although the possibility remained that these cells could be T cells with aberrant NK cell phenotype, lack of TCR $C\beta1$ rearrangement in these cells confirmed that they are actually NK cells.

In the past, Norris et al. demonstrated that in *in vitro* culture assay of 7 days, CD56+ NK cells spontaneously proliferated in response to HTLV-1. This spontaneous NK cell proliferation positively correlated with HTLV-1 proviral load, but not with the presence of HAM/TSP [7]. Besides this reactive NK cell proliferation, HTLV-1-infected NK cells were also documented; however, the HTLV-1-infected NK cells were not immortal and were phenotypically indistinguishable from their uninfected counterparts [8]. Coelho-dos-Reis et al. described a statistically significant increase, but not as magnificent as ours, of the macrophage-like subset (CD14 + CD16+) or NK cell subset in the HTLV-1-infected group with skin lesions. In their patients, high levels of proviral load were noted with an increase of NK cells [2]. By contrast, in our case, striking NK cell expansion was not associated with increased proviral load. The critical question in our case is whether these NK cells are reactive or neoplastic in nature. Ohshima et al. showed that HTLV-1-infected CD8+ and/or CD56+ cells probably confer no cytotoxic function [9]. Considering the fact that the NK cells in our case contain abundant granules, in association with barely detectable provirus load and normal karyotype, the expansion of NK cells in our case could be reactive and may play an immunoregulatory role preventing the progression of IDH to HAM/TSP. Treatment of IDH has not yet been established and there are still few treatment options [10]. In our case, we treated with a total of 12 courses of etoposide/dexamethasone. Although skin rash resolved significantly with this treatment, we hope that expanded NK cells may also act to maintain the confinement

of the HTLV-1-positive CD4+ cells in the skin and prevent the progression from IDH to the HAM/TSP stage of the disease. However, since CD4+ T cells did not coexist with NK-cells in the skin biopsy sample, this beneficial effect may be achieved through cytokines released from expanded NK cells. Although a possibility may remain that NK cells could be infected with HTLV-1 in future, as demonstrated by Steve Lo et al. [8], it is assumed that our patient clinically verifies the previously observed *in vitro* phenomenon that HTLV-1 primarily drives expansion of CD56+ NK cells.

Consent

A written informed consent was obtained from the patient for publication of this case report. A copy of the written consent is available for review.

Conflict of Interests

The authors declare that there is no conflict of interests regarding the publication of this paper.

Acknowledgment

The authors thank Dr. Atsuko Adachi, Hyogo Prefectural Kakogawa Medical Center, for referring the patient.

References

[1] A. L. Bittencourt and M. D. F. P. D. Oliveira, "Cutaneous manifestations associated with HTLV-1 infection," *International Journal of Dermatology*, vol. 49, no. 10, pp. 1099–1110, 2010.

[2] J. G. A. Coelho-dos-Reis, L. Passos, M. C. Duarte et al., "Immunological profile of HTLV-1-infected patients associated with infectious or autoimmune dermatological disorders," *PLoS Neglected Tropical Diseases*, vol. 7, no. 7, Article ID e2328, 2013.

[3] N.-K. McGill, J. Vyas, T. Shimauchi, Y. Tokura, and V. Piguet, "HTLV-1-associated infective dermatitis: updates on the pathogenesis," *Experimental Dermatology*, vol. 21, no. 11, pp. 815–821, 2012.

[4] S. J. Whittaker, Y. L. Ng, M. Rustin, G. Levene, D. H. McGibbon, and N. P. Smith, "HTLV-1-associated cutaneous diseas: a clinicopathological and molecular study of patients from the U.K," *British Journal of Dermatology*, vol. 128, no. 5, pp. 483–492, 1993.

[5] R. Okajima, J. Casseb, and J. A. Sanches, "Co-presentation of human T-cell lymphotropic virus type 1 (HTLV-1)-associated myelopathy/tropical spastic paraparesis and adult-onset infective dermatitis associated with HTLV-1 infection," *International Journal of Dermatology*, vol. 52, no. 1, pp. 63–68, 2013.

[6] L. Maragno, J. Casseb, L. M. I. Fukumori et al., "Human T-cell lymphotropic virus type 1 infective dermatitis emerging in adulthood," *International Journal of Dermatology*, vol. 48, no. 7, pp. 723–730, 2009.

[7] P. J. Norris, D. F. Hirschkorn, D. A. Devita, T.-H. Lee, and E. L. Murphy, "Human T cell leukemia virus type 1 infection drives spontaneous proliferation of natural killer cells," *Virulence*, vol. 1, no. 1, pp. 19–28, 2010.

[8] K. M. Steve Lo, E. Vivier, N. Rochet et al., "Infection of human natural killer (NK) cells with replication-defective human T cell

leukemia virus type I provirus: Increased proliferative capacity and prolonged survival of functionally competent NK cells," *Journal of Immunology*, vol. 149, no. 12, pp. 4101–4108, 1992.

[9] K. Ohshima, S. Haraoka, J. Suzumiya et al., "Absence of cytotoxic molecules in CD8- and/or CD56-positive adult T-cell leukaemia/lymphoma," *Virchows Archiv*, vol. 435, no. 2, pp. 101–104, 1999.

[10] M. Amano, M. Setoyama, A. Grant, and F. A. Kerdel, "Human T-lymphotropic virus 1 (HTLV-1) infection—dermatological implications," *International Journal of Dermatology*, vol. 50, no. 8, pp. 915–920, 2011.

Permissions

List of Contributors

Prabhath Ramakrishnan, Vijay Sylvester, Prathima Sreenivasan and Janisha Vengalath
Department of Oral Medicine and Radiology, Kannur Dental College, Anjarakandy, Kannur, Kerala 670612, India

Smruthi Valambath
Department of Physiology, SDM College of Medical Sciences, Dharwad, Karnataka 580009, India

Dietrich Barth
Hautarztpraxis Leipzig/Borna, Rudolf Virchow Straße, Borna, 04552 Leipzig, Germany

Guillermo Antonio Guerrero-González, Maira Elizabeth Herz-Ruelas, Minerva Gómez-Flores, and Jorge Ocampo-Candiani
Dermatology Department, Hospital Universitario "Dr. José Eleuterio González," Universidad Autónoma de Nuevo León, Avenida Francisco I. Madero Poniente s/n y Avenida Gonzalitos, Colonia Mitras Centro, 64460 Monterrey, NL, Mexico

Zaheer Abbas and Zahra Safaie Naraghi
Department of Dermatology, Razi Hospital, Tehran University of Medical Sciences, Vahdate Eslami Square, Vahdate Eslami Avenue, Tehran 11996, Iran

Elham Behrangi
Department of Dermatology, Rasoul-e Akram Hospital, Iran University of Medical Sciences, Tehran, Iran

Amresh Kumar Singh
Department of Microbiology, BRD Medical College, Gorakhpur, Uttar Pradesh 273013, India

Rungmei S. K.Marak, Manaswini Das and Tapan N. Dhole
Department of Microbiology, Sanjay Gandhi Post Graduate Institute of Medical Sciences, Lucknow 226014, India

Anand Kumar Maurya and Vijaya Lakshmi Nag
Department of Microbiology, All India Institute of Medical Sciences, Jodhpur 342005, India

Misbah Nasheela Ghazanfar
Department of Dermatology, Bispebjerg Hospital, 2400 Copenhagen NV, Denmark

Simon Francis Thomsen
Department of Dermatology, Bispebjerg Hospital, 2400 Copenhagen NV, Denmark
Center for Medical Research Methodology, Department of Biomedical Sciences, University of Copenhagen, 2200 Copenhagen N, Denmark

María Fernández-Ibieta
Pediatric Surgery Service, Hospital CU Virgen de la Arrixaca, El Palmar s/n, 30150 Murcia, Spain

Juan Carlos López-Gutiérrez
Vascular Anomalies Unit, Pediatric Surgery Department, Hospital La Paz, Madrid, Spain

Stephanie Nemir
Division of Plastic Surgery, Department of Surgery, University of Texas Medical Branch, Galveston, TX 77555, USA

Lindsey Hunter-Ellul and Richard Wagner
Department of Dermatology, University of Texas Medical Branch, Galveston, TX 77555, USA

Vlad Codrea
School of Medicine, University of Texas Medical Branch, Galveston, TX 77555, USA

Habib Ansarin
Department of Dermatology, Hazrat-e Rasool University Hospital, Iran University of Medical Sciences, Tehran, Iran

Hoda Berenji Ardestani
Skin and Stem Cell Research Center, Tehran University of Medical Sciences, Kamraniye Street, No. 4, Maryam Alley, Tehran 1937957511, Iran

Seyed Mehdi Tabaie
Iranian Center for Medical Laser, Academic Center for Education, Culture and Research, Tehran, Iran

Nasrin Shayanfar
Department of Pathology, Iran University of Medical Sciences, Tehran, Iran

Pelin Üstüner
Dermatology Clinic, Rize State Hospital, Eminettin Mahallesi, 53100 Rize, Turkey

Nadia Abidi, Kristen Foering and Joya Sahu
Department of Dermatology, Jefferson Medical College, Thomas Jefferson University, 833 Chestnut Street, Suite 740, Philadelphia, PA 19107, USA

Rahul Mannan, Sanjay Piplani, Harjot Kaur and Harleen Kaur
Department of Pathology, SGRDIMSR, Amritsar, Punjab 143001, India

Jasmine Kaur
Department of Oral and Maxillofacial Surgery, SGRDIMSR, Amritsar, Punjab, India

Jasleen Kaur
Department of Dermatology, SGRDIMSR, Amritsar, Punjab, India

Laura Maffeis, Lorenza Pugni, Carlo Pietrasanta, Andrea Ronchi, Monica Fumagalli and Fabio Mosca
NICU, Department of Clinical Sciences and Community Health, Fondazione IRCCS Ca' Granda Ospedale Maggiore Policlinico, University of Milan, Via della Commenda 12, 20122 Milan, Italy

Carlo Gelmetti
Pediatric Dermatology Unit, Fondazione IRCCS Ca' Granda Ospedale Maggiore Policlinico, University of Milan, Via Pace 9, 20122 Milan, Italy

Maira Elizabeth Herz-Ruelas, Minerva Gómez-Flores and Guillermo Antonio Guerrero-González
Dermatology Department, Hospital Universitario "Dr. José Eleuterio González," Universidad Autónoma de Nuevo León, Monterrey, Mexico

Joaquín Moxica-del Angel and Adriana Orelia Villarreal-Rodríguez
Christus Mugerza Sur Hospital, Monterrey, Mexico

Ivett Miranda-Maldonado
Pathology Department, Hospital Universitario "Dr. José Eleuterio González," Universidad Autónoma de Nuevo León, Monterrey, Mexico

Ilse Marilú Gutiérrez-Villarreal
School of Medicine, Universidad Autónoma de Nuevo León, Monterrey, Mexico

Beata Sosada, Katarzyna Loza and Ewelina Bialo-Wojcicka
Department of Dermatology, Miedzyleski Specialist Hospital in Warsaw, ul. Bursztynowa 2, 04-479 Warsaw, Poland

Dhiraj Jain and Stalin Viswanathan
Department of General Medicine, Indira Gandhi Medical College & RI, Pondicherry 605009, India

Chandramohan Ramasamy
Department of Cardiology, Jawaharlal Institute of Postgraduate Medical Education and Research, Pondicherry 605006, India

Andressa Gonçalves Amorim, Brunelle Batista Fraga Mendes and Antônio Chambô Filho
Department of Obstetrics and Gynecology, Santa Casa de Misericórdia Hospital, 29025-023 Vitória, ES, Brazil

Rodrigo Neves Ferreira
Pathology Department, Santa Casa de Misericórdia Hospital, Dr. João dos Santos Neves Street 143, 29025-023 Vitória, ES, Brazil

André Laureano and Jorge Cardoso
Department of Dermatology and Venereology, Hospital de Curry Cabral, Centro Hospitalar de Lisboa Central, 1069-166 Lisboa, Portugal

Fu-qiu Li, Sha Lv, and Jian-xin Xia
The Second Hospital of Jilin University, Changchun, Jilin 130000, China

Hilal Kaya Erdoğan and Işıl Bulur
Department of Dermatology, Eskisehir Osmangazi University, 26480 Eskisehir, Turkey

Zeliha Kaya
Department of Pathology, Kırsehir Ahi Evran University, 40200 Kirsehir, Turkey

Caroline Balvedi Gaiewski, Sergio Zuneda Serafini and Janyana M. D. Deonizio
Dermatology Department, Federal University of Parana, 80530-905 Curitiba, PR, Brazil

Betina Werner
Pathology Department, Federal University of Parana, 80530-905 Curitiba, PR, Brazil

Rosanna Qualizza
Allergy Service, Istituti Clinici di Perfezionamento, 20100 Milan, Italy

Eleni Makrì and Cristoforo Incorvaia
Allergy/Pulmonary Rehabilitation, Istituti Clinici di Perfezionamento, 20100 Milan, Italy

Laura Losappio
General Medicine, University of Foggia, 71100 Foggia, Italy

Asli Feride Kaptanoglu and Didem Mullaaziz
Department of Dermatology, Near East University Hospital, Lefkosa, North Cyprus, Mersin 10, Turkey

Kaya Suer
Department of Infectious Diseases and Clinical Microbiology, Near East University Hospital, Lefkosa, North Cyprus, Mersin 10, Turkey

Ambika Gupta and Harneet Singh
Department of Oral Medicine and Radiology, Pandit B.D. Sharma UHS (PGIDS), Rohtak, Haryana, India

Rikinder Sandhu, Zaw Min and Nitin Bhanot
Department of Medicine, Allegheny General Hospital, 420 East North Avenue, Allegheny Health Network, Pittsburgh, PA 15212, USA

Sama Kassira, Tarannum Jaleel, Peter Pavlidakey and Naveed Sami
Department of Dermatology, University of Alabama at Birmingham, EFH 414, 1530 3rd Avenue S, Birmingham, AL 35294, USA

Betül Ünal, Cumhur İbrahim Başsorgun, Meryem İlkay Eren Karanis and Gülsüm Özlem Elpek
School of Medicine, Department of Pathology, Akdeniz University, 07070 Antalya, Turkey

Jeyanthini Risikesan and Troels Herlin
Department of Pediatrics, Aarhus University Hospital, 8200 Aarhus N, Denmark

Uffe Koppelhus and Mette Deleuran
Department of Dermatology, Aarhus University Hospital, Aarhus C, 8000 Aarhus, Denmark

Torben Steiniche
Department of Pathology, Aarhus University Hospital, Aarhus C, 8000 Aarhus, Denmark

David Veitch, Georgios Kravvas and Christopher Bunker
Department of Dermatology, University College London Hospitals, London NW1 2BU, UK

Sian Hughes
Department of Histopathology, University College London Hospitals, London NW1 2BU, UK

Sumir Kumar, B. B. Mahajan and Amarbir Singh
GGS Medical College & Hospital, Sadiq Road, Faridkot, Punjab 151203, India

Sandeep Kaur
GGS Medical College & Hospital, Sadiq Road, Faridkot, Punjab 151203, India
Skin OPD, GGS Medical College & Hospital, OPD Block, 1st Floor, Sadiq Road, Faridkot, Punjab 151203, India

Elizabeth A. Brezinski, Maxwell A. Fung and Nasim Fazel
Department of Dermatology, Davis Health System, University of California, 3301 C Street, Suite 1400, Sacramento, CA 95816, USA

Nida Iqbal and Vinod Raina
Department of Medical Oncology, Dr. B. R. A. Institute Rotary Cancer Hospital, All India Institute of Medical Sciences, New Delhi 110029, India

Isil Bulur, Hilal Kaya Erdoğan and Zeynep Nurhan Saracoglu
Department of Dermatology and Venereology, Faculty of Medicine, Osmangazi University, Eskişehir, Turkey

Deniz ArJk
Department of Pathology, Faculty of Medicine, Osmangazi University, Eskişehir, Turkey

Hasan Tak, Gülben SarJcJ, NazlJ Dizen Namdar and Mehtap KJdJr
Department of Dermatology, Faculty of Medicine, Dumlupinar University, 43100 Kutahya, Turkey

Cengiz Koçak
Department of Pathology, Faculty of Medicine, Dumlupinar University, 43100 Kutahya, Turkey

Ferit KulalJ, Ahmet Yagmur Bas, Yusuf Kale, Istemi Han Celik and Nihal Demirel
Division of Neonatology, Etlik Zübeyde Hanim Women's Health Teaching and Research Hospital, Ankara, Turkey

Sema ApaydJn
Department of Pathology, Dr. Sami Ulus Maternity and Children Research and Training Hospital, Ankara, Turkey

Andrés González García, Ignacio Barbolla Díaz and Guadalupe Fraile
Department of Internal Medicine, University Hospital Ramón y Cajal, Madrid, Spain

Emiliano Grillo Fernández and Asunción Ballester
Department of Dermatology, University Hospital Ramón y Cajal, Madrid, Spain

Héctor Pian
Department of Pathology, University Hospital Ramón y Cajal, Madrid, Spain

Preeti Jadhav, Hassan Tariq and Giovanni Franchin
Bronx Lebanon Hospital Center, Department of Medicine, 1650 Selwyn Avenue, Suite No. 10C, Bronx, NY 10457, USA

Masooma Niazi
Bronx Lebanon Hospital Center, Department of Pathology, 1650 Grand Concourse, Bronx, NY 10457, USA

Estefânia Correia
Family Practice Unit of Pedras Rubras, Rua Divino Salvador de Moreira 160, 4470-105 Maia, Portugal

António Santos
Department of Dermatology, Portuguese Institute of Oncology, Portugal

Fabio Guerriero, Giovannoi Ricevuti, Carmelo Sgarlata, Niccolò Maurizi and Matthew Francis
Department of Internal Medicine and Medical Therapy, Section of Geriatrics, University of Pavia, 27100 Pavia, Italy
Agency for Elderly People Services, Hospital Santa Margherita, 27100 Pavia, Italy
Ambra Elektron, Associazione Italiana di Biofisica per lo Studio dei Campi Elettromagnetici in Medicina, 00186 Rome, Italy

Marco Rollone and Davide Guido
Agency for Elderly People Services, Hospital Santa Margherita, 27100 Pavia, Italy
Department of Public Health, Experimental and Forensic Medicine, Biostatistics and Clinical Epidemiology Unit, University of Pavia, 27100 Pavia, Italy

Emanuele Botarelli, Gianni Mele, Lorenzo Polo, Daniele Zoncu, Paolo Renati and Piero Mannu
Ambra Elektron, Associazione Italiana di Biofisica per lo Studio dei Campi Elettromagnetici in Medicina, 00186 Rome, Italy
Alberto Sorti Research Institute, Medicine and Metamolecular Biology, 10122 Turin, Italy

Mariangela Rondanelli and Simone Perna
Department of Public Health, Experimental and Forensic Medicine, Section of Human Nutrition, Endocrinology and Nutrition Unit, University of Pavia, 27100 Pavia, Italy

Hatice Uludag Altun, Tuba Meral and Emel Turk Aribas
Department of Clinical Microbiology, Faculty of Medicine, Turgut Ozal University, Emek, 06510 Ankara, Turkey

Canan Gorpelioglu
Department of Dermatology, Faculty of Medicine, Turgut Ozal University, Emek, 06510 Ankara, Turkey

Nilgun Karabicak
Mycology Reference Laboratory, Public Health Institution of Turkey, Sıhhıye, 06100 Ankara, Turkey

Enzo Errichetti, Giuseppe Stinco and Pasquale Patrone
Institute of Dermatology, Department of Experimental and Clinical Medicine, University of Udine, San Michele Hospital, Piazza Rodolone 1, Gemona del Friuli, 33013 Udine, Italy

Enrico Pegolo
Institute of Anatomic Pathology, Department of Medical and Biological Sciences, University of Udine, University Hospital of Santa Maria della Misericordia, Piazzale Santa Maria della Misericordia 15, 33100 Udine, Italy

Nicola di Meo and Giusto Trevisan
Institute of Dermatology and Venereology, University of Trieste, Maggiore Hospital, Piazza Ospedale 1, 34100 Trieste, Italy

Kalliopi Armyra, Anargyros Kouris, Arsinoi Xanthinaki, Alexandros Stratigos and Irene Potouridou
Department of Dermatology and Venereology, Hospital "Andreas Sygros", Ionos Dragoumi 5, 16121 Athens, Greece

Jose Maria Pereira de Godoy
Cardiology and Cardiovascular Surgery Department, Medicine School in São José do Rio Preto (FAMERP), Avenida Constituição 1306, 15025120 São José do Rio Preto, SP, Brazil

Daniel Zucchi Libanore
Research Group in Godoy Clinic, Avenida Constituição 1306, 15025120 São José do Rio Preto, SP, Brazil

Maria de Fatima Guerreiro Godoy
Medicine School in São José do Rio Preto (FAMERP) and Research Group in Godoy Clinic, Avenida Constituição 1306, 15025120 São José do Rio Preto, SP, Brazil

K. Kouakou and M. E. Dainguy
Department of Pediatrics, Training and Research Unit of Medical Sciences, Felix Houphouët Boigny University of Abidjan, Côte d'Ivoire

K. Kassi
Department of Dermatology and Infectiology, Training and Research Unit of Medical Sciences, Felix Houphouët Boigny University of Abidjan, BP 5151, Abidjan 21, Côte d'Ivoire

Hajime Deguchi, Riho Aoyama and Hideaki Takahashi
Fujita Health University School of Medicine, Toyoake, Aichi 470-1192, Japan
Department of Pathology, Fujita Health University School of Medicine, Toyoake, Aichi 470-1192, Japan

Yutaka Tsutsumi
Department of Pathology, Fujita Health University School of Medicine, Toyoake, Aichi 470-1192, Japan

Yoshinari Isobe
Isobe Clinic, Anjo, Aichi 446-0026, Japan

Seth L. Cornell
Department of Medicine, Tripler Army Medical Center, Honolulu, HI 96859, USA

Daniel DiBlasi and Navin S. Arora
Dermatology Service, Tripler Army Medical Center, Honolulu, HI 96859, USA

F. A. Sendrasoa, I.M. Ranaivo, O. Raharolahy, M. Andrianarison, L. S. Ramarozatovo, and F. Rapelanoro Rabenja
Department of Dermatology, Joseph Raseta Befelatanana Hospital, 101 Antananarivo, Madagascar

Jared Martínez-Coronado, Bertha Torres-Álvarez, and Juan Pablo Castanedo-Cázares
Department of Dermatology, Hospital Central "Dr. Ignacio Morones Prieto", Universidad Autonoma de San Luis Potosí, 2395 Venustiano Carranza Avenue, 78210 San Luis Potosí, SLP, Mexico

Michelle Fog Andersen
Department of Otorhinolaryngology, Head and Neck Surgery, Køge Hospital, Lykkebaekvej 1, 4600 Køge, Denmark

Anette Bygum
HAE Centre Denmark, Department of Dermatology and Allergy Centre, Odense University Hospital, Sdr. Boulevard 29, Entrance 142, 5000 Odense C, Denmark

Alexandra Caitlin Perel- Winkler
St. Luke's-Roosevelt Hospital Center, New York, NY 10025, USA

Chris T. Derk
Division of Rheumatology, University of Pennsylvania, One Convention Boulevard, 8th Floor Penn Tower, Philadelphia, PA 19104, USA

Pankti Jariwala, Vinay Kumar, Khyati Kothari and Dipak Dayabhai Umrigar
Department of Skin & VD, Government Medical College & New Civil Hospital, Surat, Gujarat 395001, India

Sejal Thakkar
Department of Skin & VD, GMERS Medical College & General Hospital, Gotri 202, Wings Ville 41, Arunoday Society, Alkapuri, Vadodara, Gujarat 390001, India

Adrián Imbernón-Moya, Elena Vargas-Laguna, Antonio Aguilar and Miguel Ángel Gallego
Department of Dermatology, Hospital Universitario Severo Ochoa, Avenida de Orellana, Leganés, 28911 Madrid, Spain

Claudia Vergara and María Fernanda Nistal
Department of Ophthalmology, Hospital Universitario Severo Ochoa, Avenida de Orellana, Leganés, 28911 Madrid, Spain

Rosa María Fernández-Torres and Eduardo Fonseca
Department of Dermatology, University Hospital of La Coruña, Xubias de Arriba 84, 15006 La Coruña, Spain

Susana Castro and Ana Moreno
Department of Pediatrics, University Hospital of La Coruña, Xubias de Arriba 84, 15006 La Coruña, Spain

Roberto Álvarez
Department of Pathology, University Hospital of La Coruña, Xubias de Arriba 84, 15006 La Coruña, Spain

Antonella Tammaro, Claudia Abruzzese, Alessandra Narcisi, Giorgia Cortesi, Pier Paolo Di Russo, Gabriella De Marco and Severino Persechino
NESMOS Department, UOC Dermatology, Faculty of Medicine and Psychology, University of Rome "Sapienza", 00189 Rome, Italy

Francesca Romana Parisella
Faculty of Medicine, University of Towson, Towson, MD 21204, USA

Mauro Carducci and Marcella Bozzetti
Department of Dermatologic Surgery, Centro Ortopedico di Quadrante Hospital, 28882 Omegna, Italy

Marco Spezia
Department of Orthopedics, Centro Ortopedico di Quadrante Hospital, 28882 Omegna, Italy

Giorgio Ripamonti
Department of Medicine, Centro Ortopedico di Quadrante Hospital, 28882 Omegna, Italy

Giuseppe Saglietti
Department of Metabolic Disease and Diabetology, ASL VCO, 28925 Verbania, Italy

Atiyah Patel and Shabir Lakhi
Department of Medicine, University of Zambia School of Medicine, University Teaching Hospital, Lusaka, Zambia

Victor Mudenda
Pathology Department, University Teaching Hospital, Lusaka, Zambia

Owen Ngalamika
Dermatovenereology Section, Department of Medicine, University of Zambia School of Medicine, University Teaching Hospital, Lusaka, Zambia

Shinsaku Imashuku and Naoko Kudo
Division of Hematology, Takasago Seibu Hospital, 1-10-41 Nakasuji, Takasago 676-0812, Japan

Kagekatsu Kubo
Division of Internal Medicine, Takasago Seibu Hospital, Takasago 676-0812, Japan

Kouichi Ohshima
Department of Pathology, School of Medicine, Kurume University, Kurume 830-0011, Japan

www.ingramcontent.com/pod-product-compliance
Lightning Source LLC
Chambersburg PA
CBHW070152240326
41458CB00126B/4497